Harnessing Artificial Intelligence and Pervasive Internet of Things for an Empowered Aging

Quan Z. Sheng · Yao Liu · Lina Yao

Harnessing Artificial Intelligence and Pervasive Internet of Things for an Empowered Aging

Springer

Quan Z. Sheng
Macquarie University
Sydney, NSW, Australia

Yao Liu
Northeastern University
Shenyang, China

Lina Yao
University of New South Wales
Sydney, NSW, Australia

ISBN 978-3-032-16501-5 ISBN 978-3-032-16502-2 (eBook)
https://doi.org/10.1007/978-3-032-16502-2

This Springer imprint is published by the registered company Springer Nature Switzerland AG
The registered company address is: Gewerbestrasse 11, 6330 Cham, Switzerland

To my mother for her unconditional and everlasting love. To my family for their love and support

—Quan Z. Sheng

To my family, for their love, patience, and support

—Yao Liu

For Mom and Dad, whose love is the home I return to and the compass that guides me.

—Lina Yao

Preface

Worldwide, the population in both developed and developing countries is aging due to increasing life expectancy and low birth rate. According to the World Health Organization, in 2020, about 1 billion people aged 60 years and over, outnumbering children younger than five years. By 2050, this number is projected to be doubled (2.1 billion), making up 22% of the world's population. In particular, the population aged 80 years or older is expected to triple between 2020 and 2050, reaching 426 million. Such a significant growth of the older population presents many challenges to all countries' current health systems, aged care services, and social systems. Indeed, current aged care practice and services will not be sustainable if innovation is not investigated, introduced into, and embraced by the sector. There is, therefore, an urgent need to develop innovative technologies that help the aging population remain independent and safe in their own homes or residential care, with minimal support from the decreasing number of individuals in the working-age population.

With recent developments in artificial intelligence (AI), low-cost, unobtrusive Internet of Things (IoT) sensor and networking technologies, it has become possible to develop a wide range of valuable applications that offer the potential to enhance the quality of life for the older people, afford them a greater sense of security, and facilitate independent living. For example, by monitoring the daily routines of a person with dementia, an elder assistant service can track how completely and consistently the daily routines are performed and determine when the resident needs assistance. Recognizing and understanding the activities performed by people are a fundamental research topic in this area. Unfortunately, although many approaches have been proposed, they still do not perform well outside of the laboratory and are difficult to be used in real-world applications.

This book provides a comprehensive overview of the latest research progress in addressing the challenges faced by the support for aging population. It covers a broad spectrum of technologies, including the Internet of Things (IoT) and Artificial Intelligence (AI), that are pivotal in supporting older people in their daily lives. The book delves into various domains such as human activity recognition, indoor localization, cognitive activity recognition, and AI-empowered health and identity management solutions. Additionally, it explores the integration of brain–computer interfaces and the development of intent-aware interactive robot-assisted systems, offering insights into how these cutting-edge technologies can be harnessed to enhance the quality of life for the older population.

This book is a collection of 15 chapters that summarize the decade-long research activities and results from the authors on tackling smart aging challenges. The book provides a detailed exposition of the latest research activities and technological breakthroughs in the field of smart aging and aims to bridge the gap between advanced technologies and their practical applications in enhancing the daily lives of older people. From this book, the reader will be able to gain not only a wide range of topics and the corresponding technological advancements, but also a comprehensive understanding of how various technologies can be harmonized to create effective and practical smart aging solutions.

Sydney, Australia — Quan Z. Sheng
Shenyang, China — Yao Liu
Sydney, Australia — Lina Yao
September 2025

Acknowledgements This book is a collection of the decade-long research activities from the authors, and it would not have been possible without the contribution and help of many people. We would like to extend sincere gratitude and appreciation to our research collaborators and previous research students for their contributions. In particular, we would like to mention John Bennett, Robert Boots, Kaixuan Chen, Ling Chen, Weitong Chen, Gangfeng Cui, Xiaojun Chang, Schahram Dustdar, Hsiao-Yun Hu, Chaoran Huang, Zawar Hussain, Sylvia Gustina, Tao Gu, Bin Guo, Salil Kanhere, Hanna Kurniawati, Binghao Li, Mingjie Li, Xue Li, Jiahui Luo, Feiping Nie, Guodong Long, Adnan Mahmood, Julian McAuley, Michele Ruta, Mingkui Tan, Nicole Huang, Peipei Xu, Rui Liu, Ruoyu Wang, Sen Wang, Shen Zhao, Shuai Zhang, Sira Yongchareon, Claude Sammut, Longfei Shangguan, Dalin Zhang, Feng Yuan, Tong Yu, Wen-Chih Peng, Wenjie Ruan, Xianzhi Wang, Xiang Zhang, Xiaofei Xu, Xin Zhao, Junda Wu, Lei Yang, Yi Yang, Yu Zhang, James Xi Zheng, Yunhao Liu, Zesheng Ye, Zheng Yang, Zhiwen Yu, and Zhongjie Wang. We also would like to mention Leo Zhang, who reproduced all the figures of this book. Thank you all!

We would like to sincerely thank the organizations and companies that provided financial supports to our research projects, in particular, Australian Research Council (ARC) under its Discovery Project, Linkage Project, and Linkage Infrastructure, Equipment and Facilities Project schemes, the Huawei Innovation Research Program Open Award, the NSW (New South Wales) Smart Sensing Network (NSSN) under its Grand Challenge Fund, the University of Adelaide under its Beacon Interdisciplinary Research Grant, and Macquarie University under its Start-Up Research Grant.

We would also like to thank Springer Nature's Senior Editor Susan Evans Grove for her trust and support and people at Springer Nature, in particular, Pradeep Rajasekaran, for their continuous help and assistance throughout the book-production process.

Competing Interests The authors have no competing interests to declare that are relevant to the content of this manuscript.

Contents

About the Authors

Quan Z. Sheng is Distinguished Professor and Head of School of Computing at Macquarie University, Australia. Before moving to Macquarie University, Michael spent 10 years at School of Computer Science, the University of Adelaide, serving in a number of senior leadership roles including interim Head and Deputy Head of School of Computer Science. Michael holds a Ph.D. degree in computer science from the University of New South Wales (UNSW) and did his post-doc as Research Scientist at CSIRO ICT Centre. From 1999 to 2001, Michael worked at UNSW as Visiting Research Fellow. Prior to that, he spent six years as Senior Software Engineer in industries. Distinguished Prof. Sheng is ranked by Microsoft Academic as one of the Most Impactful Authors in Services Computing (Top 5 of All Time worldwide) and in the Web of Things (ranked Top 20 All Time) in 2021 and is ranked by ScholarGPS as one of the Highly Ranked Scholars in Web Information System (Top 5 Lifetime) in 2025. He is Recipient of the AMiner Most Influential Scholar Award on IoT (2007–2017), ARC (Australian Research Council) Future Fellowship (2014), Chris Wallace Award for Outstanding Research Contribution (2012), and Microsoft Research Fellowship (2003). Distinguished Prof Michael Sheng served as Vice Chair of the Executive Committee of the IEEE Technical Community on Services Computing (IEEE TCSVC, 2022–2024) and has been Member of the Australian Computing Society (ACS) Technical Advisory Board on IoT since 2019.

Yao Liu is Lecturer and Master's Supervisor at the School of Computer Science and Engineering, Northeastern University, Shenyang, China, and Honorary Lecturer at the School of Computing, Macquarie University, Australia. He received his Ph.D. in Computer Science and Engineering from the University of New South Wales (UNSW), Australia, and later held a Postdoctoral Research Associate position at Macquarie University in 2024. Dr. Liu's research interests include artificial intelligence, computer vision, deep learning, and large language models, with a focus on spatio-temporal data modeling and analysis. His work spans application areas such as 3D point clouds, trajectory prediction, video understanding, and human action recognition. He has published in venues including IEEE TKDE, ACM TOMM,

Knowledge-Based Systems, and ACM CIKM. He has also served as Principal Investigator of a sub-topic under the National Key R&D Program of China. Before his academic career, Dr. Liu worked as Software Engineer at Huawei Technologies Co., Ltd.

Lina Yao is Science Lead in Translational Machine Learning and Senior Principal Research Scientist @ CSIRO's Data61, Conjoint Professor @ UNSW, Honorary Professor @ Macquarie University and Adjunct Professor @ University of Technology Sydney. Her research spans machine learning, data mining, information retrieval, recommender systems, and natural language processing, with a particular focus on developing robust ML systems and intelligent AI agents. She is deeply interested in explainable and personalized AI, as well as human–AI cooperation, aiming to create steerable, user-centric, and impactful systems. She is also passionate about applying AI for science and social good, leveraging cutting-edge methodologies to tackle real-world challenges and deliver meaningful societal benefits. Prof. Yao has been selected in the Clarivate Highly Cited Researcher list. She has received multiple prestigious research awards, including Australian Research Council Future Fellowship (Level 3) in 2025, Australian Research Council Discovery Early Career Research Award in 2015 and Inaugural Vice Chancellor's Women's Research Excellence Award from the University of Adelaide in 2015, Scientia Fellow in 2019 from the University of New South Wales, Inaugural Australia and New Zealand Women in AI Awards in 2021 and the CORE Outstanding Research Contribution Award (formerly named after Chris Wallace) in 2022.

List of Figures

List of Tables

Chapter 1
Introduction

"Fiona's frail 88-year-old father lives alone in a small apartment. He is making a cup of tea and his kitchen knows it. Tiny sensors monitor his every move and track each tea-making step. If he pauses for too long, a nearby computer reminds him about what to do next. Later that day, Fiona accesses a secure website and scans a checklist, which was created from the computer in her father's apartment. She finds that her father took his medicine on schedule, ate normally, and continued to manage his daily activities on his own. This puts Fiona's mind at ease."

Worldwide, the population is aging due to increasing life expectancy and decreasing fertility [18]. According to the Australian Bureau of Statistics [1], in 2022, people aged 65 and over made up 17% of Australia's population, which is projected to increase to between 25% to 27% in 2071. For the population aged 85 or over, it will double from 2.1% in 2022 to between 5.2% to 6.4% in 2071. United Nations recently reported that virtually every country in the world is experiencing growth in the number and proportion of older persons in their population. By the late 2070s, the global population aged 65 and over is projected to reach 2.2 billion, surpassing the number of children under 18. By the mid-2030s, there will be 265 million people aged 80 and older, outnumbering infants [21]. With increasing age comes increasing need for health and aged care services, particularly as dementia prevalence increases with aging.

The significant growth in older population presents many challenges to every government's health and aged care services, demanding improvements and reforms to the aged care system with aim of increased consumer choice and control, more affordable and easier access of services, and improved and expanded home care and support [5]. Consumer directed care (CDC) has been implemented in both home and residential (nursing home) settings. Optimizing older people's wellbeing and independence, however poses challenges for the aged care system including an increasing demand for aged care services as the proportion and numbers of older people increases, as expectations on aged care provision changes, and as the number of formal and informal carers (the backbone of the aged care support system) decreases due to socio-economic changes in society [2, 5, 18].

Q. Z. Sheng et al., *Harnessing Artificial Intelligence and Pervasive Internet of Things for an Empowered Aging*, https://doi.org/10.1007/978-3-032-16502-2_1

Current practices and services in aging and aged care will not be sustainable if innovation is not investigated, introduced and embraced by the sector [10]. Indeed, COVID-19 aged care death rates around the world (e.g., Victoria in Australia [22]) serve as an alarming "wake-up call" to the vulnerability of this sector and there is an urgent need to develop innovative technical solutions to improve aged care services. Optimizing the way care is provided is of high priority. Organizations are looking for new, efficient and cost-effective ways to address client needs that help older people, including those with dementia, live longer independently and safely in their own homes or residential care with minimum support from decreasing working-age population [18].

With the development of low-cost, unobtrusive Internet of Things (IoT) sensors, along with data analytics and artificial intelligence (AI) technologies, there is now a significant opportunity to apply the new technologies to the aged care field [14, 17, 18, 20, 24]. These technologies have the potential to reduce the formal and informal personal carer burden, thus reducing public expenditure outlays while optimizing the ability of older people to remain at home and to improve their quality of life. For example, by monitoring the daily routines of an old person with dementia, an elder assistant service can track how completely and consistently the daily routines are performed, and determine when the resident needs assistance.

However, despite decades' active research, the techniques still largely remain in laboratories and are difficult to use in real-world applications [6, 9, 12, 18, 25, 27].

1.1 Motivations and Objectives of This Book

The global demographic landscape is undergoing a profound transformation, with populations aging at unprecedented rates across developed and developing nations. This demographic shift represents a fundamental challenge that demands innovative technological solutions to support healthy aging, independent living, and sustainable healthcare delivery [5, 18, 26]. The convergence of artificial intelligence (AI) and pervasive Internet of Things (IoT) technologies creates unprecedented opportunities for developing intelligent environments that can adapt to the evolving needs of aging populations [19, 28].

The integration of AI and IoT represents a paradigm shift from traditional reactive healthcare models toward proactive, predictive, and personalized systems. Unlike conventional approaches that rely on episodic care delivery, smart aging technologies enable continuous monitoring, real-time analysis, and adaptive responses that support aging in place while maintaining dignity, autonomy, and quality of life. This technological convergence creates ambient intelligence environments where everyday objects become sensing platforms, data streams provide insights into health and behavior patterns, and AI algorithms translate these insights into actionable support mechanisms.

This monograph presents a systematic approach demonstrating how AI-empowered IoT solutions can work synergistically to create comprehensive support ecosystems for older populations. These systems must balance multiple requirements: maintaining privacy while enabling monitoring, preserving autonomy while providing assistance, ensuring reliability while remaining cost-effective, and supporting diverse user capabilities while maintaining ease of use.

This book provides a comprehensive overview of the latest research progress in addressing the challenges faced by the support of aging population. It covers a broad spectrum of technologies, including the Internet of Things (IoT) and Artificial Intelligence (AI), that are pivotal in supporting older people in their daily lives. The book delves into various domains such as human activity recognition, indoor localization, cognitive activity recognition, and AI-driven health and identity management solutions. Additionally, it explores the integration of brain-computer interfaces and the development of intent-aware interactive robot-assisted systems, offering insights into how these cutting-edge technologies can be harnessed to enhance the quality of life for the older population.

The purpose of this book is to provide a detailed exposition of the latest research activities and technological breakthroughs in the field of empowered aging. It aims to bridge the gap between advanced technologies and their practical applications in enhancing the daily lives of older people. By showcasing a collection of research findings on topics such as human activity recognition, cognitive activity tracking, assistive robotics, and AI-empowered health management, the book seeks to contribute to the development of innovative solutions that can address the unique challenges faced by the aging population. The ultimate goal is to foster a deeper understanding of how these technologies can be effectively utilized to create safer, healthier, and more supportive living environments for the older people.

1.2 Technological Foundations

The technological foundation for AI-empowered IoT solutions in smart aging encompasses advanced sensing technologies, machine learning methodologies, and human-computer interaction paradigms that enable the creation of intelligent, adaptive, and user-centered aging support systems.

Environmental and Wearable Sensing Integration. Modern smart aging systems leverage diverse sensing technologies that capture comprehensive information about human activities, health status, and environmental conditions without imposing significant burden on users. Environmental sensing approaches enable unobtrusive monitoring by strategically placing sensors in the environment rather than requiring individuals to wear specific devices [8, 11, 16]. These systems address privacy concerns while providing continuous monitoring capabilities for detecting behavioral changes and identifying potential health risks.

Wearable sensing technologies complement environmental approaches by providing detailed physiological and behavioral information through voluntarily adopted sensors [3, 13]. The integration of both environmental and wearable sensing creates comprehensive monitoring ecosystems that adapt to individual preferences while maintaining robust coverage of relevant health and behavior indicators.

Artificial Intelligence Methodologies. The transformation of sensor data into actionable insights requires sophisticated AI methodologies that handle the complexity, variability, and uncertainty inherent in human behavior and health data. Semi-supervised and unsupervised learning techniques address the challenge of limited labeled data in healthcare contexts [4, 29]. Advanced neural network architectures, including transformer networks and attention mechanisms, provide the computational foundation for understanding complex temporal patterns and multi-modal data fusion [6, 23, 25, 31].

Personalized machine learning approaches enable systems to learn individual patterns while maintaining robustness to gradual changes in physical capabilities and cognitive function. These adaptive capabilities ensure that smart aging systems remain effective throughout the aging process.

Human-Computer Interaction and Accessibility. The success of smart aging technologies depends on their ability to provide meaningful value while remaining accessible and trustworthy. This requires careful consideration of interaction principles that account for the diverse capabilities and limitations of aging populations. Multiple interaction modalities, from voice interfaces to brain-computer interfaces, provide alternative approaches that accommodate different physical and cognitive capabilities while maintaining consistent functionality [7, 12, 15, 30].

1.3 Contributions and Book Organization

In this book, the foundational understanding begins with aging challenges and smart living paradigms (Chap. 2) and essential technical backgrounds in AI, IoT, and robotics (Chap. 3).

The main technical contributions of this monograph are organized into four interconnected parts that progressively build from foundational sensing technologies to comprehensive AI-empowered solutions for smart aging applications (see Fig. 1.1). Each part addresses distinct technical challenges while contributing to an overarching framework for creating intelligent, adaptive, and user-centered aging support systems.

Part I: Device-free Sensing and Environmental Intelligence. The foundation of ambient intelligence rests on understanding human activities and spatial patterns without requiring active participation from users. This part consists of two chapters. Device-free localization and tracking systems leverage environmental sensing to determine spatial positions and predict movement patterns (Chap. 4). Advanced activity recognition approaches demonstrate how environmental intelligence can replace wearable sensors while preserving user privacy and enabling natural interactions (Chap. 5). These systems provide unobtrusive monitoring of daily activities, fall detection, and behavioral pattern analysis.

Part II: Wearable Sensing and Physiological Monitoring. Wearable sensing technologies enable detailed monitoring of physiological states and behavioral patterns essential for comprehensive health assessment. This part consists of two chapters. Physical activity recognition addresses challenges including insufficient labeled training data and distribution shifts across users (Chap. 6). Cognitive activity recognition represents a critical frontier in brain-computer interactions, enabling direct communication between cognitive states and external devices (Chap. 7). This integration provides comprehensive understanding of both behavioral patterns and mental states, and the necessary support of the cognitive and physical health of older people.

Part III: Interactive and Cooperative Ambient Intelligence Systems. Environmental and wearable sensing integrate with interactive technologies to create cooperative intelligent environments that understand, predict, and respond to human needs. This part consists of three chapters. Web-based interactive ambient intelligence provides comprehensive IoT management frameworks (Chap. 8). Intent-aware interactive systems combine intent recognition with semantic reasoning and robotic actuation (Chap. 9). Brain-computer interface integration enables direct brain-to-device communication for cognitive control of ambient intelligence systems (Chap. 10). These innovations represent a significant leap forward in creating adaptive environments that respond to the intentions and cognitive states of older people, thereby improving their quality of life through personalized and supportive interactions.

Part IV: AI-empowered IoT Solutions. Artificial intelligence integration with IoT systems creates comprehensive solutions for smart aging applications. This part consists of four chapters exploring AI-driven solutions for aging-related applications. More specifically, personal health management leverages sophisticated data mining approaches for health insight extraction (Chap. 11). Advanced identity management provides multimodal biometric authentication for enhanced security (Chap. 12). Conversational AI interfaces utilize large language models for natural language interactions (Chap. 13). Emergent capabilities of large foundation models enable intelligent navigation and adaptive assistance through vision-language understanding and weakly-supervised learning paradigms (Chap. 14). These AI-empowered solutions are specifically designed to address the unique challenges faced by the aging population, enhancing their health and security in an increasingly connected world.

Finally, future directions and comprehensive synthesis of these technologies are presented in the concluding chapter (Chap. 15).

1.4 Cross-Cutting Themes and Integration

As depicted in Fig. 1.1, several fundamental themes guide the design and implementation of AI-empowered IoT solutions for smart aging throughout this monograph.

Privacy-Preserving Intelligence. A critical consideration in smart aging systems is balancing comprehensive monitoring capabilities with individual privacy and autonomy. This book demonstrates approaches that minimize invasive data collection while maximizing useful insights. Device-free sensing approaches avoid capturing identifiable information, while advanced machine learning techniques enable local processing that keeps sensitive data within controlled environments. Edge computing

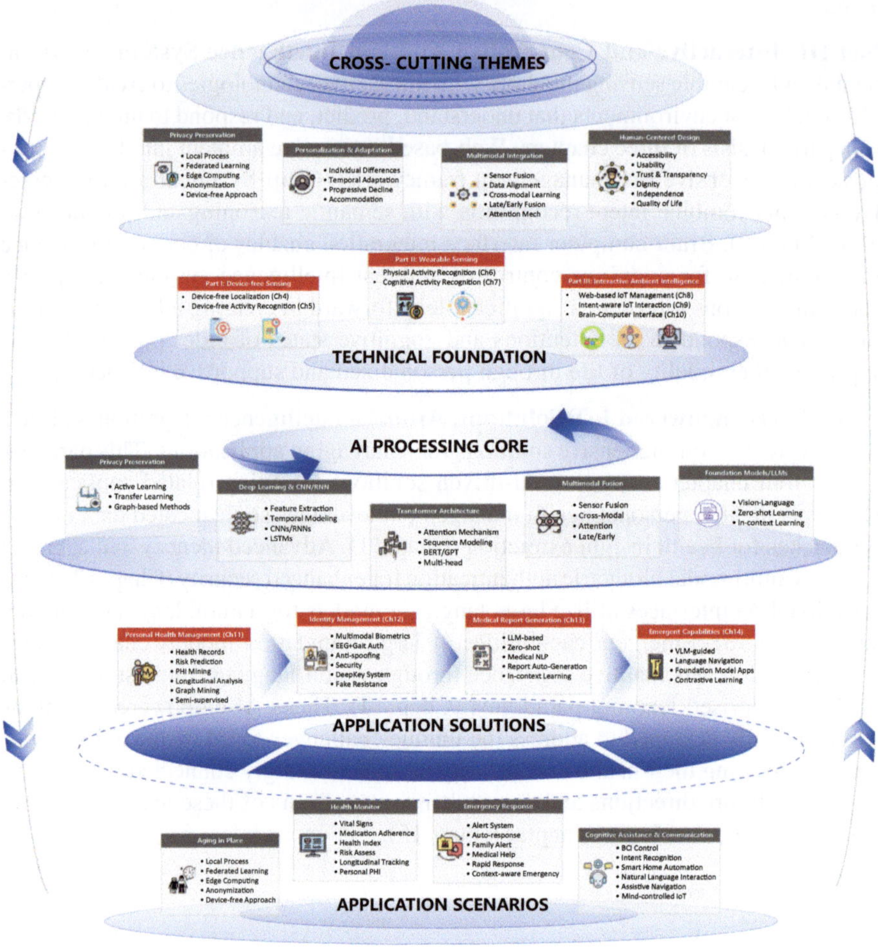

Fig. 1.1 The main themes and the organization of the book

capabilities, federated learning approaches, and differential privacy techniques provide pathways for creating intelligent systems that learn and adapt while maintaining strict privacy controls.

Adaptive and Personalized Systems. Aging is a highly individual process characterized by diverse trajectories and capabilities. Effective smart aging systems must adapt to individual differences while maintaining robust performance across diverse user populations. This book demonstrates multiple approaches for creating adaptive systems, from personalized machine learning models to interface designs that accommodate diverse capabilities. The temporal dimension of adaptation ensures systems continue providing value as users' capabilities evolve over time.

Multimodal Integration and Sensor Fusion. The complexity of human behavior and health requires comprehensive sensing approaches that integrate information from multiple sources. Advanced machine learning approaches, including attention mechanisms and graph neural networks, provide the computational foundation for effectively integrating diverse data streams while maintaining interpretability and reliability. These techniques enable systems to adapt their reliance on different sensor modalities based on availability, quality, and context.

Human-Centered Design. The fundamental principle underlying all smart aging technologies presented in this book is human-centered design, which places older adults' needs, preferences, and capabilities at the core of system development. This approach recognizes that technology serves people, not the reverse, and that successful aging support systems must respect user autonomy while providing meaningful assistance. Throughout this monograph, human-centered design manifests in multiple dimensions: unobtrusive sensing that maintains dignity and privacy, adaptive interfaces that accommodate diverse physical and cognitive capabilities, and personalized systems that learn individual patterns rather than imposing standardized behaviors. The integration of multiple interaction modalities, from voice commands to brain-computer interfaces, demonstrates responsiveness to varied user abilities and preferences. This design philosophy ensures that technological sophistication translates into practical benefit, creating systems that enhance quality of life while remaining accessible, trustworthy, and respectful of individual autonomy.

1.5 Conclusion

This monograph summarizes the decade-long research activities and results from the authors on tackling aging population support challenges by exploiting advanced technologies including the pervasive Internet of Things (IoT) and artificial intelligence. It provide a comprehensive overview of the latest research progress in addressing the challenges faced by the support for aging population, and presents a systematic exploration of how AI and IoT technologies can be integrated to address these complex challenges. Through the four interconnected technical parts spanning environmental sensing, wearable computing, interactive ambient intelligence, and AI-empowered solutions, this book demonstrates the technical feasibility and practical value of creating intelligent systems that support healthy aging and independent living.

The technological contributions establish both the foundation and pathway for creating smart aging ecosystems capable of understanding human needs, adapting to individual differences, and providing appropriate support while maintaining privacy, autonomy, and dignity. The integration of advanced sensing technologies, sophisticated machine learning methodologies, and user-centered design principles creates a framework for ambient intelligence that enhances human wellbeing throughout the aging process. All technical chapters are supported by rigorous research findings and practical implementations, making this book an essential reference for researchers and practitioners in the field of empowered active aging.

References

1. Australian Bureau of Statistics: Population Projections, Australia 2022 (Base)-2071. https://www.abs.gov.au/statistics/people/population/population-projections-australia/latest-release (2023)
2. Australian Institute of Health and Welfare: Older Australians. https://www.aihw.gov.au/reports/older-people/older-australians/contents/health/health-care-gps-specialists. Accessed 09 Sept 2025
3. Chen, K., Yao, L., Zhang, D., Chang, X., Long, G., Wang, S.: Distributionally robust semi-supervised learning for people-centric sensing. In: Proceedings of the Thirty-Third AAAI Conference on Artificial Intelligence (AAAI-19). AAAI Press (2019)
4. Chen, K., Yao, L., Zhang, D., Guo, B., Yu, Z.: Multi-agent attentional activity recognition. In: Proceedings of the Twenty-Eighth International Joint Conference on Artificial Intelligence (IJCAI-19). IJCAI (2019)
5. Douglas, H., Georgiou, A., Tariq, A., Prgomet, M., Warland, A., Armour, P., Westbrook, J.: Implementing information and communication technology to support community aged care service integration: lessons from an Australian aged care provider. Int. J. Integr. Care **17**(1), 9 (2017)
6. Fernandes, J.M., Silva, J.S., Rodrigues, A., Boavida, F.: A survey of approaches to unobtrusive sensing of humans. ACM Comput. Surv. **55**(2), 41:1–41:28 (2023)
7. Huang, C., Yao, L., Wang, X., Sheng, Q.Z., Dustdar, S., Wang, Z., Xu, X.: Intent-aware interactive internet of things for enhanced collaborative ambient intelligence. IEEE Internet Comput. **26**(5), 68–75 (2022)
8. Hussain, Z., Sheng, Q.Z., Zhang, W.E.: A review and categorization of techniques on device-free human activity recognition. J. Netw. Comput. Appl. **167**, 102738 (2020)
9. Jeste, D.V., Alexopoulos, G.S., Blazer, D.G., Lavretsky, H., Sachdev, P.S., Reynolds, C.F.: Wisdom, resilience, and well-being in later life. Annu. Rev. Clin. Psychol. **21**, 33–59 (2025)
10. Jones, C.H., Dolsten, M.: Healthcare on the brink: navigating the challenges of an aging society in the United States. npj Aging **10**(1), 22 (2024)
11. Kim, E., Helal, S., Cook, D.J.: Human activity recognition and pattern discovery. IEEE Pervasive Comput. **9**(1), 48–53 (2010)
12. Lu, J., Tian, Y., Zhang, Y., Sheng, Q.Z., Zheng, X.: LGL-BCI: a motor-imagery-based brain-computer interface with geometric learning. Proc. ACM Interact. Mob. Wearable Ubiquitous Technol. **9**(1), (2025)
13. Lu, J., Zheng, X., Sheng, M., Jin, J., Yu, S.: Efficient human activity recognition using a single wearable sensor. IEEE Internet Things J. **7**(11), 11137–11146 (2020)

14. Ma, B., Yang, J., Wong, F.K.Y., Wong, A.K.C., Ma, T., Meng, J., Zhao, Y., Wang, Y., Lu, Q.: Artificial intelligence in elderly healthcare: a scoping review. Ageing Res. Rev. **83**, 101808 (2023)
15. Mallick, M., Kodeswaran, P., Sen, S., Kokku, R., Ganguly, N.: TSFS: an integrated approach for event segmentation and ADL detection in IoT enabled smart-homes. IEEE Trans. Mob. Comput. **18**(11), 2686–2700 (2019)
16. Mennicken, S., Vermeulen, J., Huang, E.M.: From today's augmented houses to tomorrow's smart homes: new directions for home automation research. In: Proceedings of the 2014 ACM International Joint Conference on Pervasive and Ubiquitous Computing (UbiComp '14), pp. 105–115. ACM (2014)
17. Qin, Y., Sheng, Q.Z., Falkner, N.J.G., Dustdar, S., Wang, H., Vasilakos, A.V.: When things matter: a survey on data-centric internet of things. J. Netw. Comput. Appl. **64**, 137–153 (2016)
18. Rashidi, P., Mihailidis, A.: A survey on ambient-assisted living tools for older adults. IEEE J. Biomed. Health Inform. **17**(3), 579–590 (2013)
19. Sheng, Q.Z.: AIoT sensing for smart aging: research activities and future directions. In: The 33rd IEEE/ACM International Symposium on Quality of Services (IWQoS 2025). https://iwqos2025.ieee-iwqos.org/program/keynotes (2025). Accessed 01 Sept 2025
20. Sheng, Q.Z., Li, X., Zeadally, S.: Enabling next-generation RFID applications: solutions and challenges. Computer **41**(9), 21–28 (2008)
21. United Nations: Ageing. https://www.un.org/en/global-issues/ageing. Accessed 09 Sept 2025
22. Warriner, J.: Victoria was a wake-up call. So is the aged care system ready for a coronavirus outbreak? https://www.abc.net.au/news/2020-08-04/coronavirus-in-victoria-a-wake-up-call-so-is-aged-care-ready/12519628. Accessed 09 Sept 2025
23. Xia, Y., Yongchareon, S., Lutui, R., Sheng, Q.Z.: Dynamic self-attention gated spatial-temporal graph convolutional network for skeleton-based human activity recognition. In: Proceedings of International Conference on Neural Information Processing, pp. 197–211 (2025)
24. Xiao, F., Miao, Q., Xie, X., Sun, L., Wang, R.: SHMO: a seniors health monitoring system based on energy-free sensing. Comput. Netw. **132**, 108–117 (2018)
25. Xiao, J., Li, H., Wu, M., Jin, H., Deen, M.J., Cao, J.: A survey on wireless device-free human sensing: application scenarios, current solutions, and open issues. ACM Comput. Surv. **55**(5), (2022)
26. Xu, H., Xie, B., Chang, C.H.: Empowering the care of older adults through the use of technology. Work Aging Retire. **10**(1), 1–5 (2023)
27. Yamout, Y., Yeasar, T.S., Iqbal, S., Zulkernine, M.: Beyond smart homes: an in-depth analysis of smart aging care system security. ACM Comput. Surv. **56**(2), 45:1–45:35 (2024)
28. Yao, L., Sheng, Q.Z., Benatallah, B., Dustdar, S., Wang, X., Shemshadi, A., Kanhere, S.S.: WITS: an Iot-endowed computational framework for activity recognition in personalized smart homes. Computing **100**(4), 369–385 (2018)
29. Yao, L., Sheng, Q.Z., Li, X., Wang, S., Gu, T., Ruan, W., Zou, W.: Freedom: online activity recognition via dictionary-based sparse representation of RFID sensing data. In: IEEE International Conference on Data Mining (ICDM 2015), pp. 1087–1092. IEEE (2015)
30. Zhang, X., Yao, L., Huang, C., Gu, T., Zhang, D., Sheng, Q.Z.: Mindid: person identification from brain waves through attention-based recurrent neural network. In: ACM International Joint Conference on Pervasive and Ubiquitous Computing (UbiComp). ACM (2018)
31. Zhang, X., Yao, L., Huang, C., Sheng, Q.Z., Gu, T.: Multi-modality sensor data classification with selective attention. In: Proceedings of the 27th International Joint Conference on Artificial Intelligence (IJCAI), pp. 3111–3117. IJCAI (2018)

Chapter 2
Aging Challenges and Smart Living

2.1 The Global Aging Challenge

The twenty-first century faces an unprecedented demographic transformation as world populations experience rapid aging. This shift challenges existing healthcare systems, social structures, and economic models, creating urgent needs for innovative solutions to support independent living and quality aging.

Population aging occurs at different rates globally, with developed nations leading the transition while developing countries face accelerated changes with fewer resources [62]. This demographic shift transforms societies from having large working-age populations supporting smaller elderly populations to the reverse, creating sustainability challenges for traditional care models. The scale and complexity of this transformation demand technological innovations that go beyond traditional approaches to care delivery and monitoring.

Aged care becomes one of the fastest growing industries worldwide due to increased aging of the population and decrease in working-age population [62]. Australia, which enjoys one of the highest life expectancies in the world, generates $38+ billion a year in revenue from its aged care sector [53]. China, according to a recent United Nations report, will be one of the countries with the largest increase in share of older persons between 2019 and 2050. Due to its "one-child policy" implemented during 1979–2015, the booming aged care market in China presents enormous opportunities, estimated to be worth $2.6 trillion by 2030 [41, 63].

The proliferation of low-cost, unobtrusive sensor devices and Internet of Things (IoT) technologies creates unprecedented opportunities to address aging challenges through ubiquitous monitoring and intelligent assistance systems [30]. These technologies have the potential to reduce the number of personal carers (both formally and informally) thus reducing public expenditure outlays and burden on carers, while optimizing the opportunity for older people to remain at home independently and safely as long as possible and for as long as they wish. However, the deployment

Q. Z. Sheng et al., *Harnessing Artificial Intelligence and Pervasive Internet of Things for an Empowered Aging*, https://doi.org/10.1007/978-3-032-16502-2_2

of these technologies in aging contexts requires careful consideration of the unique technical and social challenges that distinguish older adult populations from other user groups.

Cultural contexts significantly influence aging experiences and technology acceptance. Eastern societies often emphasize family-based care responsibilities, while Western models rely more heavily on institutional and formal support systems [63]. Understanding these variations is essential for developing appropriate technological interventions that align with cultural expectations and preferences. The development of cognitive Internet of Things systems must accommodate these diverse cultural contexts while providing universal benefits for aging populations [66].

The evolution from simple connectivity to intelligent, cognitive systems represents a fundamental paradigm shift necessary for addressing aging challenges. Traditional Internet of Things approaches focus primarily on connecting devices and collecting data, but aging applications require systems capable of learning, thinking, and understanding complex human behaviors and needs [68]. This cognitive capability becomes essential for processing the noisy, sparse, and variable data characteristic of aging environments.

The technical challenges of implementing smart aging solutions mirror broader challenges in sensor-based human activity recognition, where traditional machine learning approaches often prove insufficient for the complexity and variability of real-world aging scenarios [12]. The success of smart aging initiatives depends on addressing fundamental issues, including feature extraction from ambiguous sensor data, annotation scarcity for rare but critical events, and distribution discrepancies across diverse aging populations.

The convergence of artificial intelligence (AI), Internet of Things, and ambient intelligence technologies offers transformative potential for creating comprehensive smart living environments. These integrated systems must seamlessly bridge physical monitoring capabilities with social and cognitive support services, providing proactive, personalized, and scalable solutions that adapt to the progressive nature of aging-related changes [8]. Figure 2.1 depicts an overview of this chapter.

2.2 Core Challenges of Aging

Having established the global context and technological opportunities, it is essential to examine the specific challenges that aging populations face, which drive the requirements for intelligent technological interventions [63]. These challenges span multiple domains and create complex interdependencies that smart aging systems must address comprehensively. Indeed, developing the applicability of innovative technology to aged care cannot be adequately addressed without understanding and integrating expertise and knowledge from different disciplines. Furthermore, it is important that end users, designers, and manufacturers of new technologies are

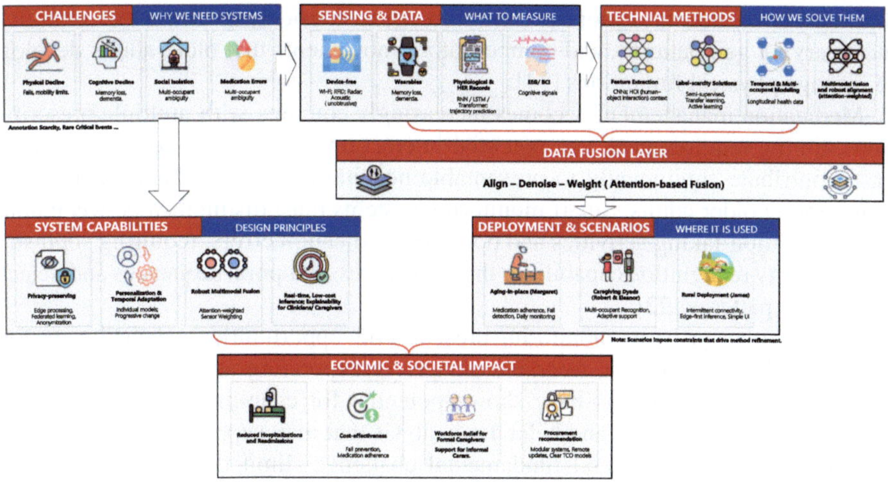

Fig. 2.1 Overview: core aging challenges, sensing modalities, technical methods, system design principles, and representative real-world scenarios. This chapter focuses on problem-driving sensing and practical deployment constraints

enabled to work together to ensure that products are tailored to need. At present, there is a significant gap with new technologies being developed without this co-design.

2.2.1 Physical Health and Functional Decline

Aging involves progressive changes in physiological systems that affect functional capacity and increase vulnerability to chronic conditions. Multiple chronic conditions become increasingly common, with most older adults managing several health issues simultaneously. These conditions affect activities of daily living and instrumental activities such as medication management, financial tasks, and home maintenance [63].

Mobility limitations represent a primary barrier to independent living, affecting increasing percentages of older adults as they age. These limitations impact personal care, household activities, and community participation. Falls constitute a particularly serious concern, often triggering cascades of functional decline and institutionalization. Fear of falling can lead to activity restriction, creating cycles of deconditioning and further vulnerability.

The complexity of physical health monitoring in aging populations presents unique challenges for sensor-based recognition systems. Age-related movement patterns exhibit significant inter-activity similarity, where activities such as walking and shuffling may appear nearly identical to automated recognition systems [39].

This similarity becomes more pronounced when considering the use of mobility aids, varying gait patterns, and compensatory movements that older adults develop to manage physical limitations [34].

Medication management becomes increasingly complex with multiple prescriptions, timing requirements, and potential interactions. Errors in medication adherence contribute significantly to preventable hospitalizations and health complications among older adults. Smart monitoring systems must distinguish between normal medication-taking activities and potential medication errors, requiring sophisticated activity recognition capabilities that can process temporal sequences and detect anomalous patterns [22].

Wearable sensor-based monitoring presents both opportunities and challenges for aging populations. Modern wearable devices incorporating accelerometers, gyroscopes, and magnetometers have shown potential for enabling continuous health monitoring, fall detection, and behavior analysis that may support independent living [6, 15]. However, several fundamental challenges limit their effectiveness in aging contexts, including insufficient labeled training data, intra-class variability in how activities are performed by different individuals, and distribution shifts across users due to diverse biological conditions and behavior patterns [24, 34, 60]. These challenges may be particularly pronounced in aging populations where individual differences in physical capabilities and health conditions can significantly affect movement patterns and sensor data characteristics.

The sensor-based monitoring of physical health challenges traditional activity recognition approaches due to the highly personalized nature of age-related functional decline. Individual variations in mobility, chronic condition management, and adaptive behaviors create substantial distribution discrepancy challenges that must be addressed through personalized learning approaches [35]. Healthcare applications demand robust systems that can adapt to progressive changes in physical capabilities while maintaining accurate monitoring and emergency detection capabilities [37].

Device-free localization and tracking technologies offer particularly promising solutions for aging populations by eliminating the burden of carrying specific devices or actively participating in monitoring processes [54, 71]. These approaches detect environmental disturbances caused by human presence and movement through various sensing modalities, providing more comfortable and dignified monitoring solutions in residential spaces. However, real-world deployment in cluttered home environments presents substantial challenges, as radio signals experience heavy obstruction from furniture and metallic appliances, reducing localization accuracy compared to optimal conditions.

Advanced personal health management systems leveraging data mining and machine learning techniques have shown considerable potential for addressing the challenges of comprehensive health monitoring in aging populations. These systems can analyze vast amounts of Electronic Health Records (EHRs) collected from annual geriatric medical examinations to predict personal health status and identify individuals at risk [13, 18]. Personal Health Indexing (PHI) systems demonstrate the capability to evaluate health status from-cradle-to-grave by processing hundreds of examination parameters and their longitudinal progression [17]. Such approaches address the manually impossible task of exploring correlations among test results, their temporal changes, and relationships to similar participants with comparable health development patterns.

Modern health examination data present unique challenges, including heterogeneity and sparsity, particularly relevant for aging populations with varying health conditions and irregular examination schedules. Semi-supervised learning approaches utilizing heterogeneous graph construction have demonstrated potential for risk prediction from longitudinal health examination records, effectively handling the predominantly unlabeled nature of health data where participants' conditions may vary greatly from healthy to very-ill without clear ground truth differentiation. These systems require careful validation in diverse aging populations to establish their reliability and clinical utility [18].

2.2.2 Cognitive and Social Challenges

Cognitive aging encompasses both normal age-related changes and pathological conditions affecting memory, decision-making, and executive function. While some cognitive changes are part of normal aging, dementia represents a growing global challenge requiring innovative intervention approaches. Early-stage cognitive changes can affect safety, financial management, and medication adherence before formal diagnosis occurs. The progressive nature of cognitive decline creates unique challenges for technology deployment. Annotation scarcity becomes particularly acute when attempting to collect labeled data for cognitive assessment activities, as these behaviors are often subtle, highly variable between individuals, and difficult to observe consistently [69]. Traditional machine learning approaches struggle with the temporal dynamics of cognitive changes, where behavioral patterns evolve gradually over extended periods.

Brain-computer interface (BCI) technologies offer promising avenues for cognitive monitoring and assistance in aging populations. EEG-based systems, in particular, provide non-invasive approaches to understanding cognitive activities and intentions, potentially enabling direct communication pathways for individuals with motor disabilities or communication difficulties [67]. However, EEG signals face inherent challenges, including noise from physiological activities, ambiguous correlations between brain signals and cognitive intentions, and the need for personalized adaptation to individual neural patterns [26, 58]. While laboratory studies have shown promising results, translation to real-world aging contexts may require careful validation and adaptation to accommodate individual differences in neural patterns and varying capabilities among older adults.

Advanced BCI-IoT integration technologies demonstrate considerable potential for enabling direct human-thing cognitive interactivity in smart aging environments. These systems establish communication pathways between the human brain and IoT devices, eliminating the need for traditional physical interactions that may be challenging for aging populations with motor limitations [61, 64]. BCI technologies can enable mind-controlled operation of smart home appliances, assistive devices, and communication systems, offering enhanced independence for individuals with diverse interaction needs [5, 75]. However, brain signal processing faces fundamental challenges, including low signal-to-noise ratios, susceptibility to environmental factors, and insufficient spatial or temporal resolution that currently limit practical deployment [25, 52].

The inherent privacy characteristics of brain activity present unique advantages for aging populations, as neural signals remain invisible and impossible to observe or replicate externally, providing secure authentication and interaction capabilities [48]. BCI systems also offer real-time interaction convenience, allowing users to control devices through thought processes rather than physical movements, which may prove particularly valuable for aging individuals with mobility limitations or dexterity challenges [47]. While current cognitive recognition systems achieve approximately 70–80% accuracy, advancement toward the reliability levels necessary for practical aging applications requires continued development of sophisticated signal processing and machine learning approaches.

Social isolation significantly impacts physical health, cognitive function, and overall well-being among aging populations. Multiple factors contribute to isolation, including mobility limitations, transportation barriers, sensory impairments, and loss of social networks through retirement or bereavement. Environmental safety concerns arise as homes and communities often lack age-friendly design features [63]. The detection and monitoring of social isolation present complex multi-occupant activity recognition challenges. Smart systems must distinguish between chosen solitude and problematic isolation while respecting privacy boundaries [22]. Social interaction patterns vary significantly across cultural contexts, creating distribution discrepancy issues when deploying technology solutions across diverse populations.

Advanced trajectory prediction capabilities complement basic localization by enabling intelligent systems to anticipate needs, detect anomalies in movement patterns, and prevent potential hazards. These predictive capabilities must address three key challenges: incorporating social interaction information as human movement is influenced by the presence and behavior of others, adapting to dynamic environments where individuals can enter or exit at any time, and handling the inherent multi-modality of human movement where future trajectories encompass numerous possibilities based on individual decisions [56].

Cognitive IoT systems offer promising approaches to address these challenges by moving beyond simple connectivity to intelligent understanding of social and cognitive contexts [68]. These systems must integrate perception-action cycles that can adapt to changing cognitive capabilities while providing appropriate levels of support without overwhelming users with complex interfaces [2]. The development of intuitive, voice-based interaction systems becomes crucial for accommodating users with varying levels of technological familiarity and cognitive capacity [50].

Finally, time-series data analysis becomes particularly important for cognitive and social monitoring, as changes often occur gradually and may be imperceptible in short-term observations. Advanced processing capabilities are required to detect patterns in noisy, sparse data that characterize aging environments [59].

2.2.3 Technology Implementation Challenges and Solutions

While technology offers tremendous potential for addressing aging challenges, implementing effective sensor-based monitoring and artificial intelligence solutions faces unique technical barriers that must be overcome for successful deployment in aging contexts [12]. In this section, we will briefly discuss some of them.

Feature extraction represents a fundamental challenge in aging-related activity recognition systems. Different activities may exhibit similar characteristics, such as the overlapping movement patterns between walking and shuffling in older adults with mobility impairments. This inter-activity similarity makes it difficult to produce distinguishable features that uniquely represent different activities, particularly when considering age-related changes in movement patterns. Traditional time-frequency transformation techniques often prove insufficient for capturing the nuanced patterns of aging-related activities [28]. Deep learning approaches offer promising solutions to these feature extraction challenges. The hierarchical nature of deep neural networks enables automatic feature learning from raw sensor data, addressing inter-activity similarity through layer-by-layer abstraction [12]. Convolutional neural networks demonstrate particular effectiveness in capturing spatial patterns in multi-sensor environments, while their translational invariance properties help accommodate the variability in aging-related movement patterns [23].

Promising technical developments include leveraging human-object interaction (HOI) contexts to enhance localization accuracy in furnished homes, where interaction events such as opening a refrigerator door or turning on a desk lamp provide valuable contextual information that complements traditional signal-based approaches [54]. Such multi-modal fusion approaches have shown potential for significant improvements in localization accuracy, with experimental studies reporting increases from 80% to over 96% accuracy when combining signal-based measurements with interaction context, though these results may require adaptation and validation for diverse aging populations in real-world environments.

Annotation scarcity poses another significant barrier, as collecting and annotating sensory activity data for aging populations is both expensive and time-consuming. The challenge intensifies when considering emergent or unexpected activities such as falls or medical emergencies, leading to severe class imbalance in training datasets. These rare but critical events are precisely those that smart aging systems must detect most reliably. Semi-supervised learning and transfer learning techniques address annotation challenges by leveraging limited labeled data more effectively [1]. Deep active learning approaches can strategically select the most informative samples for annotation, reducing the overall labeling burden while maintaining system performance [21].

Distribution discrepancy emerges from three primary sources particularly relevant to aging contexts. First, activity patterns are highly person-dependent, with significant variations between individuals based on health status, mobility levels, and personal habits. Second, activity concepts vary over time as individuals experience progressive changes in capabilities and routines. Third, diverse sensor configurations and deployment environments create substantial variability in data characteristics. Advanced neural network architectures provide mechanisms to address these challenges through attention mechanisms that can focus on relevant sensor modalities and temporal segments [46]. Recurrent neural networks and their variants effectively model temporal dependencies, enabling systems to adapt to changing behavioral patterns over time [42].

Composite activities present substantial challenges for aging support systems. Many meaningful daily routines consist of sequences of atomic activities, requiring precise data segmentation to identify temporal boundaries between component activities. Concurrent activities frequently occur in aging contexts, while multi-occupant scenarios add complexity when aging individuals live with caregivers or family members.

Identity management and secure authentication also present critical challenges in smart aging environments, where traditional security measures may prove inadequate for older adults with varying physical and cognitive capabilities. While biometric authentication technologies demonstrate considerable promise for enhancing security and personalization, their implementation in aging contexts requires careful consideration of age-related limitations [14, 74]. Physiological biometrics such as face, iris, and fingerprint recognition may face challenges due to age-related changes in skin texture, eye conditions, or hand mobility. Traditional authentication methods often prove vulnerable to spoofing attacks using specialized masks or artificial materials, necessitating more robust approaches with enhanced fake-resistance characteristics.

Multimodal biometric systems combining complementary authentication traits may offer improved security and reliability while accommodating the diverse needs of aging populations. Advanced approaches integrating Electroencephalography (EEG) signals with gait-based authentication have shown potential for achieving enhanced accuracy and reliability, as brain electromagnetic neural oscillations remain unique to individuals and are difficult to replicate [14]. Gait-based authentication leverages individual walking patterns determined by intrinsic and temporal factors, though such systems require validation across diverse aging populations with varying mobility levels and assistive device usage [10]. The effectiveness of such multimodal approaches may prove suitable for high-security applications while maintaining usability for older adults, though comprehensive validation across diverse aging contexts remains necessary.

Computational cost considerations become critical for aging applications, where systems must operate on resource-constrained devices while providing instant responses for safety-critical situations. Enhanced manufacturing capabilities enable the development of more efficient sensor systems and processing architectures [19]. Privacy concerns are particularly acute in aging contexts, as continuous monitoring systems record detailed information about personal activities, health status, and living patterns.

Finally, interpretability requirements are heightened, where sensory data must be translated into meaningful insights for healthcare providers, family members, and the older adults themselves. Attention mechanisms and other explainable AI techniques help bridge this gap by providing insights into which aspects of sensor data contribute to system decisions [32].

2.3 Smart Living Technologies and Solutions

While the challenges outlined above might appear daunting, recent advances in artificial intelligence (AI), Internet of Things (IoT), and ambient intelligence technologies offer unprecedented opportunities to address these aging-related issues comprehensively. Building upon our understanding of the core challenges, this section explores how these emerging technologies can be systematically integrated to create intelligent living environments that support successful aging in place.

Device-free activity recognition emerges as a particularly valuable paradigm for aging populations, strategically placing sensing devices in the environment (i.e., augmented environment) rather than requiring individuals to wear them (i.e., augmented person) [27, 34, 43]. This approach addresses fundamental concerns about privacy, practicality, and user acceptance that often hinder the adoption of wearable technologies among older adults. By analyzing signal variations induced by movement patterns, these systems can recognize activities without the privacy concerns of vision-based approaches or the compliance challenges associated with wearable sensors.

The integration of these technologies creates comprehensive monitoring ecosystems that can detect falls, monitor daily activities, and assess behavioral patterns that are crucial for independent living. Multiple sensing modalities including radio frequency-based systems (Wi-Fi, RFID, radar), acoustic-based recognition using Doppler effects, and depth sensor-based approaches provide complementary capabilities for different monitoring scenarios [51, 72]. These device-free systems offer potential advantages including continuous monitoring capability, low maintenance requirements, and non-intrusive operation that may better respect user dignity and privacy compared to traditional wearable approaches.

Web-based IoT management interfaces present promising opportunities for creating accessible and intuitive control systems for aging populations. These interfaces have shown potential for seamlessly integrating virtual and physical worlds to effectively manage things of interest (TOIs) in home environments, enabling residents and caregivers to monitor, control, and visualize connected devices through familiar Web browsers [3, 7]. Such approaches may be particularly valuable for smart aging applications where technology accessibility and ease of use are paramount considerations, though deployment success depends on careful attention to user interface design, technical reliability, and accommodation of diverse user capabilities.

Intent-aware interactive IoT systems represent an advanced evolution of ambient intelligence that may proactively assist aging individuals by understanding user intentions through contextual sensing and historical interaction patterns [57, 70]. These systems have demonstrated potential benefits in research settings including reduced cognitive load through automatic prediction of routine tasks, enhanced safety via anticipatory monitoring of potentially dangerous activities, and increased independence through intelligent assistance with daily activities. However, accurately interpreting human intentions from sensor data remains particularly complex when dealing with older adults who may have inconsistent interaction patterns or changing capabilities over time, requiring substantial validation in real-world aging contexts.

Recently, Large Language Models (LLMs) for healthcare documentation present transformative opportunities for reducing administrative burdens in aging care while improving communication quality between healthcare providers, caregivers, and older adults. Medical report generation systems utilizing LLMs have demonstrated potential for automatically generating comprehensive reports from medical examinations, which may be particularly valuable for aging populations who require frequent health monitoring and documentation [44]. These systems can process complex medical information and generate readable reports, potentially reducing the workload on healthcare professionals while maintaining consistent documentation quality for aging care coordination. In particular, zero-shot learning capabilities in medical reporting systems address critical challenges in aging healthcare, where resource-constrained medical facilities or specialized geriatric conditions may lack sufficient training data for traditional approaches. In-context learning methodologies enable LLMs to generate appropriate medical reports for new scenarios with minimal examples, which may prove particularly valuable for rare geriatric conditions or facilities with limited computational resources [16, 33]. However, computational efficiency, accuracy validation across diverse aging populations, and integration with existing healthcare information systems remain important considerations for practical deployment in aging care environments.

Emergent capabilities of large foundation models present transformative opportunities for intelligent navigation and assistance systems in aging environments. Vision-Language Models (VLMs) and Large Language Models (LLMs) have demonstrated remarkable zero-shot learning abilities that enable systems to understand and execute complex navigation instructions based on natural language commands without explicit task-specific training [11, 40, 77]. These emergent capabilities may prove particularly valuable for aging populations, enabling intuitive interaction with smart home systems, assistive devices, and navigation aids through natural language rather than complex interfaces that may challenge older adults with varying technological familiarity.

Visual Language Navigation (VLN) capabilities represent fundamental applications where foundation models can enable agents to navigate complex environments based on natural language instructions, potentially revolutionizing how aging individuals interact with their living spaces [20]. However, significant challenges persist when leveraging emergent capabilities for specialized aging assistance applications. The gap between general knowledge encoded in foundation models and specialized requirements of aging support systems often results in performance limitations, while computational requirements for adapting large foundation models remain prohibitive for many healthcare applications [11, 38, 40, 49, 76, 77]. These limitations highlight the need for developing approaches that can bridge general-purpose foundation models with specialized aging assistance requirements while maintaining the benefits of emergent capabilities for adaptive, personalized systems.

Technical challenges remain significant, particularly regarding signal uncertainties and environmental complexity. Device-free systems fundamentally rely on environmental signals that are inherently noisy and subject to fluctuations, requiring robust signal processing approaches such as compressive sensing and dictionary learning to extract meaningful patterns from uncertain data [55]. The dynamic nature of real-world environments, with changing conditions and multiple occupants, creates variations that recognition systems must accommodate through adaptive algorithms and multi-modal integration approaches. While laboratory studies have shown promising results, deployment in diverse aging contexts may require substantial customization and validation.

2.4 Real-World Scenarios and Technology Integration

Smart Aging in Place with Chronic Conditions. Consider Margaret, a widow living alone while managing diabetes, hypertension, and arthritis. Her daily routine involves complex medication management, health monitoring, and home maintenance while dealing with fatigue and mobility limitations. Her adult children live in distant cities, creating challenges for ongoing support and emergency response.

This scenario illustrates the critical need for integrated monitoring systems that demonstrate how technical challenges translate into real-world requirements. The annotation scarcity problem becomes evident when considering the need to recognize Margaret's unique movement patterns affected by arthritis, while distribution discrepancy challenges arise from her individual medication routines and health status variations [4]. Smart home systems must address inter-activity similarity when distinguishing between normal daily activities and potential health emergencies [31].

Advanced sensor fusion and machine learning approaches can provide continuous health indicator tracking, medication adherence support, and emergency detection while preserving privacy through edge computing and secure data transmission [36]. The system must handle concurrent activities such as taking medication while watching television, demonstrating the complexity of real-world activity recognition.

Caregiving Technology for Dual Vulnerability. Robert and Eleanor represent caregiving couples where both partners face age-related challenges. Eleanor's early-stage cognitive decline requires increasing support from Robert, who manages his own health conditions while providing care. Navigation difficulties, medication management confusion, and social isolation affect both partners.

This scenario demonstrates the multi-occupant activity recognition challenge, where systems must distinguish between caregiver and care recipient activities while adapting to progressive cognitive changes [9]. The temporal variability in Eleanor's capabilities requires adaptive learning systems that can accommodate changing behavioral patterns over time.

Cognitive IoT frameworks become essential for providing intelligent decision-making support that can assist both partners [2]. Natural language processing capabilities enable intuitive interaction for users with varying cognitive abilities, while personalized intervention strategies adapt to both partners' evolving needs [50].

Rural Technology Deployment Challenges. James lives alone on rural property with limited connectivity and transportation options. His chronic respiratory condition requires careful monitoring, while geographic isolation compounds challenges accessing healthcare and emergency services. Limited technology familiarity and infrastructure create additional barriers to receiving appropriate support.

Rural scenarios highlight computational cost and resource constraints that are fundamental to practical deployment [19]. Systems must operate reliably with intermittent connectivity while maintaining local processing capabilities for emergency detection. The interpretability challenge becomes acute when family members and healthcare providers need clear, actionable insights from sensor data despite limited technical expertise.

Edge computing architectures enable robust operation in resource-constrained environments, while simplified user interfaces accommodate varying levels of technology familiarity [30]. Ambient intelligence systems can provide seamless monitoring without requiring active user engagement or complex device management.

2.5 Economic and Social Impacts

Healthcare expenditures represent the most visible economic impact of population aging, with costs for older adults typically being substantial. Long-term care costs continue rising faster than general inflation, creating affordability challenges for individuals and families. Emergency department visits and hospital readmissions are particularly expensive, often resulting from preventable complications. Workforce shortages in long-term care threaten service availability and quality. High turnover rates and recruitment challenges create gaps in formal care provision, increasing reliance on family caregivers. The economic value of informal caregiving represents a substantial hidden subsidy supporting current care systems while placing significant burdens on working-age adults.

The computational and infrastructure costs of implementing comprehensive smart aging solutions present both challenges and opportunities. Resource-intensive processing requirements for real-time sensor data analysis, machine learning model training, and continuous monitoring systems demand significant initial investments in hardware and software infrastructure [1]. However, these costs must be balanced against the potential for dramatic reductions in healthcare utilization and delayed institutionalization. Privacy protection measures add additional economic complexity, requiring investments in secure data transmission, encrypted storage systems, and compliance mechanisms [21]. The cost of ensuring robust privacy protection while maintaining system functionality creates trade-offs that must be carefully managed in resource-constrained environments.

The economic benefits of addressing technical challenges through advanced sensor systems and artificial intelligence become apparent through improved care efficiency and prevention of costly complications. Early detection of health deterioration, fall prevention systems, and medication adherence monitoring demonstrate favorable cost-effectiveness ratios by preventing expensive emergency interventions and hospitalizations [31, 37].

These economic pressures highlight the need for technological solutions including Internet of Things (IoT) sensing, artificial intelligence analytics, and ambient intelligence systems that can improve care efficiency, prevent costly complications, and support both formal and informal caregivers in providing effective assistance.

2.6 Evidence and Effectiveness

Research demonstrates significant benefits of technology interventions across multiple aging-related challenges. Remote monitoring systems reduce hospitalizations among older adults with chronic conditions, while smart home technologies decrease emergency service calls related to preventable incidents.

The effectiveness of sensor-based human activity recognition systems in aging contexts has been demonstrated across multiple domains. Smart home applications utilizing ambient sensors show promise for monitoring daily living activities and detecting deviations from normal routines that may indicate health changes [31]. Healthcare monitoring systems demonstrate substantial improvements in chronic disease management through continuous physiological and activity tracking [37].

Deep learning approaches have shown particular effectiveness in addressing the complex challenges of aging-related activity recognition. The ability of deep neural networks to automatically extract hierarchical features from sensor data addresses the inter-activity similarity challenges that are common in aging populations [42]. Convolutional neural networks excel at capturing spatial patterns in multi-sensor data, while recurrent architectures effectively model temporal dependencies in longitudinal health monitoring [23]. Advanced machine learning techniques also demonstrate effectiveness in handling the data scarcity and distribution challenges inherent in aging applications. Semi-supervised learning approaches enable systems to learn from limited labeled data while incorporating abundant unlabeled observations from continuous monitoring [46]. Transfer learning techniques allow models trained on existing datasets to be adapted for aging-specific patterns, addressing the annotation scarcity challenge.

Enhanced manufacturing and processing capabilities enable the development of sophisticated sensor systems specifically designed for aging populations [19]. Wearable devices with improved comfort, battery life, and ease of use demonstrate higher acceptance rates among older adults, leading to more consistent data collection and better system performance. Fall detection systems demonstrate ability to reduce injury severity through faster emergency response. Medication adherence support systems show significant improvements in adherence rates among older adults with complex regimens, translating to better health outcomes and reduced healthcare utilization [32].

Cost-effectiveness analyses demonstrate favorable economic returns through reduced healthcare utilization, delayed nursing home placement, and improved caregiver productivity. Technology interventions targeting high-risk individuals with multiple chronic conditions show particularly strong economic returns.

User acceptance research identifies key factors influencing adoption: perceived usefulness, ease of use, privacy concerns, and integration with existing routines. Older adults demonstrate strong acceptance of technologies providing clear benefits without requiring significant behavior changes or learning investments [45].

2.7 The Smart Living Paradigm

Smart living environments integrate multiple technologies and services to create comprehensive support ecosystems addressing the full spectrum of the aging challenges. These environments combine environmental monitoring, health tracking, social connectivity, safety systems, and emergency response in seamless platforms requiring minimal user interaction while providing maximum support value.

The evolution from traditional Internet of Things (IoT) approaches to cognitive-enabled smart living represents a fundamental paradigm shift. While conventional IoT systems focus primarily on connectivity and basic data collection, smart aging environments must possess the capability to learn, think, and understand both physical and social contexts [68]. This transformation addresses a critical limitation: without comprehensive cognitive capability, IoT systems are insufficient for the complex, nuanced requirements of aging support.

Drawing inspiration from the operational processes of human cognition, effective smart living systems must integrate five fundamental cognitive tasks [8]. First, perception-action cycles enable continuous monitoring and responsive interventions. Second, massive data analytics transform sensor streams into meaningful patterns and insights. Third, semantic derivation and knowledge discovery extract actionable intelligence from complex, multimodal data. Fourth, intelligent decision-making capabilities enable proactive and personalized interventions. Finally, on-demand service provisioning ensures appropriate and timely support delivery.

The cognitive framework addresses several critical challenges unique to aging contexts. Traditional connected systems often fail to handle the temporal dynamics and individual variability characteristic of aging populations. The noisy, sparse, and heterogeneous nature of data from aging environments requires sophisticated processing capabilities that go beyond simple connectivity [59]. Time-series data analysis becomes particularly crucial for detecting gradual changes in health status, activity patterns, and cognitive function that may indicate emerging needs or risks.

Smart living environments must seamlessly bridge the physical world—with its sensors, devices, and environmental constraints—and the social world—with its human demands, behavioral patterns, and care relationships [66]. This integration enables enhanced resource allocation, automatic system operation, and intelligent service provisioning that adapts to changing needs and preferences over time.

The technical foundation requires sophisticated cognitive radio network principles for efficient spectrum utilization and device coordination [29], while semantic-oriented approaches enable meaningful interpretation of sensor data within aging contexts [65]. Autonomous network operation capabilities reduce the burden on aging users while maintaining robust performance under varying conditions [73].

The conceptual foundations for smart living are increasingly well-established, with growing recognition of the potential for integrated technological approaches to support aging in place. Remaining challenges relate primarily to integration, customization, privacy protection, and cost optimization, rather than fundamental technology feasibility.

2.8 Conclusion

Population aging presents profound challenges and exciting opportunities for societies worldwide. Addressing these requires a paradigm shift from traditional care models to intelligent, technology-driven solutions that empower older adults to live independently, safely, and with dignity. This chapter has highlighted how AI, IoT, and ambient intelligence are converging to create smart living environments that are proactive, personalized, and scalable.

The evidence demonstrates that smart aging technologies can improve health outcomes, reduce costs, and enhance quality of life. However, successful deployment depends on interdisciplinary collaboration, robust privacy protection, and continuous innovation. As the monograph progresses, subsequent chapters will detail the technical foundations, integration strategies, and real-world implementations that are shaping the future of an empowered aging.

References

1. Akbari, A., Jafari, R.: Transferring activity recognition models for new wearable sensors with deep generative domain adaptation. In: Proceedings of the 18th International Conference on Information Processing in Sensor Networks, IPSN, pp. 85–96. ACM (2019)
2. Ashton, K.: That 'internet of things' thing in the real world, things matter more than ideas. RFID J. (2009)
3. Atzori, L., Iera, A., Morabito, G.: The internet of things: a survey. Comput. Netw. **54**(15), 2787–2805 (2010)

4. Azar, S.M., Atigh, M.G., Nickabadi, A., Alahi, A.: Convolutional relational machine for group activity recognition. In: Proceedings of the IEEE Conference on Computer Vision and Pattern Recognition, CVPR, pp. 7892–7901. IEEE (2019)
5. Bandaru, J., Kiran, M.S., Rajalakshmi, P.: A novel system architecture for brain controlled iot enabled environments. In: 19th IEEE International Conference on e-Health Networking, Applications and Services (HealthCom), pp. 1–5. IEEE (2017)
6. Bao, L., Intille, S.S.: Activity recognition from user-annotated acceleration data. In: Ferscha, A., Mattern, F. (eds.) Pervasive Computing, Pervasive 2004. Lecture Notes in Computer Science, vol. 3001, pp. 1–17. Springer, Berlin, Heidelberg (2004)
7. Barnaghi, P.M., Sheth, A.P., Henson, C.A.: From data to actionable knowledge: big data challenges in the web of things. IEEE Intell. Syst. **28**(6), 6–11 (2013)
8. Brock, D.L.: The electronic product code (epc): a naming scheme for physical objects. White Paper Auto-ID Center (2001)
9. Bulling, A., Blanke, U., Schiele, B.: A tutorial on human activity recognition using body-worn inertial sensors. ACM Comput. Surv. **46**(3), 33 (2014)
10. Callisaya, M.L., Blizzard, L., Schmidt, M.D., McGinley, J.L., Lord, S.R., Srikanth, V.K.: A population-based study of sensorimotor factors affecting gait in older people. Age Ageing **38**(3), 290–295 (2009)
11. Chen, J., Lin, B., Xu, R., Chai, Z., Liang, X., Wong, K.K.: Mapgpt: map-guided prompting for unified vision-and-language navigation (2024). arXiv:2401.07314
12. Chen, K., Zhang, D., Yao, L., Guo, B., Yu, Z., Liu, Y.: Deep learning for sensor-based human activity recognition: overview, challenges, and opportunities. ACM Comput. Surv. **54**(4), (2021)
13. Chen, L., Li, X., Wang, S., Hu, H.Y., Huang, N., Sheng, Q.Z., Sharaf, M.A.: Mining personal health index from annual geriatric medical examinations. In: Proceedings of the IEEE 14th International Conference on Data Mining (ICDM), pp. 761–766. IEEE (2014)
14. Chuang, J., Nguyen, H., Wang, C., Johnson, B.: I think, therefore i am: usability and security of authentication using brainwaves. In: Financial Cryptography and Data Security—FC Workshops 2013, pp. 1–16. Springer (2013)
15. Clarkson, B., Pentland, A.: Unsupervised clustering of ambulatory audio and video. In: Proceedings of the 1999 IEEE International Conference on Acoustics, Speech, and Signal Processing (ICASSP), vol. 6, pp. 3037–3040. IEEE (1999)
16. Dong, Q., Li, L., Dai, D., Zheng, C., Wu, Z., Chang, B., Sun, X., Xu, J., Sui, Z.: A survey on in-context learning (2022). arXiv:2301.00234
17. Eichelberg, M., Aden, T., Riesmeier, J., Dogac, A., Laleci, G.B.: A survey and analysis of electronic healthcare record standards. ACM Comput. Surv. **37**(4), 277–315 (2005)
18. Ghalwash, M.F., Radosavljevic, V., Obradovic, Z.: Extraction of interpretable multivariate patterns for early diagnostics. In: Proceedings of the 2013 IEEE 13th International Conference on Data Mining, pp. 201–210. IEEE (2013)
19. Grzeszick, R., Lenk, J.M., Rueda, F.M., Fink, G.A., Feldhorst, S., ten Hompel, M.: Deep neural network based human activity recognition for the order picking process. In: Proceedings of the 4th International Workshop on Sensor-based Activity Recognition and Interaction, iWOAR, p. 14. ACM (2017)
20. Gu, J., Stefani, E., Wu, Q., Thomason, J., Wang, X.E.: Vision-and-language navigation: a survey of tasks, methods, and future directions (2022). arXiv:2203.12667
21. Gudur, G.K., Sundaramoorthy, P., Umaashankar, V.: Activeharnet: towards on-device deep bayesian active learning for human activity recognition. In: Proceedings of the 3rd International Workshop on Embedded and Mobile Deep Learning, EMDL '19, p. 6. ACM (2019)
22. Ha, S., Yun, J.M., Choi, S.: Multi-modal convolutional neural networks for activity recognition. In: 2015 IEEE International Conference on Systems, Man, and Cybernetics, SMC, pp. 3017–3022. IEEE (2015)
23. Hammerla, N.Y., Halloran, S., Plötz, T.: Deep, convolutional, and recurrent models for human activity recognition using wearables. In: Proceedings of the Twenty-Fifth International Joint Conference on Artificial Intelligence, IJCAI, pp. 1533–1540 (2016)

24. Hammerla, N.Y., Halloran, S., Pltz, T.: Deep, convolutional, and recurrent models for human activity recognition using wearables. In: Proceedings of the Twenty-Fifth International Joint Conference on Artificial Intelligence (IJCAI), pp. 1533–1540 (2016)
25. Haselsteiner, E., Pfurtscheller, G.: Using time-dependent neural networks for EEG classification. IEEE Trans. Rehabil. Eng. **8**(4), 457–463 (2000)
26. Heydari, E., Shahbakhti, M.: Adaptive wavelet technique for EEG de-noising. In: Proceedings of the 8th Biomedical Engineering International Conference (BMEiCON), pp. 1–4. IEEE (2015)
27. Hussain, Z., Sheng, Q.Z., Zhang, W.E.: A review and categorization of techniques on device-free human activity recognition. J. Netw. Comput. Appl. **167**, 102738 (2020)
28. Huynh, T., Schiele, B.: Analyzing features for activity recognition. In: Proceedings of the 2005 Joint Conference on Smart Objects and Ambient Intelligence: Innovative Context-Aware Services: Usages and Technologies, pp. 159–163. ACM (2005)
29. Mitola III J., Maguire, G.Q.: Cognitive radio: making software radios more personal. IEEE Pers. Commun. **6**(4), 13–18 (1999)
30. International Telecommunication Union (ITU): Itu internet reports 2005: the internet of things. Technical Report, International Telecommunication Union (2005)
31. Ishimaru, S., Hoshika, K., Kunze, K., Kise, K., Dengel, A.: Towards reading trackers in the wild: detecting reading activities by EOG glasses and deep neural networks. In: Proceedings of the 2017 ACM International Joint Conference on Pervasive and Ubiquitous Computing and Proceedings of the 2017 ACM International Symposium on Wearable Computers, pp. 704–711. ACM (2017)
32. Ito, C., Cao, X., Shuzo, M., Maeda, E.: Application of CNN for human activity recognition with FFT spectrogram of acceleration and gyro sensors. In: Proceedings of the 2018 ACM International Joint Conference on Pervasive and Ubiquitous Computing and Proceedings of the 2018 ACM International Symposium on Wearable Computers, pp. 1503–1510. ACM (2018)
33. Jin, H., Che, H., Lin, Y., Chen, H.: Promptmrg: diagnosis-driven prompts for medical report generation. In: Proceedings of the AAAI Conference on Artificial Intelligence, vol. 38, pp. 2607–2615 (2024)
34. Kim, E., Helal, S., Cook, D.J.: Human activity recognition and pattern discovery. IEEE Pervasive Comput. **9**(1), 48–53 (2010)
35. Lane, N.D., Georgiev, P.: Can deep learning revolutionize mobile sensing? In: Proceedings of the 16th International Workshop on Mobile Computing Systems and Applications, HotMobile, pp. 117–122. ACM (2015)
36. Lara, O.D., Labrador, M.A.: A survey on human activity recognition using wearable sensors. IEEE Commun. Surv. Tutorials **15**(3), 1192–1209 (2013)
37. Li, X., Zhang, Y., Li, M., Marsic, I., Yang, J., Burd, R.S.: Deep neural network for RFID-based activity recognition. In: Proceedings of the 8th Workshop on Wireless of the Students, by the Students, and for the Students, S3@MobiCom, pp. 24–26. ACM (2016)
38. Lin, B., Nie, Y., Wei, Z., Chen, J., Ma, S., Han, J., Xu, H., Chang, X., Liang, X.: Navcot: boosting llm-based vision-and-language navigation via learning disentangled reasoning (2024). arXiv:2403.07376
39. Lin, J., Keogh, E., Lonardi, S., Chiu, B.: A symbolic representation of time series, with implications for streaming algorithms. In: Proceedings of the 8th ACM SIGMOD Workshop on Research Issues in Data Mining and Knowledge Discovery, pp. 2–11. ACM (2003)
40. Long, Y., Li, X., Cai, W., Dong, H.: Discuss before moving: visual language navigation via multi-expert discussions. In: 2024 IEEE International Conference on Robotics and Automation, ICRA, pp. 17380–17387. IEEE (2024)
41. Mathe, M.: Age and health in China: what can we learn from the world's largest population of older people? https://www.prb.org/wp-content/uploads/2020/07/TRA39-2020-health-aging-China.pdf (2020). Population Reference Bureau, 39. Accessed 9 Sept 2025
42. Mathur, A., Zhang, T., Bhattacharya, S., Veličković, P., Joffe, L., Lane, N.D., Kawsar, F., Liò, P.: Using deep data augmentation training to address software and hardware heterogeneities in wearable and smartphone sensing devices. In: Proceedings of the 17th International Conference on Information Processing in Sensor Networks, IPSN, pp. 200–211. IEEE (2018)

43. Mennicken, S., Vermeulen, J., Huang, E.M.: From today's augmented houses to tomorrow's smart homes: new directions for home automation research. In: Proceedings of the 2014 ACM International Joint Conference on Pervasive and Ubiquitous Computing (UbiComp '14), pp. 105–115. ACM (2014)
44. Messina, P., Pino, P., Parra, D., Soto, A., Besa, C., Uribe, S., Andía, M., Tejos, C., Prieto, C., Capurro, D.: A survey on deep learning and explainability for automatic report generation from medical images. ACM Comput. Surv. **54**(10s), 1–40 (2022)
45. Moxley, J., Sharit, J., Czaja, S.J.: The factors influencing older adults' decisions surrounding adoption of technology: quantitative experimental study. JMIR Aging **5**(4), e39890 (2022)
46. Murahari, V.S., Plötz, T.: On attention models for human activity recognition. In: Proceedings of the 2018 ACM International Symposium on Wearable Computers, ISWC, pp. 100–103. ACM (2018)
47. Nakamura, T., Goverdovsky, V., Mandic, D.: In-ear EEG biometrics for feasible and readily collectable real-world person authentication. IEEE Trans. Inf. Forensics Secur. **13**(3), 648–661 (2018)
48. Nguyen, B., Nguyen, D., Ma, W., Tran, D.: Investigating the possibility of applying EEG lossy compression to EEG-based user authentication. In: International Joint Conference on Neural Networks (IJCNN), pp. 79–85. IEEE (2017)
49. Pan, B., Panda, R., Jin, S., Feris, R., Oliva, A., Isola, P., Kim, Y.: Langnav: language as a perceptual representation for navigation (2023). arXiv:2310.07889
50. Pouyanfar, S., Sadiq, S., Yan, Y., Tian, H., Tao, Y., Reyes, M.P., Shyu, M.L., Chen, S.C., Iyengar, S.S.: A survey on deep learning: algorithms, techniques, and applications. ACM Comput. Surv. **51**(5), 92 (2018)
51. Pu, Q., Gupta, S., Gollakota, S., Patel, S.N.: Whole-home gesture recognition using wireless signals. In: Proceedings of the 19th Annual International Conference on Mobile Computing and Networking (MobiCom '13), pp. 27–38. ACM (2013)
52. Rahman, M.A., Ahmad, M.: A straight forward signal processing scheme to improve effect size of fNIR signals. In: International Conference on Informatics, Electronics and Vision (ICIEV), pp. 439–444 (2016)
53. Richardson, A.: Aged care residential services in Australia–Market Research Report (2015–2030). https://www.ibisworld.com/australia/industry/aged-care-residential-services/5531/. Accessed 9 Sept 2025
54. Ruan, W., Sheng, Q.Z., Yao, L., Gu, T., Ruta, M., Shangguan, L.: Device-free indoor localization and tracking through human-object interactions. In: 17th IEEE International Symposium on A World of Wireless, Mobile and Multimedia Networks, WoWMoM 2016, Coimbra, Portugal, June 21–24, 2016, pp. 1–9. IEEE Computer Society (2016)
55. Ruan, W., Yang, L., Sheng, Q.Z., Gu, T., Xu, P., Shangguan, L.: Making sense of doppler effect for multi-modal hand motion detection. IEEE Trans. Mob. Comput. **17**(9), 2087–2100 (2018)
56. Rudenko, A., Palmieri, L., Herman, M., Kitani, K.M., Gavrila, D.M., Arras, K.O.: Human motion trajectory prediction: a survey. Int. J. Robotics Res. **39**(8), (2020)
57. Shemshadi, A., Sheng, Q.Z., Qin, Y., Sun, A., Zhang, W.E., Yao, L.: Searching for the internet of things: where it is and what it looks like. Pers. Ubiquit. Comput. **21**(6), 1097–1112 (2017)
58. Sun, S., Zhou, J.: A review of adaptive feature extraction and classification methods for eeg-based brain-computer interfaces. In: Proceedings of the 2014 International Joint Conference on Neural Networks (IJCNN), pp. 1746–1753. IEEE (2014)
59. Sundmaeker, H., Guillemin, P., Friess, P., Woelfflé, S.: Vision and challenges for realising the internet of things. Technical Report, European Commission Information Society and Media (2010)
60. Tapia, E.M., Intille, S.S., Larson, K.: Activity recognition in the home using simple and ubiquitous sensors. In: Pervasive Computing. Lecture Notes in Computer Science. Springer (2004)
61. Teles, A., Antunes, M., Luz, P., ao Paulo, J.: Using brain–computer interface and internet of things to improve healthcare for wheelchair users. In: Proceedings of the 11th International Conference on Mobile Ubiquitous Computing, Systems, Services and Technologies (UBICOMM), pp. 92–94 (2017)

62. United Nations: Ageing. https://www.un.org/en/global-issues/ageing. Accessed 9 Sept 2025
63. United Nations: World Population Ageing 2019. https://www.un.org/en/development/desa/population/publications/pdf/ageing/WorldPopulationAgeing2019-Report.pdf. Accessed 9 Sept 2025
64. Vallabhaneni, A., Wang, T., He, B.: Brain–computer interface. In: Neural Engineering, pp. 85–121. Springer, Boston, MA, USA (2005)
65. Vermesan, O., Friess, P., Guillemin, P., et al.: Internet of things strategic research roadmap. Technical Report, The Cluster of European Research Projects (2009)
66. Vlacheas, P., Giaffreda, R., Stavroulaki, V., et al.: Enabling smart cities through a cognitive management framework for the internet of things. IEEE Commun. Mag. **51**(6), 102–111 (2013)
67. WAhnang, H., Li, Y., Long, J., Yu, T., Gu, Z.: An asynchronous wheelchair control by hybrid EEG–EOG brain-computer interface. Cogn. Neurodynamics **8**(5), 399–409 (2014)
68. Wu, Q., et al.: Cognitive internet of things: a new paradigm beyond connection. IEEE Internet Things J. **1**(2), 129–143 (2014)
69. Yang, J., Nguyen, M.N., San, P.P., Li, X.L., Krishnaswamy, S.: Deep convolutional neural networks on multichannel time series for human activity recognition. In: Proceedings of the Twenty-Fourth International Joint Conference on Artificial Intelligence, IJCAI, pp. 3995–4001 (2015)
70. Yao, L., Sheng, Q.Z., Falkner, N.J.G., Ngu, A.H.H., et al.: WITS: an IoT-endowed computational framework for activity recognition in personalized smart homes. Computing **100**(4), 369–385 (2018)
71. Youssef, M., Mah, M., Agrawala, A.K.: Challenges: device-free passive localization for wireless environments. In: Proceedings of the 13th Annual International Conference on Mobile Computing and Networking, MOBICOM 2007, Montréal, Québec, Canada, September 9–14, 2007, pp. 222–229. ACM (2007)
72. Zhang, D., Zhou, J., Guo, M., Cao, J., Li, T.: TASA: tag-free activity sensing using RFID tag arrays. IEEE Trans. Parallel Distrib. Syst. **22**(4), 558–570 (2011)
73. Zhang, M., Zhao, H., Zheng, R., et al.: Cognitive internet of things: concepts and application example. Int. J. Comput. Sci. Issues **9**(3), 151–158 (2012)
74. Zhang, X., Yao, L., Kanhere, S.S., Liu, Y., Gu, T., Chen, K.: MindID: person identification from brain waves through attention-based recurrent neural network. Proc. ACM Interact. Mob. Wearable Ubiquitous Technol. **2**(3), 149:1–149:23 (2018)
75. Zhang, X., Yao, L., Sheng, Q.Z., Kanhere, S., Gu, T., Zhang, D.: Converting your thoughts to texts: enabling brain typing via deep feature learning of EEG signals. In: IEEE International Conference on Pervasive Computing and Communications (PerCom), pp. 1–10. IEEE Computer Society (2018)
76. Zheng, D., Huang, S., Zhao, L., Zhong, Y., Wang, L.: Towards learning a generalist model for embodied navigation. In: Proceedings of the IEEE/CVF Conference on Computer Vision and Pattern Recognition, CVPR, pp. 13624–13634. IEEE (2024)
77. Zhou, G., Hong, Y., Wu, Q.: Navgpt: explicit reasoning in vision-and-language navigation with large language models. In: Proceedings of the AAAI Conference on Artificial Intelligence, pp. 7641–7649. AAAI (2024)

Chapter 3
Technical Background

3.1 Artificial Intelligence for Smart Aging

Artificial intelligence serves as the cognitive foundation that transforms sensor data into meaningful insights and actionable interventions for aging populations. The unique characteristics of aging-related applications—sparse and noisy data, individual variability, temporal dynamics, and safety-critical requirements—necessitate specialized AI approaches that prioritize interpretability, robustness, and adaptability. The application of artificial intelligence to aging contexts faces distinctive challenges that differentiate it from traditional machine learning applications. Human activity recognition in aging populations requires sophisticated approaches to handle inter-activity similarity, where different activities may exhibit nearly identical sensor patterns due to age-related movement changes [12]. The development of effective AI systems for aging support demands careful consideration of annotation scarcity, distribution discrepancy, and the need for real-time processing in resource-constrained environments.

3.1.1 Machine Learning Paradigms for Aging Applications

The application of machine learning to aging contexts requires careful consideration of data scarcity, user diversity, and deployment constraints specific to elderly populations. Advanced paradigms address these challenges through specialized architectures and training methodologies.

Semi-supervised and Active Learning. Semi-supervised learning techniques address the fundamental challenge of limited labeled data in healthcare contexts, where expert annotation is expensive and time-consuming [25]. Graph-based methods, co-training approaches, and generative models enable systems to learn from limited labeled examples while incorporating information from abundant unlabeled

Q. Z. Sheng et al., *Harnessing Artificial Intelligence and Pervasive Internet of Things for an Empowered Aging*, https://doi.org/10.1007/978-3-032-16502-2_3

observations. Variational autoencoders (VAEs) and generative adversarial networks (GANs) show particular promise for learning compact representations of behavioral and physiological patterns while enabling data augmentation for rare events.

Advanced semi-supervised approaches for aging applications include robust methods that extract intrinsic shared structures from activities to handle intra-class variability while utilizing both labeled and unlabeled data effectively [4]. These methods use techniques such as $\ell_{2,1}$ minimization to resist outliers in noisy sensor data, integrating shared structure discovery with graph-based manifold regularization. Distributionally robust semi-supervised learning models address distribution shifts between labeled and unlabeled data in people-centric sensing applications, reducing person-specific discrepancy while preserving task-specific consistency [22]. While these approaches have shown promise in controlled studies, their effectiveness in diverse aging populations may require additional validation and customization.

Deep active learning approaches strategically select the most informative samples for annotation, addressing the critical challenge of class imbalance in aging-related datasets where emergency events are rare but essential to detect accurately [25]. These methods substantially reduce labeling costs while maintaining system performance, particularly important for aging applications where domain expertise is limited and expensive.

Data Mining and Machine Learning for Personal Health Management. Personal health management systems for aging populations require sophisticated data mining approaches to handle the complexity and heterogeneity of electronic health records (EHRs) and health examination data. These systems must address fundamental challenges including the sparsity and heterogeneity of health examination records, where participants may have irregular examination schedules and sparse abnormal results, while test items naturally fall into different categories with varying semantic contributions to risk identification.

Advanced graph-based approaches for health data analysis demonstrate potential for addressing the predominantly unlabeled nature of health examination datasets, where participants' conditions may vary greatly from healthy to very-ill without clear ground truth differentiation. Semi-supervised heterogeneous graph construction methods can effectively model the natural heterogeneity in health examination items while leveraging both labeled and unlabeled data for risk prediction [23]. These approaches require careful validation in diverse aging populations to establish their reliability and clinical utility across different health conditions and demographic groups.

Personal Health Indexing (PHI) systems utilize data mining methodologies to predict health status from comprehensive medical examination records, addressing the manually impossible task of exploring correlations among hundreds of test results, their longitudinal progression, and relationships to participants with similar health development patterns [20]. Machine learning approaches for processing Electronic Health Records (EHRs) from annual geriatric medical examinations enable systems to analyze vast amounts of health data collected over years, supporting from-cradle-to-grave health evaluation through sophisticated temporal modeling and feature extraction techniques [13]. However, these systems require careful consideration of data privacy, clinical validation, and adaptation to diverse aging populations with varying health conditions and examination patterns.

Deep Learning Architectures. Deep neural networks demonstrate remarkable effectiveness for aging-related tasks, particularly medical image analysis and temporal pattern recognition. The hierarchical nature of deep learning architectures enables automatic feature extraction from raw sensor data, addressing the inter-activity similarity challenge through layer-by-layer abstraction from simple to complex patterns [12].

Convolutional neural networks (CNNs) excel at spatial pattern extraction and demonstrate translational invariance properties that accommodate the variability in aging-related movement patterns [27]. Their local connectivity features enable effective processing of multimodal sensory data common in smart aging environments. Recurrent neural networks (RNNs) and their variants, including Long Short-Term Memory (LSTM) networks, effectively analyze temporal sequences in physiological signals and behavioral data, capturing the temporal dependencies crucial for aging-related pattern recognition [37].

Transformer architectures and attention mechanisms provide enhanced capabilities for processing complex temporal dependencies and multi-modal data fusion while offering improved interpretability through attention visualization [39]. These advanced architectures enable sophisticated processing of long-term behavioral patterns essential for detecting gradual changes in aging populations.

Multi-agent attention frameworks treat activity recognition as collaborative decision-making problems, deploying multiple intelligent agents that independently select informative sensor modalities while sharing information to coordinate their selection policies [11]. These approaches consider spatially-temporally varying salience of sensor features and relationships between activities and corresponding body part motions, providing explainable insights through attention visualization that enhance system interpretability for practical deployments.

The modular and composable nature of deep learning systems enables integration of specialized techniques including transfer learning for domain adaptation across different aging populations and environments [1]. This flexibility addresses the distribution discrepancy challenge inherent in diverse aging contexts, while enabling efficient adaptation to individual user characteristics.

Reinforcement Learning. Reinforcement learning enables adaptive aging support systems that learn optimal interve ntion strategies through interaction with users and environments. Multi-armed bandit algorithms provide efficient frameworks for personalizing interventions such as medication reminders and exercise recommendations, while deep reinforcement learning approaches enable sophisticated decision-making in complex environments including robotic assistance and smart home automation.

The application of reinforcement learning to aging contexts requires careful consideration of safety constraints and gradual adaptation to changing user capabilities. Safe exploration strategies ensure that learning algorithms do not compromise user safety while discovering optimal intervention policies.

3.1.2 *Natural Language Processing for Aging Interfaces*

Natural language processing (NLP) technologies enable intuitive communication between elderly users and smart systems, while accommodating age-related changes in speech patterns and cognitive processing. Automatic speech recognition systems must handle reduced articulation clarity and altered vocal characteristics common in aging populations [46].

Conversational AI systems require careful design to provide appropriate social interaction without patronizing language. Large language models offer powerful capabilities for natural interaction but require domain-specific fine-tuning and careful attention to factual accuracy and bias mitigation in healthcare contexts. The development of voice-based interfaces becomes particularly crucial for accommodating users with varying levels of technological familiarity and cognitive capacity [58].

Large Language Models (LLMs) for medical applications have demonstrated significant potential for automated report generation and clinical documentation, particularly relevant for aging populations who frequently require comprehensive health monitoring. Medical report generation utilizing LLMs employs encoder-decoder architectures where the decoder's capacity to process lengthy sequences becomes crucial due to the extensive nature of medical reports [38]. Modern approaches have evolved from initial LSTM-based decoders to Transformer-based variants, including memory-driven, knowledge-enhanced, and contrastive learning paradigms [14, 15, 28, 32, 34].

Zero-shot learning capabilities in medical report generation address the substantial challenge of collecting large amounts of paired medical image-report data, particularly relevant for resource-constrained healthcare facilities and specialized aging-related conditions where sample sizes may be inherently limited. In-context learning (ICL) approaches leverage the emergent capabilities of LLMs to generate reports for new scenarios with minimal examples, though computational inefficiency when processing lengthy medical reports remains a significant limitation [19, 30]. Advanced techniques such as multi-modal context vector approaches have shown potential for improving efficiency while maintaining generation quality, though validation in diverse aging populations and rare geriatric conditions requires further investigation.

Brain-computer interface technologies extend natural language processing capabilities by enabling direct communication pathways between the brain and smart systems. EEG-based intention recognition systems have shown promising results through sophisticated spatio-temporal neural network architectures that convert 1D EEG sequences to 2D spatial meshes preserving correlations between brain regions [6, 49]. However, deployment in aging contexts may require careful consideration of signal processing challenges, including noise from physiological activities and the need for personalized adaptation to individual neural patterns. The effectiveness of these approaches in diverse aging populations remains to be fully validated in real-world settings.

Advanced deep learning frameworks for brain-computer interfaces offer potential for enabling human-thing cognitive interactivity through unified end-to-end processing of brain signals. These frameworks typically incorporate specialized techniques including replicate and shuffle processes for enhancing feature representation, selective attention mechanisms for identifying informative signal segments, and weighted averaging approaches for improved classification stability [40, 42]. While experimental studies have reported accuracy rates exceeding 90%, translation to practical aging applications may require careful validation of signal quality, user adaptation, and long-term reliability considerations across diverse older adult populations where neural patterns and signal characteristics may vary.

Cross-modal learning approaches enable systems to understand relationships between different modalities of data, such as brain signals and visual stimuli, showing potential for comprehensive cognitive monitoring applications [31]. Self-supervised cross-modal learning paradigms can retrieve visual matching for EEG signals evoked by visual stimuli, though their effectiveness in aging populations may require further validation and adaptation to age-related changes in cognitive processing.

3.1.3 Privacy-Preserving Monitoring

It is important that non-intrusive comprehensive monitoring is not at the cost of giving up privacy. Activity recognition systems must handle aging-related movement patterns including reduced mobility and assistive device usage. The challenge of recognizing activities in aging populations requires specialized approaches to handle symbolic representation of movement patterns and time-frequency transformation of collected data [29, 39].

Advanced signal processing techniques such as compressive sensing and dictionary learning offer opportunities to extract meaningful patterns from noisy signals, addressing fundamental challenges of signal uncertainty in device-free systems. These approaches enable compact and informative representations of activities using unsupervised subspace decomposition, facilitating efficient recognition despite streaming and unstable sensor signals [57]. Such methods have shown promise for passive RFID-based activity recognition scenarios, where signal strength indicators suffer from high uncertainties due to environmental factors, though adaptation for aging-specific movement patterns may require additional validation.

Acoustic-based recognition systems leverage Doppler effects and echo analysis to detect hand movements and gestures using built-in speakers and microphones, transforming standard devices into active sonar systems. These approaches have shown promising multi-modal detection capabilities in controlled environments, recognizing not only gesture types but also estimating continuous attributes such as movement duration, speed, and range [50]. This may enable fine-grained control interfaces that could prove suitable for smart aging environments where intuitive interaction mechanisms are essential, though user acceptance and accuracy considerations require further investigation across diverse aging populations.

Privacy-preserving approaches include edge processing, anonymization techniques, and alternative sensing modalities such as depth cameras that provide functional information without identifiable visual details. Federated learning enables collective improvement while maintaining local data processing and privacy protection, addressing the distributed nature of aging support systems across multiple homes and care facilities.

3.1.4 Multimodal Biometric Authentication Architectures

Multimodal biometric authentication systems for aging populations require sophisticated deep learning architectures that can effectively combine multiple biometric modalities while accommodating age-related physiological changes. These systems must balance security requirements with usability considerations specific to older adults, addressing challenges including noise susceptibility, environmental variations, and the need for robust fake-resistance characteristics.

Advanced deep learning frameworks for biometric authentication integrate complementary modalities such as EEG signals and gait patterns to achieve enhanced security and reliability for aging applications. EEG-based authentication leverages the unique electromagnetic neural oscillations of brain activity, which remain individual-specific and difficult to replicate, providing inherent security advantages [17]. However, EEG signal processing requires sophisticated architectures to handle low signal-to-noise ratios, environmental interference, and individual neural pattern variations that may be particularly pronounced in aging populations.

Attention-based recurrent neural networks demonstrate potential for processing multimodal biometric data by selectively focusing on the most discriminative features across different modalities and temporal segments. These architectures can effectively decode distinctive patterns in brain activities and behavioral characteristics while providing improved classification stability through attention mechanisms that identify informative signal components [17]. Gait-based authentication systems leverage deep learning approaches to analyze individual walking patterns determined by intrinsic temporal and kinematic factors, though their effectiveness across diverse aging populations with varying mobility levels and assistive device usage requires careful validation [9].

The integration of multiple biometric modalities through deep fusion architectures enables systems to achieve higher accuracy and reliability while accommodating the specific limitations of older adults. These approaches require careful consideration of computational efficiency, real-time processing requirements, and adaptive capabilities to handle progressive changes in biometric characteristics that may occur with aging. Advanced authentication systems must also incorporate privacy protection mechanisms and fail-safe procedures to ensure reliable operation across diverse aging contexts while maintaining user dignity and independence [62].

3.2 Internet of Things Architectures

Building upon the artificial intelligence foundations discussed above, the implementation of smart aging solutions requires sophisticated Internet of Things architectures that can seamlessly integrate diverse sensing modalities, processing capabilities, and service delivery mechanisms [41, 51, 56]. The evolution from traditional connectivity-focused IoT to cognitive-enabled systems represents a fundamental paradigm shift essential for addressing the complex requirements of aging support applications.

The Cognitive Internet of Things (CIoT) paradigm elevates traditional IoT architecture by integrating cognitive capabilities—learning, reasoning, and autonomous decision-making—into distributed sensing and actuation systems for smart aging environments [7, 54]. CIoT systems serve as intelligent bridges between the physical and social worlds, forming intelligent physical-cyber-social (iPCS) systems that adapt to user needs with minimal human intervention.

3.2.1 Cognitive IoT Architecture

The CIoT architecture consists of four major layers:

- *Sensing Control Layer*: Interfaces directly with the physical environment, using diverse sensors (motion, physiological, environmental) and actuators to collect and respond to stimuli. Advanced sensors such as smart flooring and wearables enable detailed activity and health monitoring, prioritizing user comfort and privacy [26, 55].
- *Data-Semantic-Knowledge Layer*: Processes heterogeneous, noisy, high-dimensional data using techniques for massive data analytics, including distributed and parallel processing, nonlinear modeling, and semantic derivation. This layer transforms raw data into meaningful semantic information and actionable knowledge [2, 18, 43].
- *Decision-Making Layer*: Employs intelligent algorithms (e.g., reinforcement learning, multi-agent reasoning) to plan, select, and adapt actions based on semantic knowledge, supporting both service provision and adaptive control in dynamic environments [59, 61].

- *Service Evaluation Layer*: Interfaces with social networks and users, providing on-demand services (e.g., Sensing-as-a-Service, Everything-as-a-Service) and evaluating system performance using novel metrics, feeding results back to optimize cognition and service quality [3, 5].

3.2.2 Massive Data Analytics and Semantic Reasoning

CIoT environments generate massive, heterogeneous data streams from distributed sources. Key technical challenges include:

- *Heterogeneous Data Processing*: Integrating multimodal data (sensor, image, audio, physiological) with robust preprocessing and fusion algorithms [2, 43].
- *Nonlinear and High-Dimensional Modeling*: Applying deep learning and dimensionality reduction to extract patterns from complex, noisy data [18].
- *Distributed and Parallel Analytics*: Leveraging edge computing and federated learning for privacy-preserving, scalable analytics across homes and care facilities [54, 61].
- *Semantic Derivation and Knowledge Discovery*: Using context-aware reasoning, ontologies, and semantic standardization to enable intelligent understanding and decision support [18].

3.2.3 Technical Challenges and Solutions

CIoT systems autonomously adapt to user states and environmental changes through intelligent decision-making. Reinforcement learning and multi-agent systems enable personalized interventions, emergency response, and resource allocation. On-demand service provisioning supports flexible, user-centric care models [5, 59]. Major challenges in CIoT for smart aging include:

- *Privacy and Security*: Ensuring data protection through edge processing, anonymization, and federated learning [54].
- *Interoperability*: Integrating diverse devices and platforms using standards and middleware [52, 53].
- *Scalability*: Managing massive data and device populations with distributed architectures and efficient resource allocation [2, 43].
- *User Acceptance*: Designing unobtrusive, adaptive systems that respect user preferences and comfort [55].

The CIoT framework provides a comprehensive, multi-layered architecture for smart aging environments, integrating advanced sensing, massive data analytics, semantic reasoning, and intelligent decision-making to deliver adaptive, privacy-preserving, and user-centric solutions [3, 5, 18, 54, 59, 61].

Furthermore, Web-based IoT management systems offer accessible interfaces for controlling and monitoring smart aging environments through familiar browser-based interactions. These systems provide layered frameworks for managing information produced by physical devices and rule-based approaches to aggregate individual components for building context-aware, personalized services [16, 45]. The integration of Web technologies with IoT has shown potential for intuitive visualization and control of connected devices, potentially reducing the technical barriers that often prevent older adults from effectively utilizing smart home technologies. However, successful deployment requires careful attention to user interface design, system reliability, and accessibility considerations specific to aging populations, with validation needed across diverse user groups and home environments.

3.3 Robotics for Aging Assistance

Robotic systems for smart aging are increasingly deployed in real-world environments, providing not only physical assistance but also intelligent support for daily living, health management, and social engagement. Modern cognitive robots leverage AI and IoT to autonomously learn, model environments, reason semantically, and collaborate with humans. These systems are now being integrated into smart homes, rehabilitation centers, and community care settings, where they support medication management, mobility, fall detection, and companionship [37, 59]. Recent advances include multimodal sensing, adaptive interaction, and privacy-preserving data processing, reflecting the latest trends in robotics for aging populations.

The evolution of device-free monitoring technologies enables robots to operate in environments where traditional sensor placement may be impractical or intrusive. Radio frequency-based systems, including Wi-Fi, RFID, and radar technologies, have shown potential for detecting human activities by analyzing signal fluctuations without requiring body-worn sensors [47, 60]. These approaches may provide continuous monitoring capabilities while operating in various lighting conditions and offering accessible, cost-effective solutions for robotic perception systems, though their effectiveness in diverse aging environments requires ongoing evaluation.

Deep learning architectures, particularly transformers and point cloud-based networks, offer enhanced capabilities for robotic perception and interaction recognition. Two-stream multi-level dynamic point transformers have demonstrated ability to process depth video data for recognizing complex interactions between individuals while preserving privacy, potentially providing robots with sophisticated understanding of social behaviors in monitoring environments [48]. These advances may enable robots to interpret social contexts and adapt their assistance strategies accordingly, though translation to real-world aging care scenarios requires careful validation and ethical consideration.

Intent-aware robotic systems integrate with IoT networks to enable collaborative ambient intelligence that can anticipate user needs and provide proactive assistance. The Internet of Robotic Things (IoRT) paradigm enables robots to gain environmental awareness and adapt their actions based on contextual information from distributed sensors and smart devices [36, 56]. Advanced reinforcement learning methodologies for robotic assistants can exploit both successful and failed experiences to expedite learning, though deployment in aging contexts requires careful consideration of safety constraints and individual adaptation requirements [8]. While laboratory studies have shown promising results, real-world validation in diverse aging environments remains an important area for continued research.

Emergent capabilities of large foundation models present transformative opportunities for intelligent robotic navigation and assistance in aging environments. Vision-Language Models (VLMs) and Large Language Models (LLMs) have demonstrated remarkable zero-shot learning abilities, enabling robots to understand and execute complex navigation instructions based on natural language commands without explicit task-specific training [10, 35, 64]. These emergent capabilities arise from complex interactions within large-scale neural architectures, allowing models to perform tasks beyond their initial training objectives. Visual Language Navigation (VLN) represents a fundamental application domain where foundation models can enable agents to navigate complex environments based on natural language instructions [24].

However, significant challenges persist when leveraging emergent capabilities for specialized applications such as aging assistance. The gap between general knowledge encoded in foundation models and specialized requirements of aging support systems often results in performance limitations [10, 35, 64]. Computational requirements for fine-tuning large foundation models remain prohibitive for many healthcare applications, while pre-trained visual perception backbones may struggle with dynamic scenarios inherent in aging assistance tasks [21, 33, 44, 63]. These limitations highlight opportunities for developing novel approaches that can bridge the gap between general-purpose foundation models and specialized aging assistance requirements while maintaining the benefits of emergent capabilities for adaptive, personalized assistance systems.

Cognitive Service Robots and Multimodal Perception. Cognitive service robots integrate visual, speech, tactile, and other multimodal sensors to comprehensively perceive home environments, user behaviors, and health status. Based on deep learning and semantic reasoning, robots can detect abnormal behaviors (e.g., falls, unusual activities), understand user intentions, and proactively adjust service strategies. Mobile manipulation platforms combine SLAM and semantic mapping to support navigation and task execution in complex environments [39, 59].

Human-Robot sCollaboration and Personalized Interaction. Intelligent robots utilize natural language processing, emotion recognition, and active learning to achieve personalized interaction with elderly users. Multimodal interfaces (voice, gesture, touch, vision) enhance interaction flexibility, adapting to diverse cognitive and physical abilities. Social robots not only provide companionship, but also promote mental health and social connection through semantic understanding and emotional feedback [5, 46].

Safety, Ethics, and Privacy Protection. Robots operating in safety-critical environments require multi-layered safety mechanisms: intrinsic safety design, sensor fusion for collision detection, emergency stop, and fault recovery. Ethical design emphasizes autonomy preservation, ensuring robots assist rather than replace human decision-making, and respecting user privacy and data security. Distributed data processing and federated learning effectively reduce privacy risks [18, 54].

Technical Challenges and Future Directions. Cognitive robots face challenges such as environmental complexity, user diversity, real-time response, and long-term adaptation. Future directions include multi-agent collaboration, cross-domain knowledge transfer, enhanced explainability, and deep integration with CIoT, aiming for truly personalized, intelligent, and safe aging assistance systems [18, 59, 61].

3.4 Integration and System Architectures

The deep integration of AI, IoT, and robotic systems is essential for realizing intelligent aging environments. Integrated architectures must address multi-source data interoperability, system complexity, reliability, and scalability to ensure seamless collaboration among subsystems and support personalized services [52, 53, 61].

Architecture Design and Interoperability. Integrated systems adopt layered architectures, combining cloud-edge-end collaboration to enable efficient data acquisition, processing, storage, and intelligent decision making. Standardized communication protocols (e.g., Matter), middleware, and semantic interoperability platforms support seamless integration of multi-vendor devices and heterogeneous data. In healthcare, standards such as FHIR facilitate data sharing and intelligent analysis [18, 52].

Scalability and Performance Optimization. Hybrid cloud-edge architectures enhance system scalability and real-time performance. Container orchestration platforms (e.g., Kubernetes) enable automatic deployment, elastic scaling, and fault recovery. Distributed resource management and cost optimization ensure comprehensive functionality and economic efficiency. Federated learning and edge intelligence technologies balance privacy protection and performance requirements [54, 61].

Technical Challenges and Future Directions. Integrated systems face challenges such as device heterogeneity, data security, real-time response, and long-term maintenance. Future developments include cross-domain knowledge fusion, intelligent central platforms, enhanced explainability, and adaptive optimization, aiming to realize truly intelligent, reliable, and sustainable aging support environments [18, 59, 61].

3.5 Conclusion

The convergence of artificial intelligence (AI), Internet of Things (IoT), and robotics is revolutionizing the landscape of smart aging. By integrating advanced sensing, intelligent decision making, and adaptive support systems, these technologies are empowering older adults to maintain independence, safety, and well-being in diverse environments. This chapter has provided a technical roadmap for understanding and implementing these solutions, with a focus on real-world impact and future innovation. Figure 3.1 summarizes the main topics covered in this chapter.

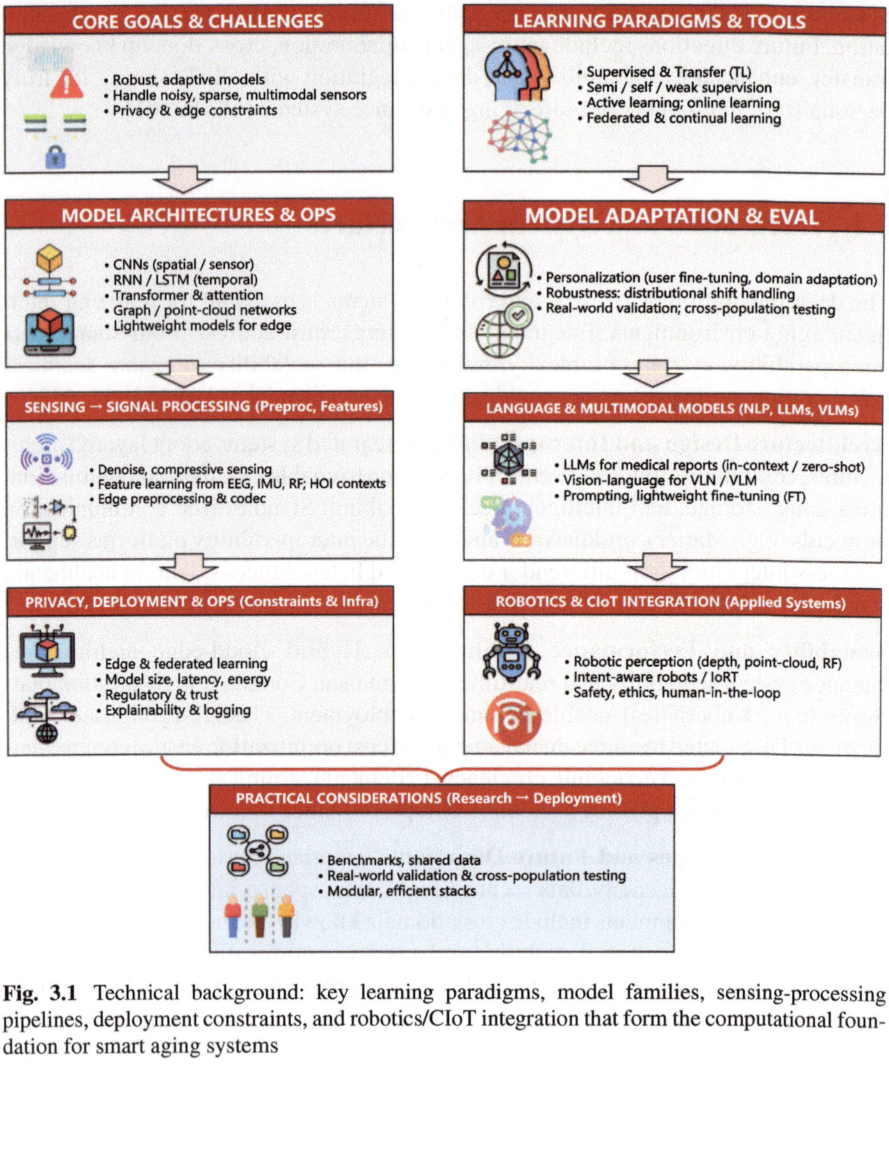

Fig. 3.1 Technical background: key learning paradigms, model families, sensing-processing pipelines, deployment constraints, and robotics/CIoT integration that form the computational foundation for smart aging systems

Moving forward, the monograph will explore practical integration strategies, deployment challenges, and case studies that exemplify the transformative potential of smart aging technologies. Continued research, cross-disciplinary collaboration, and user-centered design will be essential to realize the full promise of intelligent, connected living for aging populations.

References

1. Akbari, A., Jafari, R.: Transferring activity recognition models for new wearable sensors with deep generative domain adaptation. In: Proceedings of the 18th International Conference on Information Processing in Sensor Networks, IPSN, pp. 85–96. ACM (2019)
2. Atzori, L., Iera, A., Morabito, G.: The internet of things: a survey. Comput. Netw. **54**(15), 2787–2805 (2010)
3. Banerjee, P., Friedrich, R., Bash, C., et al.: Everything as a service: powering the new information economy. Computer **44**(3), 36–43 (2011)
4. Bhattacharya, S., Nurmi, P., Hammerla, N., Plötz, T.: Using unlabeled data in a sparse-coding framework for human activity recognition. Pervasive Mob. Comput. **15**, 242–262 (2014)
5. Bimschas, D., Hasemann, H., Hauswirth, M., et al.: Semantic-service provisioning for the internet of things. Electron. Commun. EASST **37**, (2011)
6. Bright, D., Nair, A., Salvekar, D., Bhisikar, S.: EEG-based brain controlled prosthetic arm. In: Proceedings of the Conference on Advances in Signal Processing (CASP), pp. 479–483. IEEE (2016)
7. Brock, D.L.: The electronic product code (EPC): a naming scheme for physical objects. White Paper, Auto-ID Center (2001)
8. Brockman, G., Cheung, V., Petzke, L., Schulman, J., Yiyang, S., et al.: Openai gym (2016). arXiv:1606.01540
9. Callisaya, M.L., Blizzard, L., Schmidt, M.D., McGinley, J.L., Lord, S.R., Srikanth, V.K.: A population-based study of sensorimotor factors affecting gait in older people. Age Ageing **38**(3), 290–295 (2009)
10. Chen, J., Lin, B., Xu, R., Chai, Z., Liang, X., Wong, K.K.: Mapgpt: map-guided prompting for unified vision-and-language navigation (2024). arXiv:2401.07314
11. Chen, K., Yao, L., Wang, X., Zhang, D., Gu, T., Yu, Z., Yang, Z.: Interpretable parallel recurrent neural networks with convolutional attentions for multi-modality activity modeling. In: 2018 International Joint Conference on Neural Networks (IJCNN), pp. 3016–3021. IEEE (2018)
12. Chen, K., Zhang, D., Yao, L., Guo, B., Yu, Z., Liu, Y.: Deep learning for sensor-based human activity recognition: overview, challenges, and opportunities. ACM Comput. Surv. **54**(4), (2021)
13. Chen, L., Li, X., Wang, S., Hu, H.Y., Huang, N., Sheng, Q.Z., Sharaf, M.A.: Mining personal health index from annual geriatric medical examinations. In: Proceedings of the IEEE 14th International Conference on Data Mining (ICDM), pp. 761–766. IEEE (2014)
14. Chen, Z., Shen, Y., Song, Y., Wan, X.: Cross-modal memory networks for radiology report generation. In: Proceedings of the 59th Annual Meeting of the Association for Computational Linguistics, Association for Computational Linguistics, pp. 5904–5914 (2021)
15. Chen, Z., Song, Y., Chang, T., Wan, X.: Generating radiology reports via memory-driven transformer. In: Proceedings of the 2020 Conference on Empirical Methods in Natural Language Processing, pp. 1439–1449. Association for Computational Linguistics (2020)
16. Christophe, B., Verdot, V., Toubiana, V.: Searching the 'web of things'. In: Proceedings of the 5th IEEE International Conference on Semantic Computing (ICSC 2011), pp. 308–315. IEEE Computer Society (2011)

17. Chuang, J., Nguyen, H., Wang, C., Johnson, B.: I think, therefore I am: usability and security of authentication using brainwaves. In: Financial Cryptography and Data Security—FC Workshops 2013, pp. 1–16. Springer (2013)
18. Dey, A.K., Abowd, G.D., Salber, D.: A conceptual framework and a toolkit for supporting the rapid prototyping of context-aware applications. Hum. Comput. Interact.**16**(2–4), 97–166 (2001)
19. Dong, Q., Li, L., Dai, D., Zheng, C., Wu, Z., Chang, B., Sun, X., Xu, J., Sui, Z.: A survey on in-context learning (2022). arXiv:2301.00234
20. Eichelberg, M., Aden, T., Riesmeier, J., Dogac, A., Laleci, G.B.: A survey and analysis of electronic healthcare record standards. ACM Comput. Surv. **37**(4), 277–315 (2005)
21. Fan, L., Zhou, J., Xing, X., Wu, Y.: Active open-vocabulary recognition: let intelligent moving mitigate clip limitations. In: Proceedings of the IEEE/CVF Conference on Computer Vision and Pattern Recognition, CVPR, pp. 16394–16403. IEEE (2024)
22. Ganin, Y., Ustinova, E., Ajakan, H., Germain, P., Larochelle, H., Laviolette, F., Marchand, M., Lempitsky, V.: Domain-adversarial training of neural networks. J. Mach. Learn. Res. **17**(1), 2096–2103 (2016)
23. Ghalwash, M.F., Radosavljevic, V., Obradovic, Z.: Extraction of interpretable multivariate patterns for early diagnostics. In: Proceedings of the 2013 IEEE 13th International Conference on Data Mining, pp. 201–210. IEEE (2013)
24. Gu, J., Stefani, E., Wu, Q., Thomason, J., Wang, X.E.: Vision-and-language navigation: a survey of tasks, methods, and future directions (2022). arXiv:2203.12667
25. Gudur, G.K., Sundaramoorthy, P., Umaashankar, V.: Activeharnet: Towards on-device deep bayesian active learning for human activity recognition. In: Proceedings of the 3rd International Workshop on Embedded and Mobile Deep Learning, EMDL '19, p. 6. ACM (2019)
26. Guinard, D., Trifa, V., Karnouskos, S., et al.: Interacting with the soa-based internet of things: discovery, query, selection, and on-demand provisioning of web services. IEEE Trans. Serv. Comput. **3**(3), 223–235 (2010)
27. Hammerla, N.Y., Halloran, S., Plötz, T.: Deep, convolutional, and recurrent models for human activity recognition using wearables. In: Proceedings of the Twenty-Fifth International Joint Conference on Artificial Intelligence, IJCAI, pp. 1533–1540 (2016)
28. Huang, Z., Zhang, X., Zhang, S.: KIUT: Knowledge-injected U-transformer for radiology report generation. In: Proceedings of the IEEE/CVF Conference on Computer Vision and Pattern Recognition, pp. 19809–19818 (2023)
29. Huynh, T., Schiele, B.: Analyzing features for activity recognition. In: Proceedings of the 2005 Joint Conference on Smart Objects and Ambient Intelligence: Innovative Context-Aware Services: Usages and Technologies, pp. 159–163. ACM (2005)
30. Jin, H., Che, H., Lin, Y., Chen, H.: Promptmrg: diagnosis-driven prompts for medical report generation. In: Proceedings of the AAAI Conference on Artificial Intelligence, vol. 38, pp. 2607–2615 (2024)
31. Kingma, D.P., Mohamed, S., Rezende, D.J., Welling, M.: Semi-supervised learning with deep generative models. In: Advances in Neural Information Processing Systems, NeurIPS, vol. 27, pp. 3581–3589 (2014)
32. Li, M., Liu, R., Wang, F., Chang, X., Liang, X.: Auxiliary signal-guided knowledge encoder–decoder for medical report generation. World Wide Web **26**(1), 253–270 (2023)
33. Lin, B., Nie, Y., Wei, Z., Chen, J., Ma, S., Han, J., Xu, H., Chang, X., Liang, X.: Navcot: boosting llm-based vision-and-language navigation via learning disentangled reasoning (2024). arXiv:2403.07376
34. Lin, Z., Zhang, D., Shi, D., Xu, R., Tao, Q., Wu, L., He, M., Ge, Z.: Contrastive pre-training and linear interaction attention-based transformer for universal medical reports generation. J. Biomed. Inform. **138**, 104281 (2023)
35. Long, Y., Li, X., Cai, W., Dong, H.: Discuss before moving: visual language navigation via multi-expert discussions. In: 2024 IEEE International Conference on Robotics and Automation, ICRA, pp. 17380–17387. IEEE (2024)

36. Mahieu, C., Ongenae, F., Backere, F.D., Bonte, P., Turck, F.D., Simoens, P.: Semantics-based platform for context-aware and personalized robot interaction in the internet of robotic things. J. Syst. Softw. **149**, 138–157 (2019)
37. Mathur, A., Zhang, T., Bhattacharya, S., Veličković, P., Joffe, L., Lane, N.D., Kawsar, F., Liò, P.: Using deep data augmentation training to address software and hardware heterogeneities in wearable and smartphone sensing devices. In: Proceedings of the 17th International Conference on Information Processing in Sensor Networks, IPSN, pp. 200–211. IEEE (2018)
38. Messina, P., Pino, P., Parra, D., Soto, A., Besa, C., Uribe, S., Andía, M., Tejos, C., Prieto, C., Capurro, D.: A survey on deep learning and explainability for automatic report generation from medical images. ACM Comput. Surv. **54**(10s), 1–40 (2022)
39. Murahari, V.S., Plötz, T.: On attention models for human activity recognition. In: Proceedings of the 2018 ACM International Symposium on Wearable Computers, ISWC, pp. 100–103. ACM (2018)
40. Nakamura, T., Goverdovsky, V., Mandic, D.: In-ear EEG biometrics for feasible and readily collectable real-world person authentication. IEEE Trans. Inf. Forensics Secur. **13**(3), 648–661 (2018)
41. Ngu, A.H., Gutierrez, M., Metsis, V., Nepal, S., Sheng, Q.Z.: IoT middleware: a survey on issues and enabling technologies. IEEE Internet Things J. **4**(1), 1–20 (2017)
42. Nguyen, B., Nguyen, D., Ma, W., Tran, D.: Investigating the possibility of applying EEG lossy compression to EEG-based user authentication. In: International Joint Conference on Neural Networks (IJCNN), pp. 79–85. IEEE (2017)
43. Palattella, M.R., Accettura, N., Vilajosana, X., et al.: Standardized protocol stack for the internet of (important) things. IEEE Commun. Surv. & Tutor.**15**(3), 1389–1406 (2013)
44. Pan, B., Panda, R., Jin, S., Feris, R., Oliva, A., Isola, P., Kim, Y.: Langnav: language as a perceptual representation for navigation (2023). arXiv:2310.07889
45. Pintus, A., Carboni, D., Piras, A.: Paraimpu: A platform for a social web of things. In: Mille, A., Gandon, F., Misselis, J., Rabinovich, M., Staab, S. (eds.) Proceedings of the 21st World Wide Web Conference (WWW 2012)–Companion, pp. 401–404. ACM (2012)
46. Pouyanfar, S., Sadiq, S., Yan, Y., Tian, H., Tao, Y., Reyes, M.P., Shyu, M.L., Chen, S.C., Iyengar, S.S.: A survey on deep learning: algorithms, techniques, and applications. ACM Comput. Surv. **51**(5), 92 (2018)
47. Pu, Q., Gupta, S., Gollakota, S., Patel, S.N.: Whole-home gesture recognition using wireless signals. In: Proceedings of the 19th Annual International Conference on Mobile Computing and Networking (MobiCom '13), pp. 27–38. ACM (2013)
48. Pu, Q., Gupta, S., Gollakota, S., Patel, S.N.: Whole-home gesture recognition using wireless signals. In: 19th Annual International Conference on Mobile Computing and Networking (MobiCom 2013), Miami, FL, USA, pp. 27–38. ACM (2013)
49. Qiu, S., Li, Z., He, W., Zhang, L., Yang, C., Su, C.: Brain-machine interface and visual compressive sensing-based teleoperation control of an exoskeleton robot. IEEE Trans. Fuzzy Syst. **25**(1), 58–69 (2017)
50. Ruan, W., Yang, L., Sheng, Q.Z., Gu, T., Xu, P., Shangguan, L.: Making sense of doppler effect for multi-modal hand motion detection. IEEE Trans. Mob. Comput. **17**(9), 2087–2100 (2018)
51. Sheng, Q.Z., Li, X., Zeadally, S.: Enabling next-generation RFID applications: solutions and challenges. Computer **41**(9), 21–28 (2008)
52. Sundmaeker, H., Guillemin, P., Friess, P., Woelfflé, S.: Vision and challenges for realising the internet of things. European Commission Information Society and Media, Technical Report (2010)
53. Vermesan, O., Friess, P., Guillemin, P., et al.: Internet of things strategic research roadmap. Technical report, The Cluster of European Research Projects (2009)
54. Vlacheas, P., Giaffreda, R., Stavroulaki, V., et al.: Enabling smart cities through a cognitive management framework for the internet of things. IEEE Commun. Mag. **51**(6), 102–111 (2013)
55. Wuxi Development and Reform Commission: Wuxi sensing China (2010). Technical Report
56. Yao, L., Sheng, Q.Z., Dustdar, S.: Web-based management of the internet of things. IEEE Internet Comput. **19**(4), 60–67 (2015)

57. Yao, L., Sheng, Q.Z., Li, X., Gu, T., Tan, M., Wang, X., Wang, S., Ruan, W.: Compressive representation for device-free activity recognition with passive RFID signal strength. IEEE Trans. Mob. Comput. **17**(2), 293–306 (2018)
58. Zaib, M., Sheng, Q.Z., Zhang, W.E., Mahmood, A.: When NLP meets LLM: neural approaches to context-based conversational question answering. CRC Press (2026)
59. Zaslavsky, A., Perera, C., Georgakopoulos, D.: Sensing as a service and big data. In: International Conference on Advances in Cloud Computing, ACC, pp. 21–29 (2012)
60. Zhang, D., Zhou, J., Guo, M., Cao, J., Li, T.: TASA: Tag-free activity sensing using RFID tag arrays. IEEE Trans. Parallel Distrib. Syst. **22**(4), 558–570 (2011)
61. Zhang, M., Zhao, H., Zheng, R., et al.: Cognitive internet of things: concepts and application example. Int. J. Comput. Sci. Issues **9**(3), 151–158 (2012)
62. Zhang, X., Yao, L., Kanhere, S.S., Liu, Y., Gu, T., Chen, K.: MindID: person identification from brain waves through attention-based recurrent neural network. Proc. ACM Interact. Mob. Wearable Ubiquitous Technol. **2**(3), 149:1–149:23 (2018)
63. Zheng, D., Huang, S., Zhao, L., Zhong, Y., Wang, L.: Towards learning a generalist model for embodied navigation. In: Proceedings of the IEEE/CVF Conference on Computer Vision and Pattern Recognition, CVPR, pp. 13624–13634. IEEE (2024)
64. Zhou, G., Hong, Y., Wu, Q.: Navgpt: explicit reasoning in vision-and-language navigation with large language models. In: Proceedings of the AAAI Conference on Artificial Intelligence, pp. 7641–7649. AAAI (2024)

Part I
Device-free Localization and Activity Recognition

This part presents foundational technologies for unobtrusive monitoring in smart aging environments, where individuals should not be burdened with carrying specific devices or actively participating in sensing systems. The two chapters in this part address complementary aspects of device-free sensing: spatial tracking and activity recognition.

Chapter 4 introduces device-free localization and tracking techniques that leverage environmental sensing to determine where individuals are located and predict their future movements. This chapter particularly presents HOI-Loc, a system that enhances RFID-based localization by incorporating human-object interactions in cluttered residential environments, and A-SGTN, an attention-aware transformer network for trajectory prediction. These approaches achieve significant improvements in accuracy while maintaining privacy and enabling continuous monitoring without user intervention.

Chapter 5 explores device-free human activity recognition through three innovative approaches: (i) RFID-based compressive sensing for fine-grained activity detection, (ii) acoustic-based gesture recognition using built-in device speakers and microphones, and (iii) transformer-based interaction recognition using privacy-preserving depth sensors. Together, these systems demonstrate how environmental intelligence can replace wearable sensors while preserving user privacy and enabling natural interactions.

The technologies presented in this part establish the sensing foundation for smart aging systems, enabling unobtrusive monitoring of daily activities, fall detection, and behavioral pattern analysis. These device-free approaches overcome traditional limitations of wearable sensors by eliminating user compliance requirements while maintaining high accuracy and respecting privacy concerns, which are essential for residential deployment.

Chapter 4
Device-Free Localization and Tracking

4.1 Introduction

4.1.1 Overview of Device-Free Localization and Tracking

Device-free localization and tracking techniques are emerging as valuable technologies for indoor environments, where individuals should not be burdened with carrying specific devices or actively participating in the localization process [31]. Unlike traditional localization methods that require target subjects to carry smartphones, RFID tags, or other sensing devices, device-free approaches rely on detecting disturbances in the ambient environment caused by human presence and movement. These disturbances can be captured through various sensing modalities, including radio frequency (RF) signals, computer vision systems, and Internet of Things (IoT) sensor networks.

These techniques enable a range of essential applications, including unobtrusive monitoring, activity recognition, behavioral pattern analysis, and emergency response systems. By eliminating the need for wearable sensors or tags, device-free approaches provide more comfortable, practical, and dignified monitoring solutions in residential and public spaces.

Trajectory prediction represents another crucial capability that complements localization. Predicting the future positions and movements of individuals allows intelligent systems to anticipate needs, detect anomalies in movement patterns, and prevent potential hazards such as collisions [21]. Advanced trajectory prediction models can recognize complex social interactions, understand environmental constraints, and generate probabilistic forecasts of future positions, enabling proactive assistance and enhancing safety measures in various indoor environments.

Q. Z. Sheng et al., *Harnessing Artificial Intelligence and Pervasive Internet of Things for an Empowered Aging*, https://doi.org/10.1007/978-3-032-16502-2_4

4.1.2 Challenges and Opportunities

Despite significant advances, device-free localization and tracking in real-world residential environments still face substantial challenges. In cluttered home environments, radio signals are heavily obstructed by furniture and metallic appliances, reducing localization accuracy. Most existing device-free techniques have been tested only in clear or semi-clear spaces (empty spaces or areas with very few objects), and their performance degrades significantly in multi-room residential settings.

For trajectory prediction, three key challenges persist. First, social interaction information must be effectively incorporated, as human movement is influenced by the presence and behavior of others. Second, the dynamic nature of environments, where individuals can enter or exit at any time, creates a constantly changing context that prediction models must adapt to. Finally, the inherent multi-modality of human movement means that future trajectories encompass numerous possibilities based on individual decisions, requiring probabilistic rather than deterministic predictions.

These challenges present opportunities for innovative approaches that leverage emerging technologies. The proliferation of IoT devices in smart homes enables access to rich contextual information about human-object interactions (HOI), which can potentially reveal people's interleaved locations during daily activities. Similarly, advances in graph-based deep learning architectures and transformer networks offer new computational frameworks for modeling complex spatio-temporal relationships in human movement patterns.

4.1.3 Contributions

This chapter introduces two novel approaches to address the challenges of device-free localization and trajectory prediction with applications relevant to smart aging.

First, we present HOI-Loc, a device-free indoor localization and tracking system that enhances the performance of commercial off-the-shelf (COTS) RFID-based localization by leveraging human-object interaction contexts in furnished homes [17]. HOI-Loc introduces a Bayesian probabilistic framework to integrate both Received Signal Strength Indicator (RSSI) signals and HOI events to infer the most likely location and trajectory of individuals. The system employs three key techniques: (1) a Probabilistic Polyhedron Isolation method that robustly models the likelihood of target locations despite signal attenuation and fluctuations, (2) a Bayesian framework to fuse discrete HOI events with continuous RSSI signals, and (3) a Hidden Markov Model that quantifies continuous location transitions to mitigate the negative effects of human mobility. Experiments conducted in a residential house demonstrate that HOI-Loc achieves significant improvements in both localization accuracy and tracking precision compared to the state-of-the-art alternatives, with capabilities for multi-resident tracking and basic posture recognition that would be valuable in smart aging scenarios.

Second, we propose Attention-aware Social Graph Transformer Networks for multi-modal trajectory prediction [13]. This approach combines Graph Convolutional Networks (GCNs) and Transformer Networks through a designed stacking and interception method to generate stable resolution pseudo-images from spatio-temporal graphs. The model incorporates an attention-aware module to handle social interaction information in scenarios involving mixed pedestrian-vehicle traffic. While GCNs excel at aggregating information over arbitrary numbers of neighbors, their outputs can fluctuate with input changes. Conversely, Transformer Networks effectively process complex time-dependent data but typically require consistent inputs. Our approach achieves stable integration of both network types while preserving their respective advantages. Experimental evaluation across various benchmark datasets demonstrates the model's effectiveness, particularly for long-term prediction scenarios and in reducing collision risks in complex environments.

4.1.4 Chapter Organization

The remainder of this chapter is organized as follows. Section 4.2 reviews key research in device-free localization and trajectory prediction, establishing the theoretical foundations and current approaches in these fields. Section 4.3 presents the HOI-Loc system, a device-free indoor localization and tracking approach that leverages human-object interactions to enhance performance in cluttered residential environments. Section 4.4 introduces Attention-aware Social Graph Transformer Networks (A-SGTN) for trajectory prediction, combining graph-based models with transformer networks to forecast future movement patterns. Section 4.5 explores broader implications of these technologies for smart aging applications, including privacy considerations, implementation challenges, and future research directions.

4.2 Background and Related Work

4.2.1 Device-Free Localization

Device-free localization systems track individuals without requiring them to carry electronic devices [27, 29, 31]. These approaches detect environmental changes caused by human presence and movement. Several approaches have been developed for device-free localization:

- *Computer Vision-based*: RGB cameras [25] or depth cameras [8] offer high precision but raise privacy concerns.
- *Radio Frequency-based*: RF systems detect human presence by measuring wireless signal variations. Approaches include analyzing received signal strength (RSS) or

channel state information (CSI) in WLANs [20, 24, 29], and using RF signals reflected from human bodies [1].
- *RFID-based*: Passive RFID technology offers cost-effective and maintenance-free solutions [6, 23, 27]. However, current RFID-based techniques perform well mainly in clear spaces and struggle in cluttered environments.
- *Fusion-based*: Hybrid systems combine multiple sensing technologies. A promising direction involves integrating human-object interaction (HOI) information with traditional sensing [18, 30].

4.2.2 Trajectory Prediction for Movement Analysis

Trajectory prediction extends localization by forecasting future positions and movement patterns. This capability enables proactive assistance, accident prevention, and abnormal behavior detection [21]. The fundamental challenges in trajectory prediction include:

- *Social Interaction Information*: Human movement is influenced by surrounding agents [7].
- *Environmental Dynamics*: Varying numbers of agents entering and exiting areas require adaptive models [13].
- *Multi-modality of Trajectories*: Multiple plausible future paths exist, necessitating probabilistic predictions [21].

Trajectory prediction methods have evolved significantly:

- *Traditional Approaches*: Early methods used physics-based models. Social force models [7] modeled forces between pedestrians and obstacles.
- *Learning-based Approaches*: Modern methods leverage RNNs and LSTMs [28]. Social-LSTM [2] and Social-GAN [5] introduced interaction modeling mechanisms.
- *Graph-based Approaches*: Graph Neural Networks represent agents as nodes and relationships as edges [14]. Systems like Social-BiGAT [9] and GRIP [12] demonstrate effectiveness for trajectory prediction.
- *Transformer-based Approaches*: Recent work leverages Transformer networks' self-attention mechanisms [11]. STAR [32] combines spatio-temporal graphs with Transformer structure.

Despite these advances, challenges still remain in effectively representing both spatial relationships and temporal dependencies for long-term predictions in complex multi-agent environments.

4.2.3 *Research Gaps and Opportunities in Smart Aging Applications*

Despite significant progress in device-free localization and trajectory prediction, several research gaps remain:

- *Environmental Complexity*: Most systems are evaluated in controlled environments. Performance in cluttered residential settings remains largely unexplored.
- *Multi-modality Integration*: Effective integration of multiple sensing modalities, particularly fusion of RF signals with contextual information, presents challenges and opportunities.
- *Social Interaction Modeling*: Current models often simplify complex social dynamics in mixed pedestrian-vehicle scenarios.
- *Long-term Prediction*: Accuracy typically degrades over longer time horizons, limiting proactive assistance capabilities.
- *Privacy-Preserving Monitoring*: Balancing accurate monitoring with privacy concerns remains critical.
- *Practical Deployability*: Many systems require complex infrastructure that may be impractical in real-world settings.

This chapter addresses several gaps through two complementary approaches: (1) HOI-Loc, a device-free localization system that leverages human-object interactions for enhanced accuracy in cluttered environments, and (2) Attention-aware Social Graph Transformer Networks, a trajectory prediction framework for improved movement forecasting. Both approaches prioritize non-intrusiveness, reliability, and practical deployment considerations.

4.3 Device-Free Indoor Localization and Tracking Through Human-Object Interactions

4.3.1 *Motivation and Overview of HOI-Loc*

Device-free indoor localization faces significant challenges in cluttered residential spaces. The Received Signal Strength Indicator (RSSI) is often obstructed by furniture and metallic appliances. To address this limitation, we observe that human-object interaction (HOI) events provide valuable location context that complements traditional signal-based approaches.

The HOI-Loc system [17] integrates passive RFID technology with human-object interaction sensing to improve localization accuracy. Our approach uses passive RFID tags and ambient sensors that detect interactions with household objects. This design ensures easy deployment in real-world settings, as shown in Fig. 4.1.

The system introduces three key innovations: (1) a Probabilistic Polyhedron Isolation method robust to signal interference in cluttered spaces, (2) a Bayesian

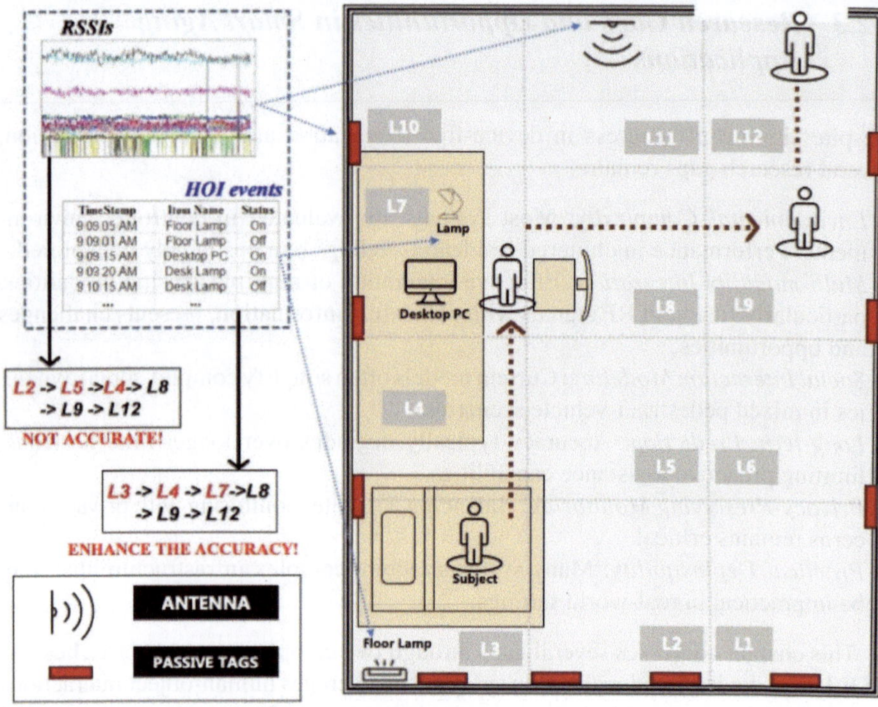

Fig. 4.1 HOI-Loc system architecture: fusion of RFID signal strength and human-object interaction events for enhanced indoor localization accuracy

framework that fuses discrete HOI events with continuous RSSI signals, and (3) a Hidden Markov Model that accounts for the variable movement patterns that can occur in residential settings.

Our experimental results demonstrate that HOI-Loc achieves 95.6% localization accuracy with average tracking error of 58cm in multi-room scenarios, significantly outperforming the existing methods. The system can track multiple occupants with 85cm average error and recognize basic living postures, enabling applications such as fall detection and activity monitoring.

4.3.2 *HOI-Loc: A Probabilistic Framework for Indoor Localization and Tracking*

In this section, we present the core methodology of HOI-Loc, our probabilistic framework that integrates Received Signal Strength Indicator (RSSI) from passive RFID tags with Human-Object Interaction (HOI) events to improve indoor localization and tracking accuracy. Our approach has three key components: (1) signal processing using Received Signal Strength Indicator (RSSI), (2) context awareness through Human-Object Interactions (HOI), and (3) a probabilistic framework that integrates both data sources for robust localization and tracking.

Passive RFID technology provides a foundation for unobtrusive monitoring. These battery-free tags harvest energy from the reader's signal through backscatter radio link. In cluttered indoor environments, RSSI signals exhibit complex, nonlinear relationships with location. We employ statistical machine learning approaches to map RSSI patterns to locations.

Human-Object Interactions provide valuable contextual information. When a person opens a refrigerator door or turns on a desk lamp, these actions reveal location information that complements RSSI data.

We divide the monitored environment into discrete zones ($\mathcal{L} = \{L_1, L_2, ..., L_J\}$) and monitor interactions with various objects ($\mathcal{C} = \{I_1, I_2, ..., I_M\}$). This allows us to address two key challenges: (1) *accurate localization*: determining the precise location of a resident at a specific moment using both RSSI measurements and detected interaction events, and (2) *continuous tracking*: following the movement trajectory through the living space over time.

Our probabilistic framework addresses these challenges through Bayesian inference, modeling the posterior distribution to find the most likely location given RSSI observations and HOI events. The framework seeks to maximize the probability of a location given both signal measurements and interaction events.

For tracking a mobile resident over time, we extend this approach to model the posterior distribution of a location sequence given continuous observations over time period T. Our probabilistic framework decomposes this complex problem using Bayesian inference, separating the computation into manageable components by combining the prior probability of being in a particular location, the RSSI probability that measures how likely specific signal patterns are observed when a person is at that location, and the HOI probability that quantifies how likely certain interaction events occur when a person is at that location.

To implement this framework, we developed two key technical components:

- *Probabilistic Polyhedron Isolation (PPI)*: For computing the RSSI probability, we developed a method that models how signal patterns cluster in high-dimensional space when a person is in specific locations. As shown in Fig. 4.2, RSSI readings from multiple tags form clusters in high-dimensional space corresponding to specific locations. Our PPI method uses k-nearest neighbor search to identify these clusters and calculates distances between new observations and established location patterns.
- *Human-Object Interaction (HOI) Matrix*: For computing the HOI probability, we developed a matrix-based approach that maps interaction events to possible locations. For example, when sensors detect that a microwave door has been opened, our algorithm assigns higher probabilities to locations near the kitchen.

For tracking mobile residents over time, we employ a Hidden Markov Model with three key components. The model incorporates emission matrices that combine both RSSI and HOI probabilities, uses a transition strategy based on adjacent movement

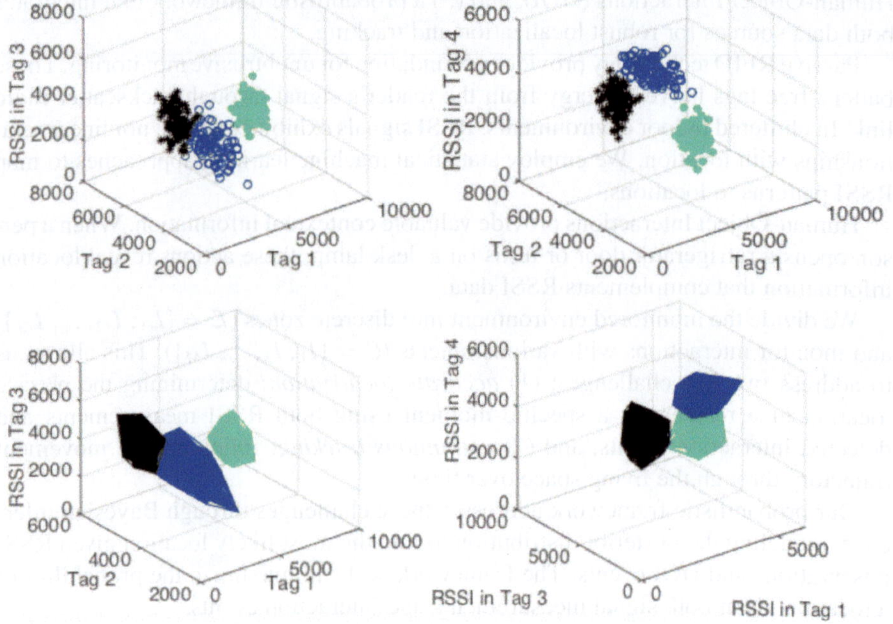

Fig. 4.2 SSIs from different locations are bounded by isolated high-dimensional polyhedrons

patterns, and employs a Viterbi searching algorithm that finds the most likely trajectory, followed by a forward calibration mechanism that addresses signal latency issues.

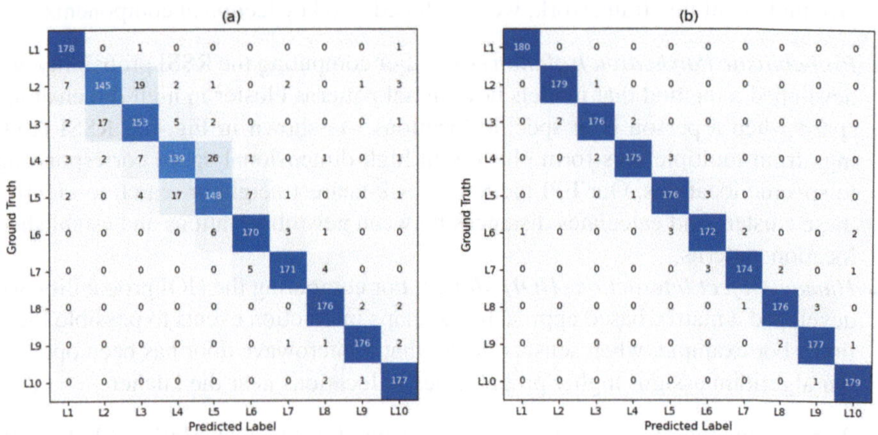

Fig. 4.3 **a** Localization result based on RSSI signal (k = 2); **b** Localization result of fusing HOI events with RSSI signal (k = 2)

This integrated approach successfully addresses the challenge of tracking individuals in cluttered indoor environments. By fusing RSSI signals with HOI events, our system achieves more than 96% localization accuracy, as illustrated in Fig. 4.3b, a significant improvement over the 80% accuracy achieved using RSSI alone (Fig. 4.3a).

4.3.3 Experimental Validation and Performance Analysis

To validate the effectiveness of HOI-Loc, we conducted extensive experiments in a real-world residential setting.

We deployed a complete system in a residential house with two bedrooms and a kitchen (see Fig. 4.4), using commercial RFID hardware including an Alien ALR-9900+ Enterprise RFID Reader, four circular antennas, and passive RFID tags

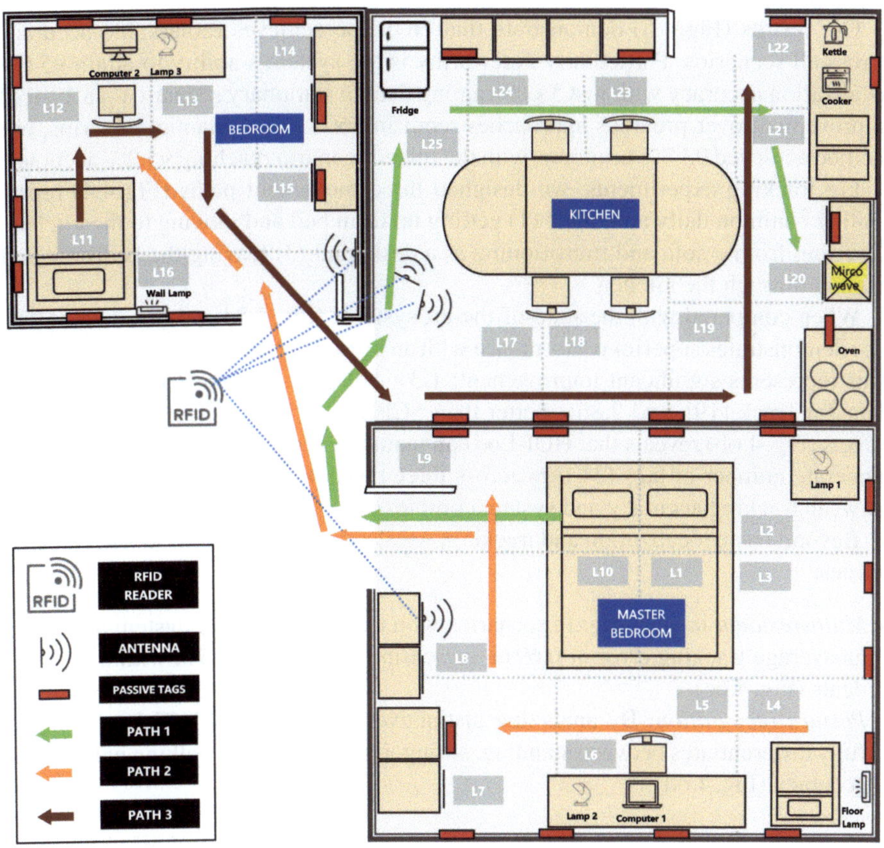

Fig. 4.4 Experiment settings and paths. *Testing Area: master bedroom:* $3.6\,m \times 4.8\,m$, *bedroom:* $3\,m \times 3.2\,m$, *kitchen:* $3.6\,m \times 4.6\,m$

attached to walls. The system was configured to sample at 2 Hz, with antennas positioned at 1.7 m height and angled to maximize tag coverage. We evaluated three key scenarios:

- *Stationary activities*: Situations where a person is sitting or standing in one location for extended periods.
- *Dynamic activities*: Active movement within a confined space, such as cooking or cleaning.
- *Mixed activities*: Combining periods of stationary and dynamic behavior, resembling actual daily living patterns.

Three participants with varying physical characteristics participated in our experiments, performing scripted activities across all 25 virtual grid locations in our test environment. For each scenario, we collected localization data and evaluated the system using standard metrics: localization accuracy (percentage of correctly identified zones) and tracking error distance (average spatial deviation between predicted and actual positions).

Our results (Fig. 4.5) demonstrate that HOI-Loc achieves remarkable accuracy across all scenarios. Particularly noteworthy is the system's ability to attain 95.6% localization accuracy with just 5 s of training data in stationary scenarios—a 12-fold improvement over previous approaches requiring 60 s. For dynamic scenarios, our method achieved 93.7% accuracy, with the mixed scenario reaching 95.2% accuracy.

For tracking experiments, we designed three movement paths (Fig. 4.4) representing common daily activities: (1) getting up from bed and moving to the kitchen, (2) rising from a sofa and transitioning to a desk, and (3) leaving the bedroom and passing through the kitchen.

When compared with the state-of-the-art systems (Fig. 4.5d and Fig. 4.6a), HOI-Loc demonstrates superior performance with an average tracking error of just 0.58 m. This represents significant improvement: 1.3× better than Twins [6], 1.86× better than TagTrack [19], and 2.86× better than SCPL [26]. Our analysis of tag density effects (Fig. 4.6b) reveals that HOI-Loc can maintain acceptable performance with a moderate number of tags (34 tags across three rooms), striking an optimal balance between tracking accuracy and system complexity.

Beyond basic localization and tracking, we also investigated two advanced capabilities:

- *Multi-resident monitoring*: In scenarios with two residents, our system maintains an average tracking error of 0.69 m, increasing slightly to 0.85 m with three residents (Fig. 4.6c).
- *Posture recognition*: By analyzing distinctive RSSI patterns, HOI-Loc successfully differentiates between standing, sitting, lying down, and walking with 94.7% accuracy (Fig. 4.6d).

4.3.4 *Summary of the HOI-Loc System*

Our experimental validation demonstrates that HOI-Loc achieves significant improvements in indoor localization and tracking accuracy without requiring residents to wear or carry devices. The system achieves up to 95.6% localization accuracy with minimal training data (5–50 s per location), representing a substantial improvement over systems requiring several minutes of training. The average tracking error of 58cm in multi-room environments demonstrates accurate movement pattern monitoring capabilities, while advanced features include multi-resident tracking with 85cm average error and posture recognition with 94.7% accuracy.

The practical advantages of HOI-Loc extend beyond performance metrics. The current implementation uses wall-mounted RFID tags and object-attached sensors that can be readily deployed in residential settings, with future integration possibilities as IoT technologies become standard in smart homes. Unlike camera-based solutions, our RFID-based approach provides location tracking and basic activity

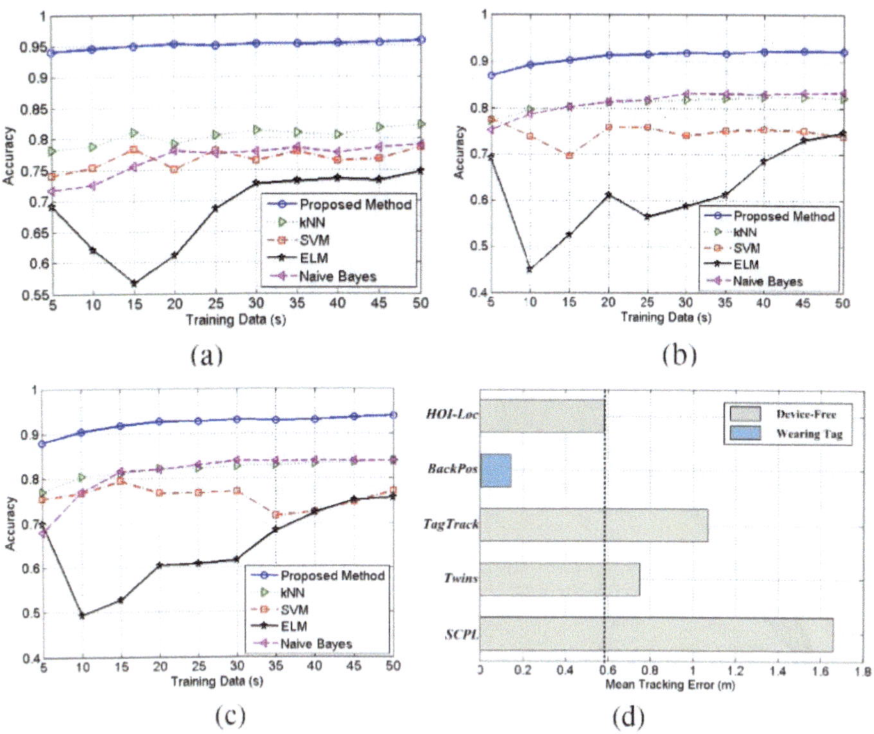

Fig. 4.5 **a** Localization result for Stationary Scenario; **b** Localization result for Dynamic Scenario; **c** Localization result for Mixed Scenario; **d** Compare tracking accuracy of *HOI-Loc* with other state-of-the-art systems

recognition while preserving dignity and privacy, making it suitable for environments where maintaining independence and comfort is essential.

By combining RFID-based localization with human-object interaction detection, HOI-Loc demonstrates how multi-modal sensing can overcome the limitations of single-technology approaches in complex indoor environments, providing a foundation for unobtrusive monitoring in residential settings.

4.4 Social Graph Transformer Networks for Trajectory Prediction

4.4.1 Motivation and Overview of A-SGTN

Accurate trajectory prediction is essential for proactive support systems and safety monitoring. Current approaches face three key challenges: (1) modeling social inter-

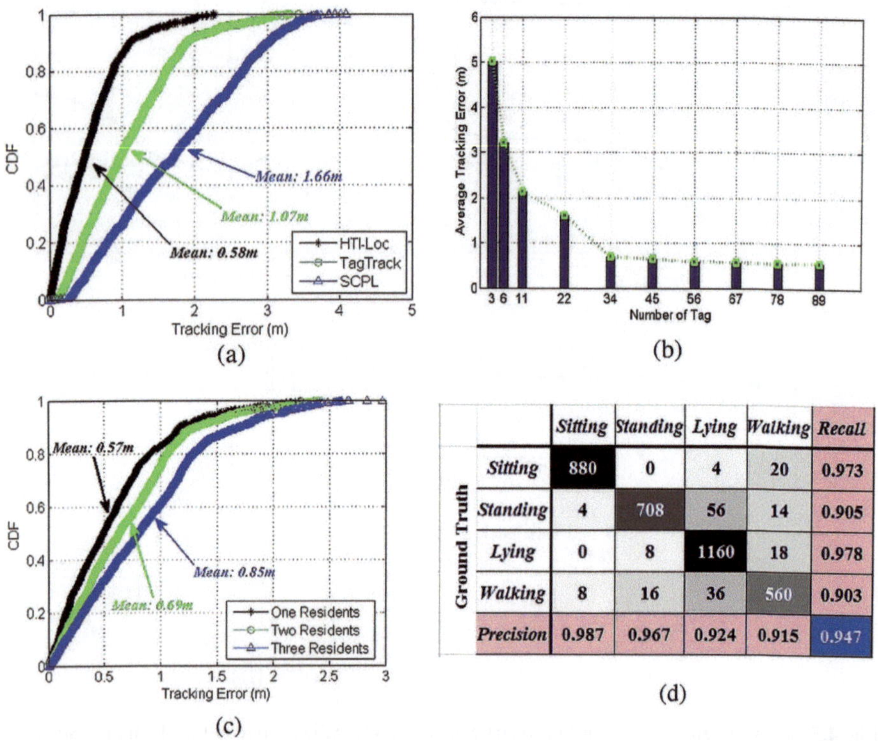

Fig. 4.6 **a** Tracking error CDF for different device-free methods; **b** Mean tracking errors using different tag numbers; **c** Tracking errors for multiple residents; **d** Confusion matrix of detecting four basic postures

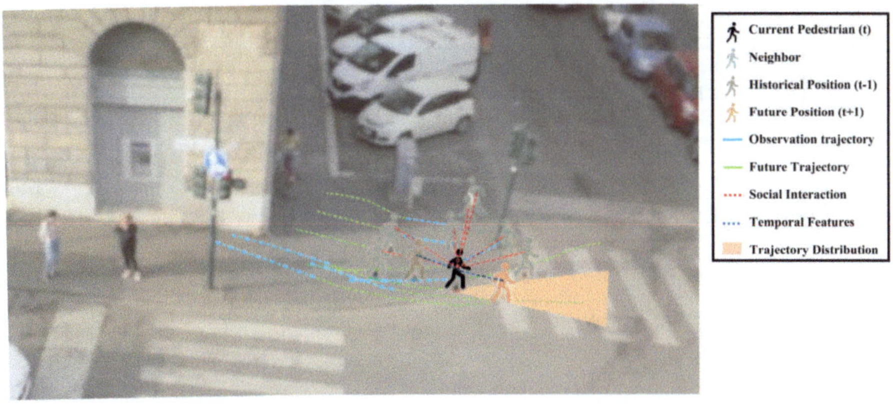

Fig. 4.7 An example of pedestrian motion trajectory in the real scenario. Pedestrian trajectory prediction needs to consider social interaction information, and pedestrian trajectories are dynamic and multi-modal

actions between individuals, (2) adapting to environmental dynamics with varying numbers of occupants, and (3) addressing the inherent multi-modality of movement patterns.

To address these challenges, we propose Attention-aware Social Graph Transformer Networks (A-SGTN) [13]. Our approach combines Graph Convolutional Networks (GCNs) with Transformer Networks through a novel stacking and interception method. The A-SGTN approach makes three key contributions:

- It integrates GCNs and Transformer Networks to predict trajectories using only coordinate data.
- It introduces a novel representation method that constructs trajectories as Social Interaction Spatio-temporal Graphs and converts them into pseudo-images.
- It significantly improves long-term trajectory prediction with a 31.7% improvement in final displacement error and reduces predicted collision rates.

Figure 4.7 illustrates pedestrian motion in a real-world scenario, highlighting the challenges of trajectory prediction that must account for social interactions while addressing the dynamic and multi-modal nature of human movement patterns.

4.4.2 A-SGTN: Framework Design and Components

Our A-SGTN approach addresses trajectory prediction with a unified framework that integrates multiple architectural innovations. Given an observed trajectory $Traj_{obs}$ from timestamp 1 to T_{obs}, we predict future paths $Traj_{pred}$ from $T_{obs}+1$ to $T_{obs}+T_{pred}$:

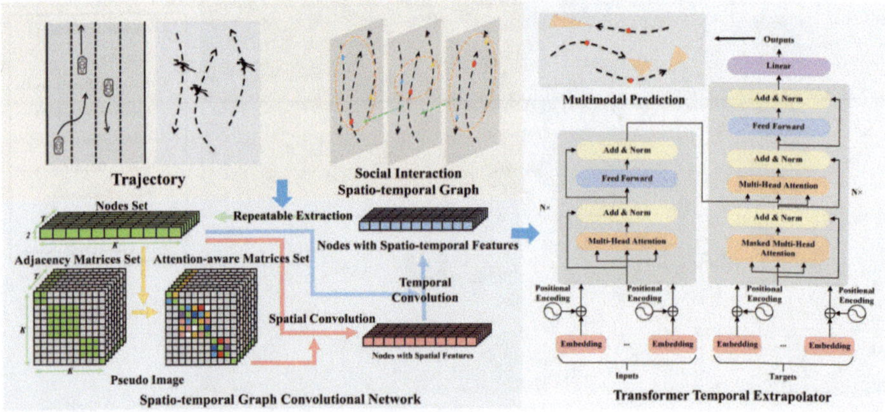

Fig. 4.8 The overview of our Attention-aware Social Graph Transformer Networks framework. The framework consists of Social Interaction Spatio-temporal Graph, Spatio-temporal Graph Convolutional Network with pseudo-image and Attention-aware module, Transformer Temporal Extrapolator, and multi-modal prediction

$$Traj_{obs} = \{p_t^n = (x_t^n, y_t^n) \mid n = f(t) \in \{1, \ldots, N\},\ t \in \{1, \ldots, T_{obs}\}\} \tag{4.1}$$

$$Traj_{pred} = \{p_t^n = (x_t^n, y_t^n) \mid n = f(t) \in \{1, \ldots, N\},\ t \in \{T_{obs} + 1, \ldots, T_{obs} + T_{pred}\}\} \tag{4.2}$$

Figure 4.8 illustrates our A-SGTN framework, which integrates three key innovations: Social Interaction Spatio-temporal Graph (SSIG), Attention-aware Module, and Transformer Temporal Extrapolator.

Social Interaction Graph Representation. We model interactions by representing each individual as a node in a graph structure, where nodes represent positions and edges capture social interactions through spatial distances. We then construct a pseudo-image representation by stacking spatio-temporal graphs, creating a structure that maintains constant resolution for stable predictions.

Attention-aware Mechanism. The attention-aware mechanism enhances standard distance-based relationships with learned attention patterns through a softmax function applied to attention scores. We also introduce a sparse attention variant that focuses only on the most significant relationships by applying a threshold to filter out weak connections.

Spatio-temporal Feature Extraction. Our Spatio-temporal Graph Convolutional Network processes the representation through spatial and temporal convolution components, effectively extracting features from both spatial relationships between individuals and temporal evolution of movement patterns.

Advanced Sequence Modeling. We employ a Transformer-based architecture for long-term dependency modeling. The self-attention mechanism calculates relationships between all points in the observed trajectory:

$$Attention(\mathbf{Q}, \mathbf{K}, \mathbf{V}) = softmax\left(\frac{\mathbf{Q} \cdot \mathbf{K}^T}{\sqrt{d_k}}\right)\mathbf{V} \tag{4.3}$$

Uncertainty-Aware Prediction. Our model generates probability distributions rather than single trajectories. Each predicted position is modeled as a bivariate Gaussian distribution with mean, standard deviation, and correlation parameters.

4.4.3 Experimental Results and Performance

We evaluated our approach on standard trajectory prediction benchmarks.

Pedestrian Trajectory Prediction. Using established datasets ETH [16] and UCY [10], we measured Average Displacement Error (ADE), Final Displacement Error (FDE), and Collision Rate (COL). The benchmark datasets encompass five scenarios: ETH, HOTEL, UNIV, ZARA1, and ZARA2, where pedestrian trajectories are collected in real-world scenarios with rich social interactions. Following the standard protocol, we observe 8 frames (3.2 s) and predict the subsequent 12 frames (4.8 s).

Our model demonstrates key advantages across all datasets, as shown in Table 4.1. The A-SGTN variant achieves state-of-the-art performance with an average FDE of 0.27 m across all datasets, representing a 31.7% improvement compared to Trajectron++ (0.41 m to 0.27 m). While Trajectron++ excels in optimizing ADE metrics, our model achieves substantially lower FDE, demonstrating superior long-term prediction capability. This indicates that LSTM-based models like Trajectron++ may make accurate predictions in the immediate future but experience growing displacement

Table 4.1 Pedestrian Trajectory Prediction Results. Values denote ADE/FDE in meters

	ETH	HOTEL	UNIV	ZARA1	ZARA2	AVG
Social-LSTM [2]	1.09/2.35	0.79/1.76	0.67/1.40	0.47/1.00	0.56/1.17	0.72/1.54
Social-GAN [5]	0.81/1.52	0.72/1.61	0.60/1.26	0.34/0.69	0.42/0.84	0.58/1.18
Social-STGCNN [15]	0.64/1.11	0.49/0.85	0.44/0.79	0.34/0.53	0.30/0.48	0.44/0.75
STAR [32]	0.36/0.65	0.17/0.36	0.26/0.55	0.22/0.46	0.31/0.62	0.26/0.53
Trajectron++ [22]	0.39/0.83	0.12/0.21	0.20/0.44	0.15/0.33	0.11/0.25	0.19/0.41
Ours (SGTN)	0.40/0.59	0.14/0.16	0.16/0.18	0.17/0.29	0.14/0.17	0.20/0.28
Ours (A-SGTN)	0.41/0.54	0.18/0.24	0.16/0.18	0.17/0.22	0.15/0.19	0.21/0.27
Ours (SA-SGTN)	0.48/0.62	0.18/0.20	0.15/0.19	0.19/0.28	0.14/0.16	0.23/0.29

Table 4.2 Mixed Agent Trajectory Prediction Results on ApolloScape Dataset. WSADE denotes weighted sum of ADE, WSFDE denotes weighted sum of FDE. Values denote displacement error in meters

Method	WSADE	ADE_v	ADE_p	ADE_b	WSFDE	FDE_v	FDE_p	FDE_b
Social-LSTM [2]	1.90	2.95	1.29	2.53	3.40	5.28	2.32	4.54
Social-GAN [5]	1.59	3.04	0.98	1.84	2.78	5.09	1.73	3.45
STAR [32]	1.55	2.56	0.95	2.17	2.86	4.63	1.80	4.04
Transformer [4]	1.28	2.23	0.73	1.84	2.40	4.03	1.43	3.48
S2TNet [3]	1.17	1.99	0.68	1.70	2.18	3.58	1.30	3.21
Ours (SGTN)	1.19	1.35	0.91	1.18	2.52	2.75	1.98	2.51
Ours (A-SGTN)	1.14	1.28	0.85	1.14	2.38	2.62	1.82	2.43
Ours (SA-SGTN)	1.14	1.25	0.90	1.15	2.40	2.59	1.95	2.46

errors over longer time horizons due to limitations in handling long-term historical memory. In contrast, our Transformer-based approach maintains consistently small errors in long-term predictions. The UNIV dataset, being the most densely populated, particularly benefits from our Social Interaction Spatio-temporal Graph, which enhances the model's ability to gather interaction information in complex scenarios. Additionally, our model achieves superior collision avoidance with 0% collision rate on the ETH dataset, demonstrating the effectiveness of our social interaction modeling.

Figure 4.9 shows a visual comparison of prediction results between our model and three other methods. Our model excels in collecting social interaction information through the adjacency matrix and optimizing Transformer performance with pseudo-images, making it particularly well-suited for long-term predictions.

Multi-Agent Scenario Performance. We extended our evaluation to mixed agent scenarios using the ApolloScape dataset [14], which includes interactions between pedestrians, vehicles, and bicyclists. The ApolloScape trajectory dataset is derived from peak-hour urban traffic data collected at traffic intersections and mixed pedestrian-vehicle roadways. The prediction task involves observing the past 6 frames and forecasting the subsequent 6 frames into the future. Following the benchmark, evaluation metrics use weighted sums of ADE (WSADE) and FDE (WSFDE): $WSADE = 0.20 \cdot ADE_v + 0.58 \cdot ADE_p + 0.22 \cdot ADE_b$ and $WSFDE = 0.20 \cdot FDE_v + 0.58 \cdot FDE_p + 0.22 \cdot FDE_b$, where 'v', 'p', and 'b' represent vehicles, pedestrians, and bicyclists respectively.

Our model achieves state-of-the-art results with only location data as input, as demonstrated in Table 4.2. Notably, our approach excels in predicting vehicle and bicyclist trajectories while relying solely on coordinate information, without additional features such as agent size, heading angle, or map images used by some competing methods. The A-SGTN and SA-SGTN variants achieve the best overall

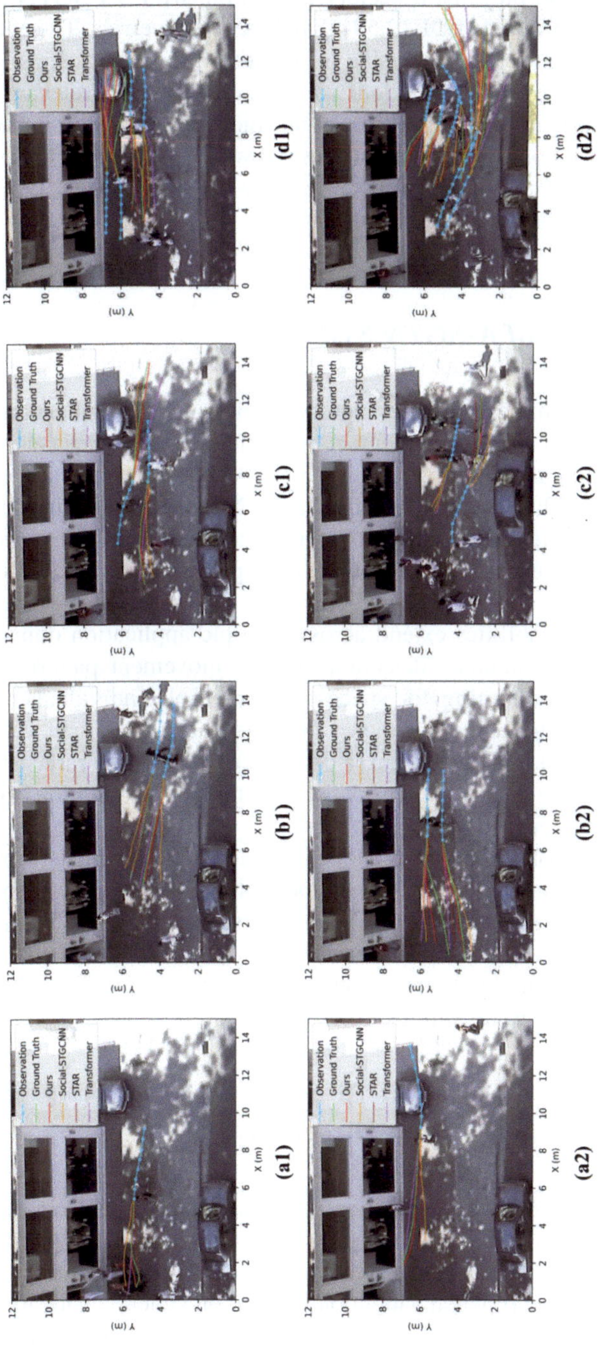

Fig. 4.9 Trajectory Prediction Visualization Comparison. (a1), (a2) for single person; (b1), (b2) for walking in the same direction; (c1), (c2) for walking in opposite directions; (d1), (d2) for mixed multi-person

WSADE of 1.14 m, outperforming other baseline methods. Our model particularly excels in vehicle and bicyclist trajectory prediction, with SA-SGTN achieving the best performance in vehicle FDE (2.59 m) and bicyclist metrics. The attention-aware mechanism proves especially valuable in mixed traffic scenarios, as it enables the model to prioritize feature-rich regions while filtering out less relevant information, which is particularly important for vehicles and bicyclists that exhibit more structured movement patterns compared to pedestrians. These results confirm the model's effectiveness in handling complex mixed scenarios with diverse agent types and strong performance across different agent categories.

4.4.4 Summary of A-SGTN System

The A-SGTN system demonstrates significant potential for enhancing monitoring applications through accurate movement prediction that balances performance with practical implementation considerations. Our experimental evaluation confirms substantial technical achievements, including a 31.7% reduction in final position error compared to the state-of-the-art methods, near-zero collision rates in multi-person environments, and successful integration of graph-based models with transformer networks for enhanced trajectory prediction accuracy.

The system's capabilities extend across multiple application domains, offering pattern analysis and anomaly detection through movement pattern analysis over time, multi-agent monitoring for spaces with multiple individuals, and privacy-preserving monitoring using abstracted position data rather than visual imagery. The trajectory-based approach focuses on movement patterns rather than personal appearance, enabling data processing at the edge to limit information exposure while maintaining high prediction accuracy.

The integration of social graph modeling with transformer networks creates a robust foundation for accurate movement prediction in complex environments. The model's effectiveness in handling diverse agent types and movement patterns, combined with its ability to maintain consistent accuracy over longer prediction horizons, positions it as a versatile solution for environments requiring sophisticated movement analysis and prediction capabilities.

4.5 Discussion and Future Directions

This chapter presented two complementary approaches to device-free localization and tracking: HOI-Loc for accurate indoor positioning through human-object interactions and A-SGTN for trajectory prediction through social graph transformer networks. While our experimental validation focused on general residential and pedestrian scenarios, these technologies offer significant potential for applications in smart environments, including contexts where unobtrusive monitoring and privacy preservation are paramount.

4.5.1 Implementation Considerations and Broader Applications

Several factors are crucial for successful deployment of these technologies in various smart environment applications. Privacy preservation remains a fundamental consideration, as both approaches provide monitoring capabilities without capturing identifiable images, offering an effective balance between safety monitoring and personal privacy. This characteristic makes them particularly suitable for environments where individuals value independence and dignity while requiring some level of monitoring support.

System integration represents another critical aspect, as these technologies should seamlessly interface with existing infrastructure and monitoring systems to maximize their utility. The modular design of both HOI-Loc and A-SGTN facilitates integration with various IoT ecosystems and smart home platforms. Additionally, deployment efficiency can be enhanced through edge computing implementation, which reduces computational costs and latency while enabling real-time processing.

The technologies presented demonstrate particular relevance for smart aging applications, where device-free monitoring can support independent living while respecting user autonomy. The HOI-Loc system's ability to track activities of daily living through object interactions provides valuable insights into behavioral patterns without requiring users to wear or carry devices. Similarly, the trajectory prediction capabilities of A-SGTN can contribute to proactive assistance systems by anticipating movement patterns and potential safety concerns.

4.5.2 Future Research Directions

Several promising research directions emerge from this work. Developing personalized trajectory models that adapt to individual movement patterns could significantly enhance prediction accuracy and enable more tailored monitoring approaches. This personalization is particularly relevant for applications where individuals have varying mobility capabilities or specific movement preferences.

Extending sensor fusion approaches to incorporate additional non-invasive sensing modalities presents opportunities for improved accuracy and robustness. Future work could explore integration with ambient sensors, environmental monitoring systems, and other unobtrusive technologies to create more comprehensive monitoring solutions. Reducing calibration requirements remains important for improving practical deployability across diverse environments. Research into self-calibrating systems and automated setup procedures could lower barriers to adoption and enable broader implementation of these technologies.

Enhancing social interaction modeling for multi-person environments represents another important direction, particularly for shared living spaces or community settings where multiple individuals interact regularly. Advanced modeling of complex social dynamics could improve both localization accuracy and trajectory prediction performance. The convergence of these technologies with emerging artificial intelligence (AI) techniques, such as federated learning and differential privacy, could further enhance their applicability in privacy-sensitive contexts while maintaining high performance standards.

In summary, the device-free localization and trajectory prediction technologies provide foundational capabilities for unobtrusive monitoring that can support various smart environment applications, with particular promise for contexts where privacy preservation, user autonomy, and non-intrusive operation are essential requirements.

References

1. Adib, F., Kabelac, Z., Katabi, D.: Multi-person localization via RF body reflections. In: 12th USENIX Symposium on Networked Systems Design and Implementation, NSDI 15, Oakland, CA, USA, May 4–6, 2015, pp. 279–292. USENIX Association (2015)
2. Alahi, A., Goel, K., Ramanathan, V., Robicquet, A., Fei-Fei, L., Savarese, S.: Social LSTM: human trajectory prediction in crowded spaces. In: 2016 IEEE Conference on Computer Vision and Pattern Recognition, CVPR 2016, Las Vegas, NV, USA, June 27–30, 2016, pp. 961–971. IEEE Computer Society (2016)
3. Chen, W., Wang, F., Sun, H.: S2tnet: spatio-temporal transformer networks for trajectory prediction in autonomous driving. In: Asian Conference on Machine Learning, ACML 2021, 17–19 November 2021, Virtual Event, Proceedings of Machine Learning Research, vol. 157, pp. 454–469. PMLR (2021)
4. Giuliari, F., Hasan, I., Cristani, M., Galasso, F.: Transformer networks for trajectory forecasting. In: 25th International Conference on Pattern Recognition, ICPR 2020, Virtual Event/Milan, Italy, January 10–15, 2021, pp. 10335–10342. IEEE (2020)
5. Gupta, A., Johnson, J., Fei-Fei, L., Savarese, S., Alahi, A.: Social GAN: socially acceptable trajectories with generative adversarial networks. In: 2018 IEEE Conference on Computer Vision and Pattern Recognition, CVPR 2018, Salt Lake City, UT, USA, June 18–22, 2018, pp. 2255–2264. Computer Vision Foundation/IEEE Computer Society (2018)
6. Han, J., Qian, C., Wang, X., Ma, D., Zhao, J., Xi, W., Jiang, Z., Wang, Z.: Twins: device-free object tracking using passive tags. IEEE/ACM Trans. Netw. **24**(3), 1605–1617 (2016)
7. Helbing, D., Molnár, P.: Social force model for pedestrian dynamics. Phys. Rev. E **51**, 4282–4286 (1995)
8. Helten, T., Müller, M., Seidel, H., Theobalt, C.: Real-time body tracking with one depth camera and inertial sensors. In: IEEE International Conference on Computer Vision, ICCV 2013, Sydney, Australia, December 1–8, 2013, pp. 1105–1112. IEEE Computer Society (2013)
9. Kosaraju, V., Sadeghian, A., Martín-Martín, R., Reid, I.D., Rezatofighi, H., Savarese, S.: Social-bigat: Multimodal trajectory forecasting using bicycle-gan and graph attention networks. In: Advances in Neural Information Processing Systems 32: Annual Conference on Neural Information Processing Systems 2019, NeurIPS 2019, December 8–14, 2019, Vancouver, BC, Canada, pp. 137–146 (2019)

10. Leal-Taixé, L., Fenzi, M., Kuznetsova, A., Rosenhahn, B., Savarese, S.: Learning an image-based motion context for multiple people tracking. In: 2014 IEEE Conference on Computer Vision and Pattern Recognition, CVPR 2014, Columbus, OH, USA, June 23–28, 2014, pp. 3542–3549. IEEE Computer Society (2014)
11. Lee, N., Choi, W., Vernaza, P., Choy, C.B., Torr, P.H.S., Chandraker, M.: DESIRE: distant future prediction in dynamic scenes with interacting agents. In: 2017 IEEE Conference on Computer Vision and Pattern Recognition, CVPR 2017, Honolulu, HI, USA, July 21–26, 2017, pp. 2165–2174. IEEE Computer Society (2017)
12. Li, X., Ying, X., Chuah, M.C.: GRIP: graph-based interaction-aware trajectory prediction. In: 2019 IEEE Intelligent Transportation Systems Conference, ITSC 2019, Auckland, New Zealand, October 27–30, 2019, pp. 3960–3966. IEEE (2019)
13. Liu, Y., Li, B., Wang, X., Sammut, C., Yao, L.: Attention-aware social graph transformer networks for stochastic trajectory prediction. IEEE Trans. Knowl. Data Eng. **36**(11), 5633–5646 (2024)
14. Ma, Y., Zhu, X., Zhang, S., Yang, R., Wang, W., Manocha, D.: Trafficpredict: trajectory prediction for heterogeneous traffic-agents. In: The Thirty-Third AAAI Conference on Artificial Intelligence, AAAI 2019, The Thirty-First Innovative Applications of Artificial Intelligence Conference, IAAI 2019, The Ninth AAAI Symposium on Educational Advances in Artificial Intelligence, EAAI 2019, Honolulu, Hawaii, USA, January 27–February 1, 2019, pp. 6120–6127. AAAI Press (2019)
15. Mohamed, A.A., Qian, K., Elhoseiny, M., Claudel, C.G.: Social-stgcnn: a social spatio-temporal graph convolutional neural network for human trajectory prediction. In: 2020 IEEE/CVF Conference on Computer Vision and Pattern Recognition, CVPR 2020, Seattle, WA, USA, June 13–19, 2020, pp. 14412–14420. Computer Vision Foundation/IEEE (2020)
16. Pellegrini, S., Ess, A., Schindler, K., Gool, L.V.: You'll never walk alone: modeling social behavior for multi-target tracking. In: IEEE 12th International Conference on Computer Vision, ICCV 2009, Kyoto, Japan, September 27–October 4, 2009, pp. 261–268. IEEE Computer Society (2009)
17. Ruan, W., Sheng, Q.Z., Yao, L., Gu, T., Ruta, M., Shangguan, L.: Device-free indoor localization and tracking through human-object interactions. In: 17th IEEE International Symposium on A World of Wireless, Mobile and Multimedia Networks, WoWMoM 2016, Coimbra, Portugal, June 21–24, 2016, pp. 1–9. IEEE Computer Society (2016)
18. Ruan, W., Sheng, Q.Z., Yao, L., Yang, L., Gu, T.: Hoi-loc: towards unobstructive human localization with probabilistic multi-sensor fusion. In: 2016 IEEE International Conference on Pervasive Computing and Communication Workshops, PerCom Workshops 2016, Sydney, Australia, March 14–18, 2016, pp. 1–4. IEEE Computer Society (2016)
19. Ruan, W., Yao, L., Sheng, Q.Z., Falkner, N.J.G., Li, X.: Tagtrack: device-free localization and tracking using passive RFID tags. In: 11th International Conference on Mobile and Ubiquitous Systems: Computing, Networking and Services, MOBIQUITOUS 2014, London, United Kingdom, December 2–5, 2014, pp. 80–89. ICST/ACM (2014)
20. Ruan, W., Yao, L., Sheng, Q.Z., Falkner, N.J.G., Li, X., Gu, T.: Tagfall: towards unobstructive fine-grained fall detection based on UHF passive RFID tags. In: Proceedings of the 12th EAI International Conference on Mobile and Ubiquitous Systems: Computing, Networking and Services, MobiQuitous 2015, Coimbra, Portugal, July 22–24, 2015, pp. 140–149. ICST/ACM (2015)
21. Rudenko, A., Palmieri, L., Herman, M., Kitani, K.M., Gavrila, D.M., Arras, K.O.: Human motion trajectory prediction: a survey. Int. J. Robotics Res. **39**(8), (2020)
22. Salzmann, T., Ivanovic, B., Chakravarty, P., Pavone, M.: Trajectron++: dynamically-feasible trajectory forecasting with heterogeneous data. In: Computer Vision—ECCV 2020—16th European Conference, Glasgow, UK, August 23–28, 2020, Proceedings, Part XVIII. Lecture Notes in Computer Science, vol. 12363, pp. 683–700. Springer (2020)
23. Sheng, Q.Z., Li, X., Zeadally, S.: Enabling next-generation RFID applications: solutions and challenges. Computer **41**(9), 21–28 (2008)

24. Wu, C., Yang, Z., Zhou, Z., Liu, X., Liu, Y., Cao, J.: Non-invasive detection of moving and stationary human with WiFi. IEEE J. Sel. Areas Commun. **33**(11), 2329–2342 (2015)
25. Xiao, J., Joseph, S.L., Zhang, X., Li, B., Li, X., Zhang, J.: An assistive navigation framework for the visually impaired. IEEE Trans. Hum. Mach. Syst. **45**(5), 635–640 (2015)
26. Xu, C., Firner, B., Moore, R.S., Zhang, Y., Trappe, W., Howard, R.E., Zhang, F., An, N.: SCPL: indoor device-free multi-subject counting and localization using radio signal strength. In: The 12th International Conference on Information Processing in Sensor Networks (Co-located with CPS Week 2013), IPSN 2013, Philadelphia, PA, USA, April 8–11, 2013, pp. 79–90. ACM (2013)
27. Yang, L., Lin, Q., Li, X., Liu, T., Liu, Y.: See through walls with COTS RFID system! In: Proceedings of the 21st Annual International Conference on Mobile Computing and Networking, MobiCom 2015, Paris, France, September 7–11, 2015, pp. 487–499. ACM (2015)
28. Yang, Z., Sun, H., Huang, J., Sun, Z., Xiong, H., Qiao, S., Guan, Z., Jia, X.: An efficient destination prediction approach based on future trajectory prediction and transition matrix optimization. IEEE Trans. Knowl. Data Eng. **32**(2), 203–217 (2020)
29. Yang, Z., Zhou, Z., Liu, Y.: From RSSI to CSI: indoor localization via channel response. ACM Comput. Surv. **46**(2), 25:1–25:32 (2013)
30. Yao, L., Sheng, Q.Z., Ngu, A.H.H., Li, X.: Things of interest recommendation by leveraging heterogeneous relations in the internet of things. ACM Trans. Internet Techn. **16**(2), 9:1–9:25 (2016)
31. Youssef, M., Mah, M., Agrawala, A.K.: Challenges: device-free passive localization for wireless environments. In: Proceedings of the 13th Annual International Conference on Mobile Computing and Networking, MOBICOM 2007, Montréal, Québec, Canada, September 9–14, 2007, pp. 222–229. ACM (2007)
32. Yu, C., Ma, X., Ren, J., Zhao, H., Yi, S.: Spatio-temporal graph transformer networks for pedestrian trajectory prediction. In: Computer Vision—ECCV 2020—16th European Conference, Glasgow, UK, August 23–28, 2020, Proceedings, Part XII, Lecture Notes in Computer Science, vol. 12357, pp. 507–523. Springer (2020)

Chapter 5
Device-Free Human Activity Recognition

5.1 Introduction

5.1.1 Overview of Device-Free Human Activity Recognition

Understanding and recognizing human activities has emerged as a fundamental research topic in ubiquitous computing with applications in various domains, including smart aging [11, 21]. Activity recognition enables fall detection, remote health monitoring, and behavior analysis that enhance the quality of people's lives. With the global aging trend, unobtrusive activity recognition systems that facilitate independent living have gained significant research attention.

Device-free human activity recognition represents an emerging paradigm that strategically places sensing devices in the environment rather than requiring subjects to wear them [8]. By analyzing signal variations induced by a subject's movements, these systems can recognize activities without the privacy concerns of vision-based approaches (e.g., using cameras to monitor individuals at home) or the practicality challenges of wearable sensors (e.g., requiring consistent device usage).

In this chapter, we present our research on three innovative device-free human activity recognition approaches. We explore compressive representation for activity recognition using passive RFID signal strength, making sense of the Doppler effect for multi-modal hand motion detection, and a two-stream multi-level dynamic point transformer for two-person interaction recognition. These approaches collectively demonstrate the potential of device-free technologies to enhance environment sensing capabilities with particular relevance to independent living applications.

The evolution of this field has been driven by advancements in several key technologies:

- *Radio Frequency-based Recognition*: Systems utilizing RF signals, including Wi-Fi [26], RFID [31, 43], and radar technologies, detect human activities by analyzing signal fluctuations. These approaches operate in various lighting conditions and provide non-intrusive monitoring capabilities.

Q. Z. Sheng et al., *Harnessing Artificial Intelligence and Pervasive Internet of Things for an Empowered Aging*, https://doi.org/10.1007/978-3-032-16502-2_5

- *Acoustic-based Recognition*: Systems leveraging acoustic signals detect subtle movements through echo patterns and Doppler shifts. By utilizing built-in speakers and microphones in everyday devices, these approaches offer accessible and cost-effective solutions.
- *Depth Sensor-based Recognition*: Systems employing depth sensors capture spatial information without detailed visual features, providing privacy-preserving alternatives to RGB cameras for environments where privacy is a concern.

The non-intrusive nature, privacy preservation, continuous monitoring capability, and low maintenance requirements of device-free systems make them valuable for various applications, including detecting emergency situations, monitoring daily activities, and supporting independent living environments.

5.1.2 Challenges and Opportunities

Despite the promising potential of device-free human activity recognition, several significant technical and practical challenges must be addressed for these systems to achieve widespread adoption:

Technical Challenges. Device-free systems fundamentally rely on environmental signals that are inherently noisy and subject to fluctuations. For instance, RFID signal strength indicators suffer from high uncertainties due to real-world conditions such as distraction, diffusion, and degradation. Similarly, acoustic signals used in Doppler-based systems can be contaminated by ambient noise. These signal uncertainties, combined with the complexity of distinguishing between similar activities or capturing subtle movements with limited signal information, necessitate robust signal processing and advanced computational approaches.

Real-world environments introduce additional complexity through their dynamic nature. Changing conditions, moving objects, and multiple occupants create variations in the sensing environment that recognition systems must accommodate. Furthermore, many existing solutions require dense deployment of sensing devices or have stringent requirements for device placement, increasing deployment costs and complexity.

Research Opportunities. The challenges in device-free activity recognition present significant opportunities for innovation. We identify several promising research directions.

First, advanced signal processing techniques such as compressive sensing and dictionary learning offer opportunities to extract meaningful patterns from noisy signals, addressing the fundamental challenge of signal uncertainty. Our work on RFID-based activity recognition demonstrates how compressive sensing can create compact and robust activity representations despite noisy signals. Second, multi-modal recognition approaches that integrate information from multiple sensing modalities or extract diverse attributes from a single modality can provide more comprehensive activity recognition. Our acoustic-based system AudioGest exemplifies how extracting multiple dimensions (gesture type, duration, speed, and range) from a single modality enhances recognition capabilities. Third, deep learning approaches, particularly transformers and point cloud-based networks, offer promising avenues for improved feature extraction and activity classification. Our two-stream multi-level dynamic point transformer for interaction recognition demonstrates the potential of these approaches in privacy-preserving contexts.

Finally, leveraging existing infrastructure or commonly available devices, such as built-in speakers and microphones or passive RFID tags, presents opportunities for cost-effective deployment. This is particularly relevant when considering applications in independent living environments, where deployment complexity and cost are important considerations.

Through our research presented in this chapter, we address these challenges and explore these opportunities, developing innovative approaches to device-free human activity recognition that balance technical performance with practical considerations for real-world deployment.

5.1.3 Contributions

This chapter makes several significant contributions to the field of device-free human activity recognition for smart aging.

We develop a compressive sensing, dictionary-based approach for activity recognition using passive RFID signal strength. Our method learns compact and informative dictionaries of activities using unsupervised subspace decomposition, enabling efficient and robust activity recognition despite noisy, streaming, and unstable RFID signals. This approach achieves more compact representation of activities while preserving richer information, with potential applications in independent living monitoring.

We present AudioGest, a device-free gesture recognition system that accurately senses hand in-air movements using only built-in speaker and microphone pairs. Our system transforms devices into active sonar systems that transmit inaudible audio signals and decode the echoes of hand movements, enabling multi-modal hand detection without requiring extra hardware or infrastructure support. AudioGest recognizes various hand gestures and estimates hand in-air duration, average moving speed, and waving range, providing fine-grained control commands with potential applications in smart aging scenarios.

We propose a Two-stream Multi-level Dynamic Point Transformer (TMDPT) for two-person interaction recognition, utilizing depth videos as the sole input to ensure privacy preservation. Our approach introduces a novel frame sampling technique called Interval Frame Sampling (IFS) and leverages a two-stream multi-level feature aggregation module to capture informative global and partial features. This system demonstrates superior performance in recognizing interactions between individuals, which could provide insights into social behaviors in various monitoring environments.

We conduct extensive real-world experiments across diverse settings to validate the effectiveness, efficiency, and robustness of our proposed approaches. Our results demonstrate the practical potential of device-free activity recognition systems to support independent living of elderly individuals and enhance their quality of life.

These contributions collectively advance the state-of-the-art in device-free human activity recognition and provide practical solutions for smart aging applications.

5.1.4 *Chapter Organization*

The remainder of this chapter is organized as follows. Section 5.2 provides a comprehensive review of related work and background in device-free human activity recognition, covering various sensing modalities and computational approaches. We also discuss research gaps and opportunities specific to smart aging applications. Section 5.3 presents our first approach to device-free activity recognition using passive RFID signal strength. We introduce a compressive representation technique that deals with noisy, streaming, and unstable RFID signals to achieve robust activity recognition. Section 5.4 explores our second approach, which leverages the Doppler effect for multi-modal hand motion detection. We detail the development of AudioGest, a system that transforms consumer electronic devices into active sonar systems using built-in speakers and microphones. Section 5.5 introduces our third approach, which utilizes a two-stream multi-level dynamic point transformer for two-person interaction recognition. We describe how this privacy-preserving approach uses depth videos to recognize complex interactions between individuals. Section 5.6 concludes the chapter with a discussion of the implications of our research for smart aging applications and outlines future directions for device-free human activity recognition.

5.2 Background and Related Work

Human activity recognition has evolved significantly over the past decades, transitioning from wearable sensor-based approaches to device-free methods that offer greater convenience and non-intrusiveness. In this section, we provide an overview of related work in activity recognition, highlighting the evolution from instrumenting people to device-free approaches.

5.2.1 Evolution of Activity Recognition Technologies

Early activity recognition systems primarily relied on wearable sensors attached to the human body. Accelerometers and gyroscopes were commonly used to recognize various activities, with systems that distributed sensors across a user's body to infer activities through movement patterns. Smartphone-based recognition leveraged built-in sensors for detecting basic movements [2]. RFID technology expanded these capabilities, with approaches combining passive RFID tags with traditional sensors to track object interactions and infer activities using machine learning algorithms. Wang et al. [36] utilized RFID radio patterns to extract spatiotemporal features for activity characterization.

Despite their effectiveness, wearable approaches face significant limitations, including user discomfort, maintenance requirements, and compliance issues. These limitations become particularly pronounced in contexts where users may have difficulty for consistently wearing or managing devices.

To overcome these limitations, device-free activity recognition has emerged as a promising alternative where sensing devices are placed in the environment rather than on individuals. This approach has developed along several technological trajectories:

- *Radio Frequency-based Recognition*: RF-based systems analyze signal fluctuations induced by human movements. Zhang et al. [43] developed noise reduction algorithms for passive RFID tag arrays, while WiFi-based solutions like WiGest [1] exploit wireless signal properties, including signal strength and Doppler shifts to detect gestures and activities.
- *Acoustic-based Recognition*: These systems transform speakers and microphones into sonar-like sensing platforms. SoundWave [6] leverages the audio Doppler effect to recognize gestures without training, while recent research has extended these capabilities to detect human movements. These approaches use standard audio hardware to detect subtle movements by analyzing echo patterns.
- *Vision and Depth Sensor-based Recognition*: Vision-based systems extract features from visual data using techniques ranging from traditional methods to more recent deep learning approaches [22]. Depth sensor-based methods have gained popularity due to their privacy advantages, with RGB-D-based interaction recognition [14] utilizing skeleton data [34, 39] or hybrid features from multiple channels. Recent transformer-based approaches such as MViT [4] have advanced the state-of-the-art in action recognition.

5.2.2 Research Gaps and Application Opportunities

Despite significant advancements in device-free activity recognition, important research gaps remain. Signal uncertainty continues to be a fundamental challenge, particularly for fine-grained activity recognition. Many existing systems require precise sensor placement or dense deployments, limiting real-world applicability. The technology has promising applications in independent living contexts for safety monitoring, continuous health assessment, and social interaction analysis while preserving privacy. Integration with ambient intelligence systems represents opportunities for holistic solutions that adapt to user needs based on recognized activities.

Our research addresses these challenges through three complementary approaches to device-free human activity recognition, each targeting different technical challenges while demonstrating practical applications across various contexts.

5.3 RFID-Based Activity Recognition with Compressive Representation

5.3.1 Motivation and Overview of RFID-Based Activity Recognition

Device-free activity recognition addresses key limitations in existing approaches: vision-based systems raise privacy concerns while wearable sensors require consistent usage, making them impractical for individuals who may forget or find it difficult to wear sensing devices regularly. Understanding and recognizing human activities is fundamental for applications including fall detection and remote health monitoring, with particular importance for the global aging population.

We present a low-cost, unobtrusive RFID-based activity recognition system that supports independent living through device-free monitoring [42]. Figure 5.1 illustrates the system setup. Our approach leverages off-the-shelf passive RFID tags with relaxed placement requirements, using compressive sensing and dictionary-based methods to handle noisy and unstable signals.

To address the inherent challenges of noisy, streaming, and unstable RFID signals, we develop a compressive sensing, dictionary-based approach that learns compact and informative dictionaries of activities through unsupervised subspace decomposition. Our approach creates more compact and robust representation of activities, enabling efficient classification despite signal uncertainties.

The system achieves approximately 95% accuracy in person-dependent validation and 70% in person-independent scenarios across 23 fine-grained activities, demonstrating practical potential for elderly care environments with advantages including ease of deployment, maintenance-free operation, low cost, and lightweight computational requirements.

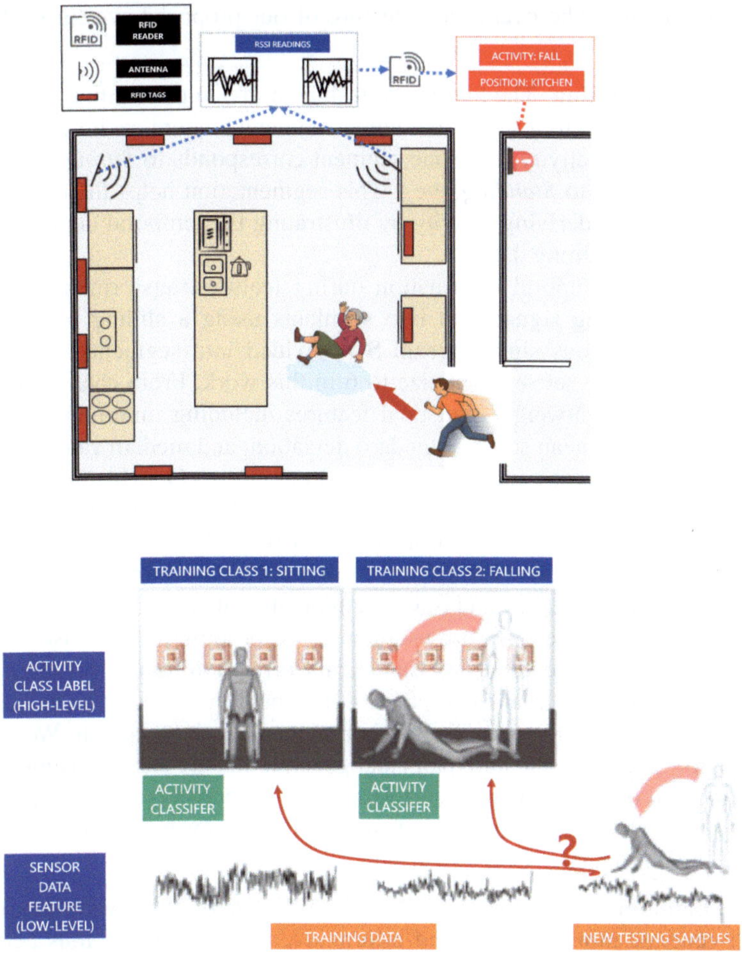

Fig. 5.1 **a** The proposed lightweight setup: A person performs different activities between the wall deployed with an RFID array and an RFID antenna. **b** The activities can be recognized by analyzing the corresponding signal strength fluctuation, Received Signal Strength Indicator (RSSI)

5.3.2 Compressive Dictionary Learning Methodology

Our proposed system for device-free activity recognition processes noisy RFID signal streaming data to perform robust activity identification. The overall architecture consists of three main stages: (1) signal processing and feature extraction, (2) activity dictionary learning, and (3) activity classification using learned dictionaries. This approach allows for efficient and accurate recognition of activities from passive RFID signals, which can be valuable for monitoring daily activities in independent living environments. The overall architecture of our proposed system is shown in Fig. 5.2.

Feature Representation. The first major task is to divide the continuous sequence of RSSI data stream into a set of individual segments, where each segment corresponds to a specific activity (e.g., one segment corresponds to *Sitting*, and another segment corresponds to *Standing*, etc.). This segmentation helps the classifier better understand the underlying activity by illustrating the temporal dependency and compressing the streaming data.

We incorporate temporal information during feature transformation by dividing the raw streaming signal data into segments using a sliding window-based method. The continuous signal stream $\mathbf{S}$ is divided into segments of equal size $\mathbf{S} = \{\mathbf{S}_1, \ldots, \mathbf{S}_n\}$. We set segment size to 6 in this work. From each segment, we extract 7 types of lightweight statistical features including minimum, maximum, mean, variance, root mean square, standard deviation, and median values.

The extraction process yields a total of m feature vectors $\mathbf{O} = \{\mathbf{o}_1, \ldots, \mathbf{o}_i\}$, where $\mathbf{o} \in \mathbb{R}^m$ with $m = 7 \times t$, with t being the number of tags. Due to the "curse of dimensionality" and the presence of irrelevant or redundant features, we employ a feature selection technique to identify the most discriminative features, which helps improve recognition accuracy and reduce computational cost.

To systematically assess feature usefulness, we propose a filter-based unsupervised feature selection method using Canonical Correlation Analysis (CCA). Unlike existing approaches that treat each feature component independently, we study the correlations between features to identify complementary information. We compute canonical correlations for feature pairs and generate feature subsets using a greedy algorithm based on these pairwise correlations. This approach assigns higher ranks to weakly correlated (complementary) feature pairs and lower ranks to strongly correlated (redundant) pairs.

Activity Dictionary Learning. A well-learned dictionary fitted with training samples can generate more compact and informative representations, thus helping to achieve better recognition performance. We learn one single dictionary for each activity, formed by a set of basis vectors learned by solving a sparse optimization

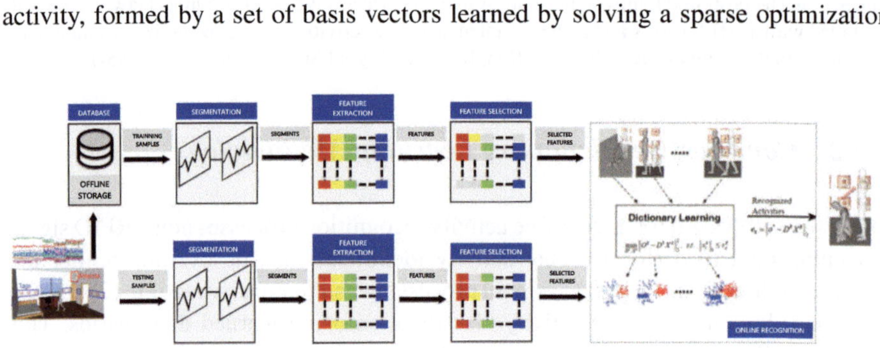

Fig. 5.2 The architecture of our proposed activity recognition system

problem. Each basis vector effectively captures part of the key structural information of the training data.

The advantages of this dictionary-based approach include: (1) each activity dictionary is learned independently from other activities, making the system flexible and scalable when new activities are added; (2) dictionaries can be trained with a small number of samples, reducing the labeling workload; and (3) the approach can effectively handle noisy, streaming signal data.

For K types of activities, we construct K dictionaries. Given training samples from activity class c^k as $\mathbf{O}^k = \{\mathbf{o}_1^k, \mathbf{o}_2^k, \ldots, \mathbf{o}_N^k\}$, we learn a dictionary matrix $\mathbf{D}^k \in \mathbb{R}^{m \times K}$ over which $\mathbf{O}^k$ has a sparse representation. We adopt the K-SVD algorithm to solve this optimization problem, performing sparse coding and dictionary updating steps iteratively until convergence.

Classification Strategies Using Dictionary Coefficients. One advantage of having class-specific dictionaries is that each class is modeled independently, avoiding the repetition of training when new activities are added. After learning individual activity-specific dictionaries, any new incoming RFID signal can be represented in terms of dictionary bases. For classification, we propose several strategies to exploit the learned sparse coefficients:

- *Reconstruction error (RE)*: Assigns the activity label corresponding to the dictionary with the smallest reconstruction error.
- *Maximal coefficient (MC)*: Associates the activity label with the dictionary having the largest absolute coefficient value.
- *Maximal mean of coefficients (MMC)*: Assigns the activity label with the maximum average of coefficients.
- *Maximal sum of coefficients (MSC)*: Uses the maximum sum of absolute coefficient values to determine the activity.
- *Concatenate coefficients (ConSVM)*: Stacks learned coefficients with original features and feeds them into an SVM classifier.

These classification strategies leverage the learned dictionaries in different ways, enabling us to identify the most effective approach for activity recognition in independent living environments. In the next section, we will present our comprehensive experimental evaluation of these proposed methods.

5.3.3 Experimental Evaluation and Implementation Results

To validate our proposed approach, we conducted extensive experiments evaluating system performance across different settings and conditions. Our evaluation focuses on performance comparison, parameter optimization, and practical considerations for real-world deployment in independent living environments.

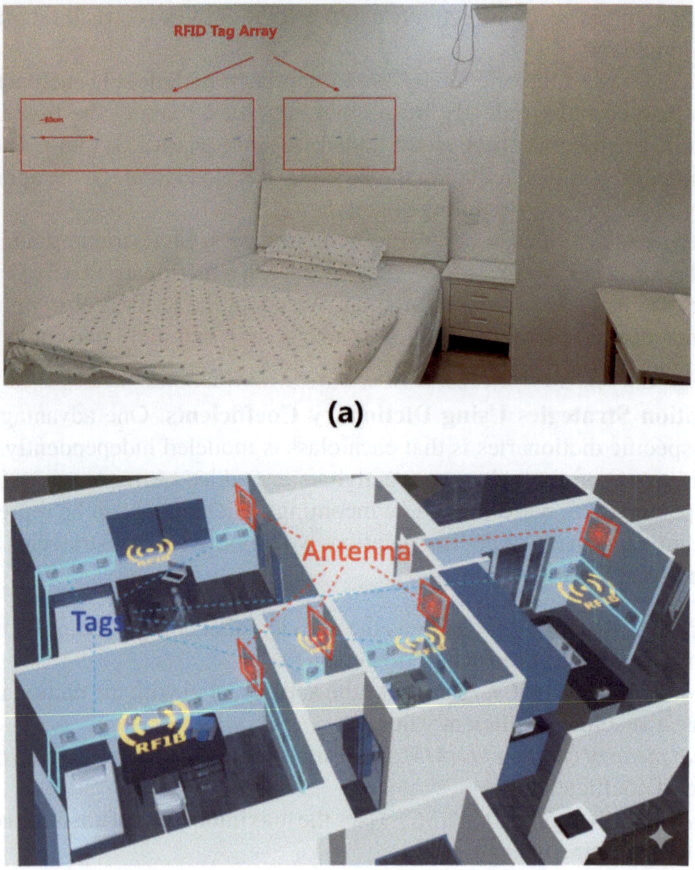

(a)

(b)

Fig. 5.3 Experimental setup: **a** bedroom setup and **b** whole house setup

Experimental Settings

Hardware Setup. We used one Alien 9,900+ RFID reader, one circular antenna and Squig inlay passive RFID tags in our experiments. Passive tags were placed on the wall at certain distances. The antenna was positioned approximately 1.3 m high from the ground, arranged at an angle of approximately 70° to ensure optimal signal coverage. Subjects stood between the wall and the antenna (approximately 1.5 to 1.8 m) and performed various predefined activities. RSSI signals were collected at a sampling rate of 0.5 s. The overall set up is shown in Fig. 5.3.

It is worth noting that commercial RFID readers and tags operate at electromagnetic frequencies in the low-energy range, effectively eliminating health risks for monitored individuals. Passive tags have no baseline electromagnetic activity and

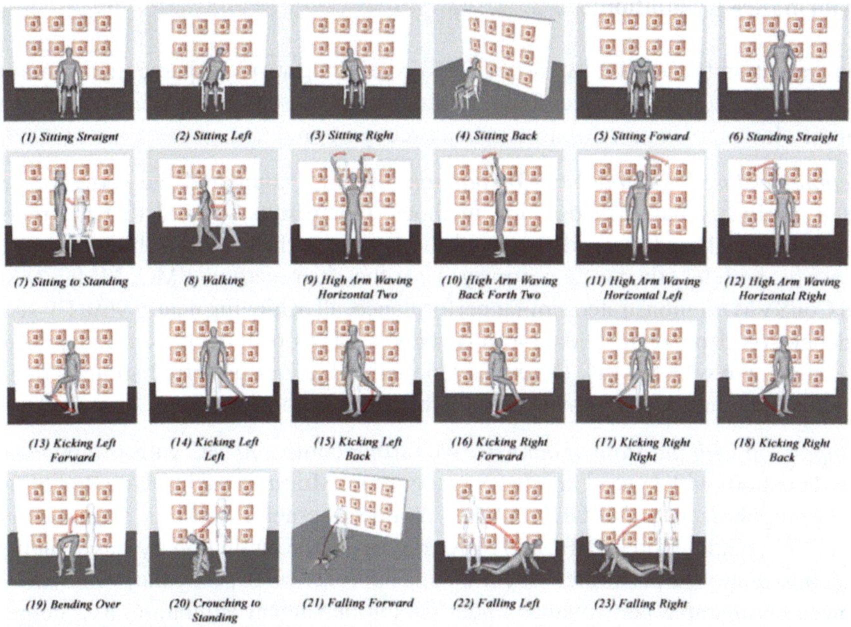
(1) Sitting Straight
(2) Sitting Left
(3) Sitting Right
(4) Sitting Back
(5) Sitting Foward
(6) Standing Straight
(7) Sitting to Standing
(8) Walking
(9) High Arm Waving Horizontal Two
(10) High Arm Waving Back Forth Two
(11) High Arm Waving Horizontal Left
(12) High Arm Waving Horizontal Right
(13) Kicking Left Forward
(14) Kicking Left Left
(15) Kicking Left Back
(16) Kicking Right Forward
(17) Kicking Right Right
(18) Kicking Right Back
(19) Bending Over
(20) Crouching to Standing
(21) Falling Forward
(22) Falling Left
(23) Falling Right

Fig. 5.4 Our proposed algorithm can detect and classify 23 postures and actions with an average accuracy of over 96%

only produce signals in response to interrogation from an RFID reader, making them suitable for long-term monitoring applications, including independent living support.

Data Collection. The data acquisition process involved six subjects (five males and one female) performing 23 fine-grained, orientation-sensitive activities (including 6 postures and 17 actions, as shown in Fig. 5.4). These activities represent common daily movements relevant to independent living monitoring. Each subject performed each activity for 120 s, and all 23 different activities performed sequentially by one subject were regarded as one set of activity data.

Validation Strategy. We validated our approach using two strategies: *person-dependent* and *person-independent*. The former uses partial samples from each subject for testing, with the remaining samples from the same participant used for training. This approach could be relevant for monitoring scenarios where systems are calibrated to specific individuals. The person-independent strategy applies a "one subject out" approach, where data from five subjects trains the algorithm while data from the left-out subject is used for testing. We report results averaged across all subjects for both strategies.

Performance Evaluation

Our evaluation focused on two aspects: (1) comparing various sparse representation dictionary-based methods and (2) comparing our proposed method with widely used generic classifiers in sensor-based activity recognition.

Dictionary-Based Approaches Comparison. We first compared the series of proposed dictionary-based recognition methods. Our results showed that the reconstruction error-based method produced the lowest performance in both validation scenarios, with less than 60% accuracy. The other four methods (MC, MMC, MSC, and ConSVM) demonstrated similar performance, all achieving nearly 96% F1-score under person-dependent validation and over 60% F1-score under person-independent validation. We selected MC (Maximal Coefficient) as our preferred strategy due to its stable recognition performance and light computational cost.

Comparison with the State of the Arts. We further compared MC with several established methods widely used in activity recognition: Multinomial Logistic Regression with ℓ_1 regularization (MLGL1), SVM with linear kernel (LSVM), k nearest neighbor (kNN), random forest (RF), and Naive Bayes (NB). Our dictionary-based method MC consistently outperformed all competing approaches. In particular, while LSVM showed comparable performance under person-dependent validation, MC demonstrated superior recognition accuracy in person-independent scenarios, indicating better ability to handle intra-class variability across different persons.

Looking at activity-specific performance, our method showed robust outcomes under person-dependent validation, correctly identifying almost all activities. Under person-independent validation, our method successfully distinguished many activities, including sitting, sitting to standing, and arm weaving with reasonably good performance, and could recognize falling with over 60% accuracy across different persons. These results suggest potential for fall detection and activity monitoring applications.

5.3.4 Summary and Conclusions for RFID-Based Activity Recognition System

Our RFID-based activity recognition system demonstrates the effectiveness of compressive sensing and dictionary learning approaches for device-free monitoring applications. The system successfully addresses fundamental challenges in RFID-based sensing, including signal noise, streaming data processing, and compact feature representation.

Key achievements include approximately 95% accuracy in person-dependent scenarios and 70% accuracy in person-independent validation across 23 fine-grained activities. The compressive dictionary learning methodology enables robust recognition despite inherent RSSI signal uncertainties, while the lightweight computational requirements and maintenance-free operation make the system practical for long-term deployment.

The system's advantages include ease of deployment with relaxed tag placement requirements, low cost using off-the-shelf components, privacy preservation without direct body monitoring, and scalability for adding new activities. These characteristics make it particularly suitable for independent living environments where unobtrusive monitoring can support fall detection and daily activity assessment.

Our experimental validation across diverse settings demonstrates the practical potential for elderly care applications, providing a foundation for continuous, non-intrusive activity monitoring that can enhance safety and independence while respecting privacy concerns.

5.4 Doppler-Based Hand Motion Detection and Recognition

5.4.1 Motivation and Overview of AudioGest System

Hand gesture interaction has emerged as an increasingly popular means of communicating with consumer electronic devices. Despite considerable advances in hand gesture recognition (HGR) systems, a fundamental challenge persists: developing a solution that works anytime (regardless of lighting conditions), anywhere (with or without network connectivity), and in a device-free manner (without wearable sensors) [10]. Existing approaches have significant limitations, including lighting dependencies, privacy concerns, additional hardware requirements, and connectivity dependencies.

We present AudioGest [29], an innovative device-free gesture recognition system that transforms standard consumer devices into active sonar systems using only their built-in speakers and microphones. The key innovation of our approach is its ability to sense hand movements without any extra hardware or infrastructure support, and without requiring training. Unlike existing solutions, AudioGest achieves true multi-modal hand detection—not only recognizing various gesture types but also reliably estimating continuous attributes like hand in-air duration, average moving speed, and waving range.

Our system operates by emitting inaudible audio signals and analyzing the reflected echoes to detect and interpret hand movements with high precision. By combining gesture type recognition with attribute estimation, AudioGest enables up to 54 distinct control commands through different combinations of gestures and their characteristics. This multi-dimensional interaction capability offers fine-grained control for various applications, including smart environment control, where users can adjust parameters or trigger functions through intuitive gestures.

We extensively evaluated AudioGest across three electronic devices under four real-world scenarios using approximately 3,900 hand gestures collected from five users. Our results demonstrate remarkable accuracy and robustness, with the system detecting six distinct hand gestures with up to 96% accuracy while precisely distinguishing differences in hand speed and moving range.

5.4.2 AudioGest System Methodology

Doppler Effect Principles

Most current hand gesture recognition (HGR) systems utilize labeled sensor readings to train classification models, lacking physical interpretation and struggling to detect contextual information such as hand moving speed and in-air duration. As shown in Fig. 5.5, our AudioGest system addresses these limitations by leveraging the Doppler Effect, which quantifies wavelength changes when wave energy travels between objects in motion.

The Doppler effect causes the received frequency to differ from the transmitted frequency when there is relative motion between source and receiver. The general equation measuring this frequency shift is:

$$\Delta f = \frac{\Delta v}{v_{wave}} f_{source}, \tag{5.1}$$

where $\Delta f = f_{receiver} - f_{source}$ represents the Doppler Frequency Shift, and $\Delta v = v_{receiver} - v_{source}$ is the relative velocity.

In our system, while the speaker (source) and microphone (receiver) remain stationary, the moving hand functions as a reflector, causing a portion of sound waves

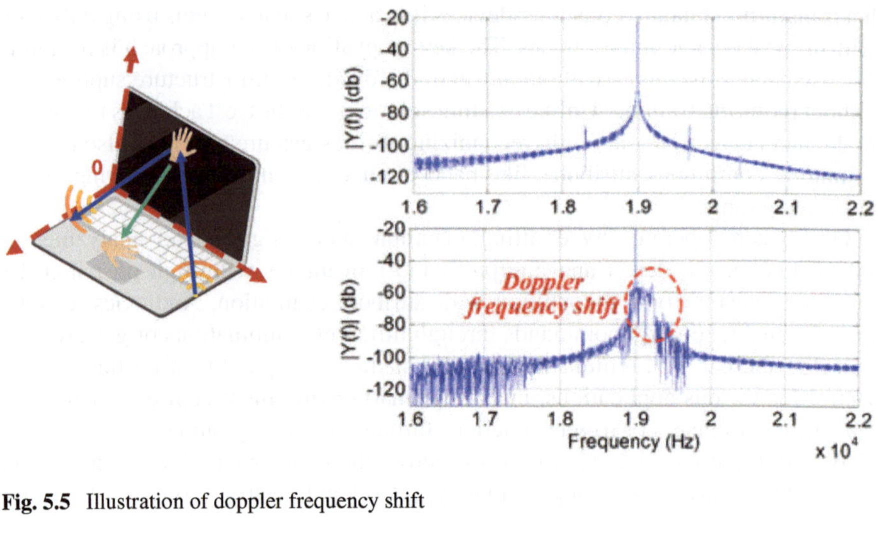

Fig. 5.5 Illustration of doppler frequency shift

to experience a Doppler frequency shift measured by:

$$f_{received} = \frac{1 + v_{rad}/v_{sound}}{1 - v_{rad}/v_{sound}} f_{sound}, \tag{5.2}$$

where v_{rad} represents the hand's radial speed relative to the microphone. This principle, widely used in radar and sonar systems, forms the foundation of our approach to detect and characterize hand movements through sound wave analysis.

System Components and Hardware

Our system transforms commercial off-the-shelf (COTS) speakers and microphones into an active sonar system for fine-grained hand gesture detection. By operating in the frequency range just above human auditory limits (approximately 18.5–19.5 kHz), we create a detection system that remains unobtrusive to users while providing high-quality hand motion data.

Modern mobile devices increasingly support high-definition audio capabilities, including extended frequency response ranges and improved sampling rates (typically 44.1 kHz or 48 kHz), making them ideal platforms for our approach. These capabilities enable the detection of subtle hand movements through precise measurement of Doppler shifts, creating new interaction possibilities for diverse user populations, including those who may benefit from more intuitive device control methods. These technical capabilities provide the foundation for AudioGest's comprehensive system design. To effectively integrate these components and deliver reliable gesture recognition, we have developed a layered architecture that systematically processes acoustic signals from raw input to final gesture classification.

System Architecture

The AudioGest system architecture comprises three conceptual layers: the gesture detection layer, the gesture categorization layer, and the application layer, as shown in Fig. 5.6.

The gesture detection layer forms the core of our system, extracting four types of gesture information: waving direction, hand's average speed, in-air duration, and waving range. This layer processes raw acoustic signals through several key steps: (1) signal cleaning through FFT normalization and background noise subtraction, (2) accurate identification of motion-induced signal segments, (3) interpretation of Doppler frequency shifts to estimate hand motion characteristics, and (4) quantification of gesture parameters.

The gesture categorization layer classifies the detected motion characteristics into semantic categories. We define six gesture directions and three intensity levels each for speed, duration, and range. This multi-modal approach enables up to 54 distinct

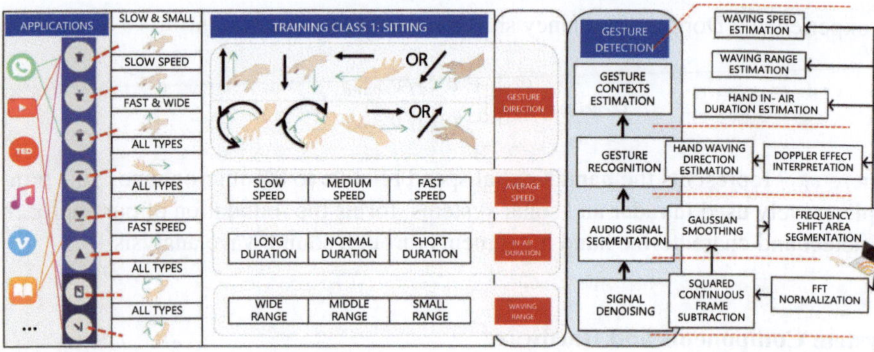

Fig. 5.6 Overview of the system for hand gesture detection

control commands from a single sensing modality, a significant advancement over previous systems that typically detect only one or two gesture contexts.

The application layer maps gestures to control commands for various applications. For example, in a media player application, an up-down hand gesture might trigger the "play" action, while moving the hand up controls volume, with the rate of change determined by gesture speed or range. This intuitive mapping can significantly improve device accessibility for users who find traditional interfaces challenging.

Technical Implementation

To implement our hand gesture recognition system, we address two fundamental challenges: *audio signal drift* and *weak echo signals*. These challenges are particularly relevant when designing systems intended for real-world deployment across diverse environments and user populations.

To manage audio signal drift (variations in signal magnitude across devices and time), we apply FFT normalization to the recorded audio signals. Our approach focuses on relative frequency patterns rather than absolute magnitudes, making the system robust to hardware variations and temporal fluctuations. This normalization process creates stable and interpretable Doppler frequency shifts regardless of device type or usage duration.

For detecting weak echo signals from hand movements, we employ a sequence of signal processing techniques. After normalizing the frequency spectrum, we apply squared continuous frame subtraction to highlight changing frequency components while suppressing static elements. We then employ Gaussian smoothing to connect discrete frequency shifts into coherent zones, followed by thresholding to identify regions of significant motion.

To interpret these processed signals, we leverage the physical relationship between hand movement and Doppler shift. The frequency shift is proportional to the hand's radial velocity (v_{rad}) toward the microphone:

$$\Delta f \propto v_{hand} \cos \theta_{hand}, \tag{5.3}$$

where θ_{hand} represents the angle between the hand's motion path and the direction to the microphone. By analyzing the temporal pattern of these shifts, we identify distinct gesture types and extract motion characteristics including direction, speed, duration, and range.

Based on these physical principles and signal processing techniques, our gesture recognition implementation utilizes a rule-based classification approach. For gesture recognition, we employ a rule-based approach derived from Doppler effect principles, eliminating the need for extensive training data. This approach not only recognizes gesture types but also quantifies motion attributes through metrics such as speed-ratio and range-ratio, providing rich interaction capabilities that can be adapted to diverse user needs and application contexts.

5.4.3 *Experimental Evaluation and Results*

We conducted extensive evaluations of the AudioGest system, beginning with controlled laboratory experiments and progressing to in-situ tests in diverse real-world environments. All tests were performed using unmodified commercial devices: a MacBook Air laptop, a GALAXY Tab-2 tablet, and a GALAXY S4 smartphone (referred to as D1, D2, and D3, respectively).

Our evaluation considered four key metrics: (1) Detection Rate, measuring the system's ability to correctly identify gesture occurrences; (2) False Detection Rate, assessing false positive errors; (3) Gesture Classification Accuracy, evaluating correct gesture type identification; and (4) Detection Accuracy, measuring the system's ability to correctly classify both gesture types and motion attributes.

Performance Results

We conducted micro-benchmark tests in a controlled laboratory environment with five participants (marked as U1, U2, U3, U4, and U5). Each participant performed each hand gesture 30 times for each of the three devices (MacBook Air laptop, GALAXY Tab-2 tablet, and GALAXY S4 smartphone), resulting in 2,700 total hand gestures collected over approximately 4.5 h of audio data.

Gesture Recognition Performance. AudioGest achieved an average 94.15% gesture classification accuracy across all users and devices. Among the participants, subject U5 achieved the highest average accuracy of 95%, while U1 achieved 90.15% mean accuracy using the tablet. The confusion matrix analysis revealed that most errors occurred in distinguishing between Right-Left/Front-Behind and Left-Right/Behind-Front gestures, which is attributable to the microphone placement characteristics of different devices.

Attribute Estimation Accuracy. The system estimated hand motion attributes with high precision, achieving average errors of 0.255 s for in-air duration, 0.242 for speed-ratio, and 0.214 for range-ratio. These results demonstrate the system's capacity for fine-grained gesture characterization beyond basic type recognition. Notably, participant U5 achieved better results in both gesture classification and attribute estimation, primarily due to having a slightly larger hand size that enhanced audio signal reflection.

System Parameters and Trade-offs. A critical design consideration involves balancing temporal and speed resolution with computational efficiency. As shown in Table 5.1, frame size selection significantly impacts system performance. Smaller frame sizes require more frequent FFT calculations and produce finer frequency bins, yielding better speed resolution but coarser time resolution. We selected a 2,048-point frame size for AudioGest, which provides 0.389 m/s speed resolution and 0.0464 s time resolution—sufficient for distinguishing three speed levels (slow, medium, fast) while maintaining reasonable calculation time (0.396 s). This resolution effectively filters false alarms from finger movements while enabling robust multi-modal gesture detection.

Our in-situ evaluation included testing in four typical daily-living environments: a living room (5 m × 3.5 m), on a public bus, in a café, and in a shared HDR (Higher Degree by Research) office space (approximately 15 m × 10 m with over 20 occupants). Two subjects (U1 and U2) collected 1,200 hand gestures across these environments (Living Room: 360, Bus: 240, Café: 240, HDR Space: 360) over a two-week testing period. Across these diverse environments, AudioGest maintained robust performance. In the living room and HDR office environments, the system performed similarly to our laboratory micro-benchmark results. However, in the most challenging condition—the public bus, which represents the most dynamic environment—performance decreased to 89.67% accuracy, primarily due to narrow space constraints and unpredictable motion influences. This resilience to environmental variations is

Table 5.1 Calculation time and resolution versus frame sizes

Frame size	Resolution of FFT (Hz)	Calculation time (s)	Resolution of speed (m/s)	In-air time resolution (s)
256	172.27	2.767	3.110	0.0058
1,024	43.07	0.733	0.777	0.0232
2,048	21.53	0.396	0.389	0.0464
4,096	10.77	0.226	0.194	0.0929
8,192	5.38	0.134	0.097	0.1858

particularly important for applications intended for diverse deployment contexts, including independent living environments.

System Robustness Evaluation. We evaluated AudioGest's robustness across four critical dimensions to assess its reliability under varying real-world conditions:

- *Device orientation*: The system maintained high accuracy (above 85%) when orientation changes were less than $\pi/4$ radians. Under a $\pi/2$ circumstance, accuracy decreased significantly to approximately 60%, which represents a limitation for future improvement.
- *Hand-device distance*: Performance remained strong at distances up to 10 cm, which accommodates typical usage scenarios for most users. We observed performance degradation when the hand waved at distances beyond 10 cm, as commercial off-the-shelf (COTS) microphones have capability limitations in capturing weak echo signals at longer ranges.
- *Environmental noise*: AudioGest showed remarkable resilience to various environmental conditions. We tested the system under five scenarios: Quiet (no audible noise and human motion), Noisy (playing music loudly), Dynamic1 (human walking approximately 4 m away), Dynamic2 (human walking approximately 2 m away), and Dynamic3 (human walking nearby, approximately 0.5 m away). The system maintained consistent performance in the first three cases, demonstrating particular resilience to audio noise. However, performance degraded in Dynamic3 due to strong interference from nearby human motion.
- *Time elapse*: With our FFT normalization technique, the system demonstrated stable performance over extended periods without parameter adjustment. We tested AudioGest at intervals of 6 h, 1 day, 3 days, 1 week, and 10 days. Comparison experiments showed that by applying FFT normalization, AudioGest achieved approximately 35–70% performance improvement when dealing with signal drifting challenges, demonstrating the effectiveness of our denoising approach for long-term deployment.

Comparison with the State of the Art

We compared AudioGest with seven state-of-the-art hand gesture recognition systems spanning various sensing modalities (WiFi, radar, audio, etc.), shown in Table 5.2. Our system offers several unique advantages:

- *Hardware requirements*: Like SoundWave, AudioGest operates using only built-in device components, eliminating the need for additional hardware.
- *Environmental robustness*: Unlike most competing systems, AudioGest was successfully tested in highly dynamic environments like moving buses.
- *Training requirements*: Our physics-based approach eliminates the need for extensive training data, unlike several machine learning-based alternatives.

- *Gesture attributes*: AudioGest uniquely captures multiple gesture dimensions (type, speed, duration, and range), enabling richer interaction than most alternatives.
- *Gesture resolution*: By combining multiple attributes, our system theoretically supports up to 54 distinct commands, exceeding the capabilities of comparable approaches.

The multi-modal nature of AudioGest makes it particularly valuable for applications requiring rich interaction without specialized hardware, including contexts where intuitive device control can enhance accessibility for users with various abilities and technological familiarity levels.

5.4.4 Summary of the AudioGest System

AudioGest represents a significant advancement in device-free hand gesture recognition by transforming standard consumer devices into sophisticated active sonar systems. The system addresses fundamental challenges in gesture recognition including environmental robustness, hardware dependency, and multi-modal attribute detection.

Our approach achieves 94.15% gesture classification accuracy across diverse real-world environments while simultaneously estimating gesture attributes with high precision. The physics-based methodology eliminates training requirements and enables operation using only built-in speakers and microphones, making the system universally deployable without additional hardware or infrastructure modifications.

Key innovations include FFT normalization for hardware-independent operation, Doppler effect-based attribute estimation for rich interaction capabilities, and robust performance across dynamic environments, including moving vehicles. The system's ability to detect up to 54 distinct control commands through gesture-attribute combinations represents a significant advancement over existing approaches.

AudioGest's environmental resilience, demonstrated through successful operation in challenging scenarios like public transportation, combined with its ability to function across diverse device types and orientations, makes it particularly valuable for accessibility applications and smart environment control, where intuitive, hardware-free interaction is essential.

Table 5.2 Comparison of typical hand gesture recognition systems

Comparison items	WiGest [1]	FineCesture [20]	AllSee [10]	SoundWave [6]	SideSwipe [45]	RadarCesture [23]	WiSee [27]	AudioGest
Measured signal	RSSI	RSS, Phase, CSI	RF signal	Audio	GSM signal	FMCW Radar	OFDM radio	Audio
Need extra hardware?	No	Yes	Yes	No	Yes	Yes	Yes	No
Test in dynamic environment? (e.g., bus)	No	Yes	No	No	No	No	No	Yes
Need training?	No	Yes (kNN)	No	No	Yes (SVM)	No	No	No
Sense gesture contexts? (e.g., speed, range)	Yes (speed)	No	No	No	No	Yes (speed and range)	No	Yes (relative speed and range)
Accuracy	96%	92%	97%	94.5%	87.2%	N/A (hand tracking)	94%	95.1%
Gesture resolution	36	25	8	5	14	N/A (hand tracking)	9	54 (randomly choose two attributes)

5.5 Transformer-Based Two-Person Interaction Recognition

5.5.1 *Motivation and Overview of the TMDPT System*

Recognizing interactions between people represents a crucial aspect of advanced human activity recognition systems and holds significant importance for smart aging applications. In potential eldercare environments, the ability to identify interactions such as handshaking, hugging, assistance with daily activities, or potential emergencies could provide valuable insights into social well-being, care needs, and safety concerns.

Traditional approaches to human activity recognition have largely focused on individual actions, but interactions between multiple people introduce additional complexity due to the interdependence between subjects, body occlusions, and the need to capture relational dynamics. Recent advancements in RGB-D-based interaction recognition have shown promise. However, existing approaches face significant limitations. Skeleton-based methods [34, 39] struggle with increased body overlaps and occlusions common in human-human interactions, while hybrid feature-based approaches that incorporate RGB data raise privacy concerns, particularly in sensitive monitoring environments.

Motivated by these challenges, we propose a novel approach designed for privacy-preserving two-person interaction recognition with applications in smart aging contexts. Our Two-stream Multi-level Dynamic Point Transformer (TMDPT) utilizes depth videos as the sole input, ensuring a higher level of personal privacy while maintaining robust recognition performance. Unlike RGB data, depth videos lack texture and color features and are insensitive to illumination, making them well-suited for privacy-sensitive applications including eldercare monitoring.

Drawing inspiration from recent advances in point cloud-based action recognition [37], we convert depth videos into point cloud videos, offering additional advantages in terms of reduced computational requirements. Our approach also addresses the frame sampling challenge through a novel Interval Frame Sampling (IFS) technique, which intelligently selects informative frames while removing redundancy from the original videos.

The TMDPT architecture effectively captures complex spatiotemporal relationships in two-person interactions through a carefully designed two-stream multi-level feature aggregation module. Extensive evaluation on standard interaction recognition datasets demonstrates the effectiveness of our approach, with TMDPT outperforming state-of-the-art methods across multiple evaluation settings.

5.5.2 TMDPT Framework and Architecture

Our Two-stream Multi-level Dynamic Point Transformer (TMDPT) comprises four main components as depicted in Fig. 5.7: a novel frame sampling scheme, a frame features learning module, a feature aggregation module, and a transformer classification module. This approach could potentially be applied to scenarios where monitoring interactions between individuals provides valuable insights.

We solely utilize depth videos as input, which could address privacy concerns in sensitive environments. First, we form 3D voxels by mapping depth values to coordinates, and convert the 3D grid into a point cloud by determining whether the voxels are occupied. Subsequently, Interval Frame Sampling (IFS) is applied to sample frames from the point cloud videos. The frame features learning module then extracts local-region features, frame spatial features, and frame temporal features from each frame. Next, a two-stream multi-level feature aggregation module combines these features into global and partial features. Lastly, the transformer classification module employs self-attention on the aggregated features and utilizes the output in conjunction with the original global feature for the final classification.

Interval Frame Sampling

We introduce a novel frame sampling technique called Interval Frame Sampling (IFS) as shown in Fig. 5.8. IFS comprises two steps: the first step executes before the training phase to sample p frames per interaction video. Given a point cloud video, we evenly separate all frames into p intervals and randomly select one frame from each interval. This balances uniform and random sampling to reduce redundancy while retaining discriminative information.

During the training phase, the second step is performed in each epoch. We apply the same sampling method again to divide the updated video from the first step into q intervals, and randomly select one frame from each interval, resulting in q frames as

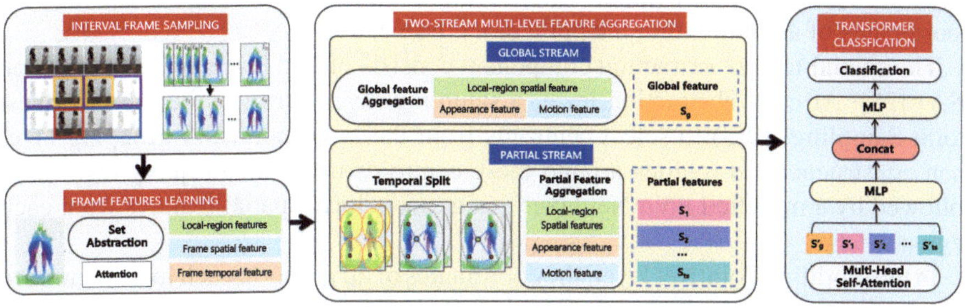

Fig. 5.7 Two-stream Multi-level Dynamic Point Transformer comprises four main components: a novel frame sampling scheme named Interval Frame Sampling, a frame features learning module, a two-stream multi-level feature aggregation module, and a transformer classification module

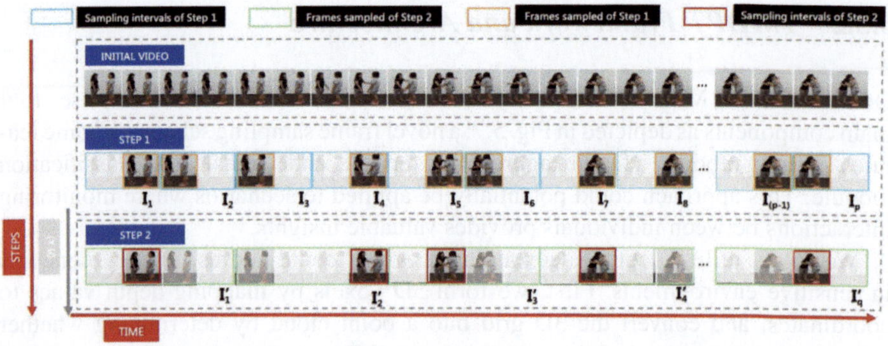

Fig. 5.8 A schematic overview of Interval Frame Sampling for two-person interaction recognition. Starting with an original interaction video, in step 1, p frames are sampled from p intervals to represent the corresponding interaction sample during the whole learning process. In step 2, q frames are further sampled from the p frames for each epoch's interaction learning

a training instance. This means the frames representing the same interaction sample vary from epoch to epoch, creating a data augmentation effect.

Our frame selection technique offers several advantages. It enables efficient access to information within the p frames, eliminates redundant information through two rounds of interval sampling, shortens processing times by only utilizing q frames per sample during training, and introduces data variation that helps the network focus on learning discriminative partial information. These advantages enhance both efficiency and performance in two-person interaction recognition, which can be valuable for various monitoring applications.

Frame Feature Learning Module

The frame features learning module outputs three types of features: local-region features, frame spatial features, and frame temporal features. This module takes a point cloud set $x_1, x_2, \ldots, x_n$ as input, where each $x_i \in \mathbb{R}^3$ represents the 3-dimensional coordinates of a point within the point cloud frame.

The spatial feature extraction component consists of two levels of set abstraction (SA) [28]. At each abstraction level, a sampling layer performs iterative Farthest Point Sampling (FPS) to select centroids from the input points. A grouping layer then constructs local regions around these centroids using a ball query algorithm, followed by a modified PointNet layer that extracts local spatial features from each region.

In the modified PointNet layer, the coordinates of all points in each local region are transformed into local coordinates relative to the centroid point. The distance between each point and its centroid is included as an additional feature to enhance performance with rotational motions. A Convolutional Block Attention Module (CBAM) [38] is applied to perform inter-feature attention on the point features in the second abstraction level.

At the end of this layer, the feature vectors are combined with the coordinates of the corresponding centroid point, forming local-region features. Subsequently, a Multi-Layer Perceptron (MLP) and Max Pooling operation capture a frame spatial feature for the entire frame, which can be formulated as:

$$FS_t = MAX\{MLP(e_j^t)\} = MAX\{MLP(SA(SA'(PC_t)))\} \tag{5.4}$$

After extracting the frame spatial features, a frame temporal feature extraction structure captures temporal clues using a sinusoidal positional encoding technique [35]. The generated temporal positional feature vectors have the same dimension as the frame spatial features and are summed together. An MLP is then applied to extract frame temporal features:

$$FT_t = MLP(FS_t + TP_t) \tag{5.5}$$

This comprehensive feature extraction process enables our system to effectively recognize interactions between individuals, providing a foundation for monitoring social activities and interpersonal dynamics in various environments.

Multi-level Feature Aggregation

With frame-level features generated, we propose a two-stream module to aggregate them into global and partial representations as illustrated in Fig. 5.9. This approach is particularly effective for recognizing complex interactions in daily living situations.

Two-Stream Feature Aggregation. Both global and partial information are important for interaction recognition. Purely focusing on global information may cause a network to overlook crucial partial details necessary for distinguishing similar interactions. To address this, we propose a two-stream feature aggregation module, comprising a global stream and a partial stream, to jointly capture global and partial information. In the partial stream, a temporal split procedure divides each video into consecutive temporal segments to obtain fine partial clues.

Multi-Level Feature Aggregation. We apply multi-level feature aggregation to simultaneously combine local-region features, frame spatial features, and frame temporal features, providing our network with more discriminative information. Under this two-stream structure, our model processes both the temporal segments and the entire video, merging features into a local-region spatial feature, an appearance feature, and a motion feature. These are concatenated into a single feature that effectively describes appearance and motion patterns jointly.

In total, our model generates one global feature and multiple partial features (corresponding to temporal segments). All these features are combined to form an

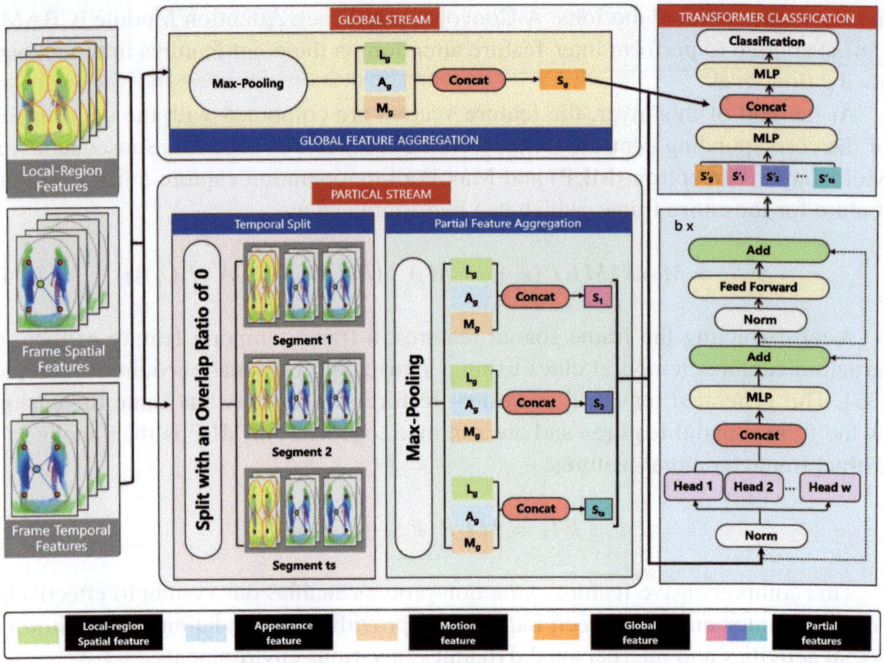

Fig. 5.9 First, a two-stream multi-level feature aggregation module merges frame-level features into global and partial features. Then, a transformer classification module performs self-attention on these aggregated features and uses the output combined with the original global feature for interaction recognition

integrated feature, enabling our network to leverage both global and fine-grained temporal information for accurate two-person interaction recognition.

The global feature S_g represents the whole video and consists of three sub-features: the global aggregated local-region spatial feature, the global appearance feature, and the global motion feature. Each partial feature also consists of three sub-partial aggregated features representing the spatial, appearance, and motion characteristics of each temporal segment. These features are then concatenated to form the integrated feature S that contains both global and partial information.

Transformer Classification

We employ a transformer to perform self-attention on the aggregated global and partial features, enhancing each feature's information by allowing them to learn important relationships from other related features. Consequently, partial features gain a global view, while the global feature captures more fine-grained motion and appearance details. The transformer uses a multi-head structure, transforming each sub-feature into key, value, and query vectors. An attention weights matrix containing relationships between each pair of sub-features is computed, and an updated feature vector is generated through matrix operations. The same calculation is performed in every head in parallel, with the final updated vector formed by concatenating all the resulting vectors.

In addition to the multi-head structure, the transformer incorporates residual connections, LayerNorms, and linear layers. Multiple identical transformer blocks are stacked to capture complex relationships within the data. Following the self-attention process, MLP layers compress the transformed features and combine them with the original global feature to predict the interaction class. This approach enables recognition of complex human interactions in various environments, where understanding relationships between individuals can provide valuable insights into social dynamics and engagement patterns.

Having established the theoretical framework and technical implementation of our TMDPT approach, we now present a comprehensive experimental evaluation to validate its effectiveness for two-person interaction recognition. Our evaluation encompasses performance comparison with state-of-the-art methods and analysis of practical deployment considerations.

5.5.3 Experimental Evaluation and Implementation Results

Datasets and Implementation. We evaluated our approach on two large-scale datasets: NTU RGB+D 60 [30] and NTU RGB+D 120 [15]. NTU RGB+D 60 contains 10,428 interaction video samples across 11 different interaction classes, while NTU RGB+D 120 extends this with additional classes and samples, containing 24,828 interaction video samples across 26 classes. Both datasets provide standard evaluation protocols including cross-subject, cross-view, and cross-setup evaluation settings.

For implementation, we set the Top and Bottom frame rates in IFS to 50 and 24 respectively. We randomly sampled 2048 points from each point cloud frame initially, then further sampled 512 points using FPS. Within the frame features learning module, we selected 128 centroids in the first abstraction level and 32 in the second. For temporal segmentation, we split each video into 6 consecutive segments with 4 frames per segment. Our transformer structure consisted of 5 stacked blocks, each with 18 heads. We trained the network for 90 epochs using Adam optimizer with an initial learning rate of 0.001 that decayed by half every 10 epochs.

This approach enables privacy-preserving monitoring of interactions without requiring wearable devices or capturing privacy-invasive RGB data, with potential applications in smart aging contexts.

Comparison with State-of-the-Art Methods. We compare our network's performance to state-of-the-art methods on two large-scale 3D two-person interaction datasets: the interaction subsets of NTU RGB+D 60 and NTU RGB+D 120. As shown in

Table 5.3 Comparison of recognition accuracy (%) on the two-person interaction subset of NTU RGB+D 60

Methods	Year	Cross-subject	Cross-view
ST-LSTM [17]	2016	83.0	87.3
GCA-LSTM [19]	2017	85.9	89.0
SPDNet [7]	2017	74.9	76.1
2S-GCA-LSTM [18]	2018	87.2	89.9
ST-GCN [40]	2018	83.3	87.1
AS-GCN [12]	2019	89.3	93.0
2S-AGCN [32]	2019	92.4	95.8
FSNET [16]	2020	74.0	80.5
MS-AGCN [33]	2020	94.1	96.7
3DV-PointNet++ [37]	2020	91.0	92.4
LSTM-IRN [25]	2021	90.5	93.5
SB-LSTM [3]	2021	93.9	95.6
GeomNet [24]	2021	93.6	96.3
SequentialPointNet [13]	2021	96.0	98.1
2s-AIGCN [5]	2022	95.3	98.0
3s-EGCN-IIG [9]	2022	**96.6**	98.7
JointContrast [44]	2023	94.1	96.8
TMDPT (Ours)	2023	**96.6**	**99.0**

Tables 5.3 and 5.4, our TMDPT method achieves impressive results, consistently outperforming most other methods across the standard evaluation settings of these challenging datasets.

Performance on NTU RGB+D 60. As Table 5.3 shows, our TMDPT achieves impressive results of 96.6 and 99.0% accuracy under the cross-subject and cross-view evaluation settings, respectively. Both results represent the best performance among all compared methods on this dataset. Notably, we achieve the same cross-subject accuracy as 3s-EGCN-IIG (96.6%) while substantially improving cross-view performance by 0.3% points over the previous best method. This demonstrates that our network is highly robust against subject and view variations for interaction recognition tasks.

Performance on NTU RGB+D 120. The NTU RGB+D 120 dataset presents even greater challenges due to its significantly higher variability in action categories (26 vs. 11 classes), subjects (106 vs. 40), camera views, and environmental setups (32 different configurations). As shown in Table 5.4, TMDPT achieves 92.7% accuracy for cross-subject evaluation, outperforming all competing methods including SequentialPointNet (91.8%) and 3s-EGCN-IIG (92.4%). For cross-setup evaluation, our method achieves 93.3% accuracy, demonstrating strong generalization across diverse environmental configurations.

Table 5.4 Comparison of recognition accuracy (%) on the two-person interaction subset of NTU RGB+D 120

Methods	Year	Cross-subject	Cross-setup
ST-LSTM [17]	2016	63.0	66.6
GCA-LSTM [19]	2017	70.6	73.7
SPDNet [7]	2017	60.7	62.1
2S-GCA-LSTM [18]	2018	73.0	73.3
ST-GCN [40]	2018	78.9	76.1
AS-GCN [12]	2019	82.9	83.7
2S-AGCN [32]	2019	86.1	88.1
FSNET [16]	2020	61.2	69.7
ST-GCN-PAM [41]	2020	83.3	88.4
MS-AGCN [33]	2020	87.7	90.5
3DV-PointNet++ [37]	2020	84.4	84.5
LSTM-IRN [25]	2021	77.7	79.6
SB-LSTM [3]	2021	83.9	83.4
GeomNet [24]	2021	86.5	87.6
SequentialPointNet [13]	2021	91.8	92.2
2s-AIGCN [5]	2022	90.7	90.7
3s-EGCN-IIG [9]	2022	92.4	**95.5**
JointContrast [44]	2023	88.2	88.9
TMDPT (Ours)	2023	**92.7**	93.3

These results demonstrate that our network is robust against subject, view, and environment variations, which is crucial for real-world applications in diverse environments. The effectiveness of our approach stems from its ability to jointly capture both global and partial information through the two-stream structure and to learn important relationships between features through the transformer mechanism.

The success of TMDPT can be attributed to several key design choices: (1) the Interval Frame Sampling technique effectively captures discriminative temporal information while reducing computational requirements, (2) the two-stream multi-level feature aggregation module enables the network to leverage both holistic context and fine-grained partial details, and (3) the transformer classification module learns complex inter-feature relationships through self-attention mechanisms. This robustness is valuable for applications where systems must work reliably across different layouts, lighting conditions, and viewing angles, with particular relevance for smart aging scenarios where monitoring social interactions can provide valuable insights into well-being and care needs.

5.5.4 *Summary of the TMDPT System*

In this study, we focused on developing a privacy-preserving approach to two-person interaction recognition that is particularly relevant for smart aging applications. Our Two-stream Multi-level Dynamic Point Transformer (TMDPT) exclusively uses depth video data, addressing privacy concerns that are especially important in home and care facility environments.

TMDPT integrates four innovative components: a unique Interval Frame Sampling technique that optimizes both accuracy and efficiency, a comprehensive frame features learning module, a two-stream multi-level feature aggregation module that captures both global and partial information, and a transformer-based classification module that learns relationships between features through self-attention.

Our extensive evaluation on large-scale datasets demonstrates the superiority of this approach, achieving state-of-the-art performance while maintaining computational efficiency and robustness to data quality variations. These characteristics make TMDPT particularly suitable for real-world smart aging applications, where systems must function reliably across diverse environments while respecting privacy concerns.

The ability to accurately recognize interactions between elderly individuals and their caregivers or family members provides valuable insights for care assessment, activity monitoring, and social engagement evaluation, all while preserving the privacy and dignity of those being monitored.

5.6 Discussion and Future Directions

5.6.1 *Summary of Technical Contributions*

This chapter has presented three innovative device-free human activity recognition approaches that address fundamental challenges in the field. The RFID-based compressive representation method achieves robust activity recognition using passive tags and dictionary learning, demonstrating 95% accuracy in controlled environments. The AudioGest system leverages Doppler effects to enable multi-modal hand gesture recognition using standard device hardware, achieving 94.15% classification accuracy across diverse real-world conditions. The TMDPT approach addresses privacy-preserving two-person interaction recognition through point cloud-based depth video analysis, outperforming state-of-the-art methods on standard datasets.

These approaches collectively demonstrate significant advances in device-free recognition technology, addressing specific technical challenges including signal uncertainty in RF-based systems, hardware diversity in acoustic-based approaches, and privacy preservation in vision-based methods. The experimental results validate the effectiveness and robustness of these approaches across various deployment scenarios.

5.6.2 Cross-Cutting Technical Challenges

Several key challenges emerge from our work that are relevant to the broader field of device-free activity recognition:

- *Signal Processing and Noise Robustness*: All three approaches address inherent signal uncertainties through different strategies. Our RFID method employs compressive sensing and dictionary learning to handle noisy RSSI signals, AudioGest uses FFT normalization to extract meaningful Doppler shifts from ambient acoustic noise, and TMDPT addresses occlusion issues through multi-level feature aggregation and transformer-based attention mechanisms.
- *Environmental Adaptability*: Real-world deployment requires systems that function across diverse conditions. AudioGest demonstrates robustness in dynamic environments, the RFID system shows insensitivity to tag placement and furniture arrangements, while TMDPT performs consistently across different camera viewpoints and lighting conditions.
- *Privacy Preservation*: Modern activity recognition systems must balance functionality with privacy protection. TMDPT exclusively uses depth data rather than RGB images, AudioGest employs acoustic signals that cannot decode personal conversations, and the RFID method avoids direct bodily monitoring through passive environmental sensing.

5.6.3 Applications and Future Directions

The unobtrusive nature of these systems makes them suitable for continuous monitoring applications where traditional wearable or camera-based approaches may be impractical or raise privacy concerns. The multi-modal capabilities demonstrated by AudioGest enable fine-grained interaction possibilities, while the privacy-preserving nature of TMDPT's depth-based approach addresses concerns about monitoring in sensitive environments.

Future research should focus on multi-modal integration, combining information from different sensing modalities to create more robust recognition systems. Additionally, developing systems capable of adapting to individual user characteristics and environmental changes over time represents an important direction for practical deployment.

5.6.4 Conclusion

Device-free human activity recognition continues to evolve towards more robust, privacy-preserving, and environmentally adaptive approaches. The three methods presented in this chapter contribute to this evolution by addressing fundamental technical challenges and demonstrating practical capabilities across diverse scenarios. Through continued innovation and empirical validation, device-free activity recognition can contribute to creating more intelligent and adaptive environments for various applications, including smart aging scenarios.

References

1. Abdelnasser, H., Youssef, M., Harras, K.A.: Wigest: a ubiquitous wifi-based gesture recognition system. In: 2015 IEEE Conference on Computer Communications (INFOCOM Kowloon, Hong Kong), pp. 1472–1480. IEEE (2015)
2. Brezmes, T., Gorricho, J., Cotrina, J.: Activity recognition from accelerometer data on a mobile phone. In: Distributed Computing, Artificial Intelligence, Bioinformatics, Soft Computing, and Ambient Assisted Living (IWANN 2009), Part II. Lecture Notes in Computer Science, vol. 5518, pp. 796–799. Springer, Berlin (2009)
3. Chiu, S., Wu, K., Tseng, Y.: Two-person mutual action recognition using joint dynamics and coordinate transformation. In: Proceedings of the 1st International Conference on AI for People: Towards Sustainable AI, CAIP 2021, p. 56. European Alliance for Innovation (2021)
4. Fan, H., Xiong, B., Mangalam, K., Li, Y., Yan, Z., Malik, J., Feichtenhofer, C.: Multiscale vision transformers. In: Proceedings of the 2021 IEEE/CVF International Conference on Computer Vision, ICCV 2021, pp. 6804–6815. IEEE (2021)
5. Gao, F., Xia, H., Tang, Z.: Attention interactive graph convolutional network for skeleton-based human interaction recognition. In: Proceedings of the IEEE International Conference on Multimedia and Expo, ICME 2022, pp. 1–6. IEEE (2022)
6. Gupta, S., Morris, D., Patel, S.N., Tan, D.S.: Soundwave: using the doppler effect to sense gestures. In: CHI Conference on Human Factors in Computing Systems (CHI 2012), pp. 1911–1914. ACM, Austin, TX, USA (2012)
7. Huang, Z., Gool, L.V.: A riemannian network for spd matrix learning. In: Singh, S., Markovitch, S. (eds.) Proceedings of the 31st AAAI Conference on Artificial Intelligence, pp. 2036–2042. AAAI Press (2017)
8. Hussain, Z., Sheng, Q.Z., Zhang, W.E.: A review and categorization of techniques on device-free human activity recognition. J. Netw. Comput. Appl. **167**, 102738 (2020)
9. Ito, Y., Kong, Q., Morita, K., Yoshinaga, T.: Efficient and accurate skeleton-based two-person interaction recognition using inter-and intra-body graphs. In: Proceedings of the 2022 IEEE International Conference on Image Processing, pp. 231–235. IEEE (2022)
10. Kellogg, B., Talla, V., Gollakota, S.: Bringing gesture recognition to all devices. In: 11th USENIX Symposium on Networked Systems Design and Implementation (NSDI 2014), pp. 303–316. USENIX Association, Seattle, WA, USA (2014)
11. Kim, E., Helal, S., Cook, D.J.: Human activity recognition and pattern discovery. IEEE Pervasive Comput. **9**(1), 48–53 (2010)
12. Li, M., Chen, S., Chen, X., Zhang, Y., Wang, Y., Tian, Q.: Actional-structural graph convolutional networks for skeleton-based action recognition. In: Proceedings of the IEEE Conference on Computer Vision and Pattern Recognition, pp. 3595–3603. Computer Vision Foundation/IEEE (2019)
13. Li, X., Huang, Q., Wang, Z., Hou, Z., Yang, T.: Sequentialpointnet: a strong parallelized point cloud sequence network for 3d action recognition (2021). arXiv:2111.08492
14. Liu, B., Cai, H., Ju, Z., Liu, H.: Rgb-d sensing based human action and interaction analysis: a survey. Pattern Recogn. **94**, 1–12 (2019)
15. Liu, J., Shahroudy, A., Perez, M., Wang, G., Duan, L., Kot, A.C.: Ntu rgb+d 120: a large-scale benchmark for 3d human activity understanding. IEEE Trans. Pattern Anal. Mach. Intell. **42**(10), 2684–2701 (2020)

16. Liu, J., Shahroudy, A., Wang, G., Duan, L., Kot, A.C.: Skeleton-based online action prediction using scale selection network. IEEE Trans. Pattern Anal. Mach. Intell. **42**(6), 1453–1467 (2020)
17. Liu, J., Shahroudy, A., Xu, D., Wang, G.: Spatio-temporal lstm with trust gates for 3d human action recognition. In: Leibe, B., Matas, J., Sebe, N., Welling, M. (eds.) Proceedings of the 14th European Conference on Computer Vision, ECCV 2016. Lecture Notes in Computer Science, vol. 9907, pp. 816–833. Springer, Berlin (2016)
18. Liu, J., Wang, G., Duan, L., Abdiyeva, K., Kot, A.C.: Skeleton-based human action recognition with global context-aware attention lstm networks. IEEE Trans. Image Process. **27**(4), 1586–1599 (2018)
19. Liu, J., Wang, G., Hu, P., Duan, L., Kot, A.C.: Global context-aware attention lstm networks for 3d action recognition. In: Proceedings of the 2017 IEEE Conference on Computer Vision and Pattern Recognition, pp. 3671–3680. IEEE Computer Society (2017)
20. Melgarejo, P., Zhang, X., Ramanathan, P., Chu, D.: Leveraging directional antenna capabilities for fine-grained gesture recognition. In: Proceedings of the 2014 ACM International Joint Conference on Pervasive and Ubiquitous Computing (UbiComp 2014), pp. 541–551. ACM, Seattle, WA, USA (2014)
21. Mennicken, S., Vermeulen, J., Huang, E.M.: From today's augmented houses to tomorrow's smart homes: new directions for home automation research. In: Proceedings of the 2014 ACM International Joint Conference on Pervasive and Ubiquitous Computing (UbiComp '14), pp. 105–115. ACM (2014)
22. Molchanov, P., Gupta, S., Kim, K., Pulli, K.: Multi-sensor system for driver's hand-gesture recognition. In: Proceedings of the 11th IEEE International Conference and Workshops on Automatic Face and Gesture Recognition (FG 2015), pp. 1–8. IEEE (2015)
23. Molchanov, P., Gupta, S., Kim, K., Pulli, K.: Short-range fmcw monopulse radar for hand-gesture sensing. In: Proceedings of the 2015 IEEE Radar Conference (RadarCon 2015), pp. 1491–1496. IEEE (2015)
24. Nguyen, X.S.: Geomnet: a neural network based on riemannian geometries of spd matrix space and cholesky space for 3d skeleton-based interaction recognition. In: Proceedings of the 2021 IEEE/CVF International Conference on Computer Vision, pp. 13359–13369. IEEE (2021)
25. Perez, M., Liu, J., Kot, A.C.: Interaction relational network for mutual action recognition. IEEE Trans. Multimedia **24**, 366–376 (2022)
26. Pu, Q., Gupta, S., Gollakota, S., Patel, S.N.: Whole-home gesture recognition using wireless signals. In: Proceedings of the 19th Annual International Conference on Mobile Computing and Networking (MobiCom '13), pp. 27–38. ACM (2013)
27. Pu, Q., Gupta, S., Gollakota, S., Patel, S.N.: Whole-home gesture recognition using wireless signals. In: 19th Annual International Conference on Mobile Computing and Networking (MobiCom 2013), pp. 27–38. ACM, Miami, FL, USA (2013)
28. Qi, C.R., Yi, L., Su, H., Guibas, L.J.: Pointnet++: Deep hierarchical feature learning on point sets in a metric space. In: Advances in Neural Information Processing Systems 30 (NeurIPS 2017), pp. 5099–5108 (2017)
29. Ruan, W., Yang, L., Sheng, Q.Z., Gu, T., Xu, P., Shangguan, L.: Making sense of doppler effect for multi-modal hand motion detection. IEEE Trans. Mob. Comput. **17**(9), 2087–2100 (2018)
30. Shahroudy, A., Liu, J., Ng, T., Wang, G.: Ntu rgb+d: a large scale dataset for 3d human activity analysis. In: Proceedings of the 2016 IEEE Conference on Computer Vision and Pattern Recognition, pp. 1010–1019. IEEE Computer Society (2016)
31. Sheng, Q.Z., Li, X., Zeadally, S.: Enabling next-generation RFID applications: solutions and challenges. Computer **41**(9), 21–28 (2008)
32. Shi, L., Zhang, Y., Cheng, J., Lu, H.: Two-stream adaptive graph convolutional networks for skeleton-based action recognition. In: Proceedings of the IEEE Conference on Computer Vision and Pattern Recognition, pp. 12026–12035. Computer Vision Foundation/IEEE (2019)
33. Shi, L., Zhang, Y., Cheng, J., Lu, H.: Skeleton-based action recognition with multi-stream adaptive graph convolutional networks. IEEE Trans. Image Process. **29**, 9532–9545 (2020)
34. Tang, Y., Liu, X., Yu, X., Zhang, D., Lu, J., Zhou, J.: Learning from temporal spatial cubism for cross-dataset skeleton-based action recognition. ACM Trans. Multimedia Comput. Commun. Appl. **18**(2), 46:1–46:24 (2022)

35. Vaswani, A., Shazeer, N., Parmar, N., Uszkoreit, J., Jones, L., Gomez, A.N., Kaiser, L., Polosukhin, I.: Attention is all you need. In: Advances in Neural Information Processing Systems 30 (NeurIPS 2017), pp. 5998–6008 (2017)
36. Wang, L., Gu, T., Xie, H., Tao, X., Lu, J., Huang, Y.: a wearable rfid system for real-time activity recognition using radio patterns. In: Mobile and Ubiquitous Systems (MobiQuitous 2013), pp. 370–383. ACM (2013)
37. Wang, Y., Xiao, Y., Xiong, F., Jiang, W., Cao, Z., Zhou, J.T., Yuan, J.: 3dv: 3d dynamic voxel for action recognition in depth video. In: Proceedings of the 2020 IEEE/CVF Conference on Computer Vision and Pattern Recognition, pp. 508–517. Computer Vision Foundation/IEEE (2020)
38. Woo, S., Park, J., Lee, J., Kweon, I.S.: Cbam: convolutional block attention module. In: Ferrari, V., Hebert, M., Sminchisescu, C., Weiss, Y. (eds.) Proceedings of the 15th European Conference on Computer Vision, ECCV 2018. Lecture Notes in Computer Science, vol. 11211, pp. 3–19. Springer , Berlin (2018)
39. Xu, C., Liu, R., Zhang, T., Cui, Z., Yang, J., Hu, C.: Dual-stream structured graph convolution network for skeleton-based action recognition. ACM Trans. Multimedia Comput. Commun. Appl. **17**(4), 120:1–120:22 (2021)
40. Yan, S., Xiong, Y., Lin, D.: Spatial temporal graph convolutional networks for skeleton-based action recognition. In: McIlraith, S.A., Weinberger, K.Q. (eds.) Proceedings of the 32nd AAAI Conference on Artificial Intelligence, AAAI-18, pp. 7444–7452. AAAI Press (2018)
41. Yang, C., Setyoko, A., Tampubolon, H., Hua, K.: Pairwise adjacency matrix on spatial temporal graph convolution network for skeleton-based two-person interaction recognition. In: Proceedings of the IEEE International Conference on Image Processing, pp. 2166–2170. IEEE (2020)
42. Yao, L., Sheng, Q.Z., Li, X., Gu, T., Tan, M., Wang, X., Wang, S., Ruan, W.: Compressive representation for device-free activity recognition with passive rfid signal strength. IEEE Trans. Mob. Comput. **17**(2), 293–306 (2018)
43. Zhang, D., Zhou, J., Guo, M., Cao, J., Li, T.: TASA: tag-free activity sensing using rfid tag arrays. IEEE Trans. Parallel Distrib. Syst. **22**(4), 558–570 (2011)
44. Zhang, J., Jia, X., Wang, Z., Luo, Y., Chen, F., Yang, G., Zhao, L.: Jointcontrast: skeleton-based interaction recognition with new representation and contrastive learning. Algorithms **16**(4), 190 (2023)
45. Zhao, C., Chen, K.Y., Aumi, M.T.I., Patel, S.N., Reynolds, M.S.: Sideswipe: detecting in-air gestures around mobile devices using actual gsm signal. In: Proceedings of the ACM Symposium on User Interface Software and Technology (UIST 2014), pp. 527–534. ACM (2014)

Part II
Wearable Sensing for Activity Recognition

This part explores advanced wearable sensing technologies that enable continuous monitoring and recognition of both physical and cognitive activities in smart aging environments. Unlike the device-free approaches in Part I, these technologies leverage sensorsworn by individuals to capture detailed physiological and behavioral information while addressing fundamental challenges in real-world deployment.

Chapter 6 focuses on physical activity recognition through wearable sensors, presenting three methodological innovations to overcome critical limitations: insufficient labeled training data, distribution shifts across different users, and intelligent sensor selection in multi-modal environments. The chapter introduces robust semi-supervised learning frameworks, distributionally robust approaches for cross-user adaptation, and multi-agent attention mechanisms for optimal sensor fusion. These methods achieve remarkable performance improvements while maintaining computational efficiency suitable for real-time deployment on resource-constrained devices.

Chapter 7 advances into cognitive activity recognition, representing a critical frontier in understanding brain-computer interactions for smart aging applications. The chapter presents three complementary approaches: EEG-based intention recognition using novel spatio-temporal neural networks, adversarial variational embedding for semi-supervised learning with limited labeled data, and self-supervised cross-modal learning for visual retrieval from brain activities. These technologies enable direct communication between cognitive states and external devices, opening newpossibilities for assistive technologies and personalized healthcare.

Together, these chapters establish comprehensive wearable sensing capabilities that complement the environmental intelligence from Part I. The combination of robust physical activity recognition and advanced cognitive monitoring provides the foundation for intelligent systems that can understand both behavioral patterns and mental states, which is essential for supporting independent living and early detection of health changes in aging populations.

Chapter 6
Wearable Sensor-Based Physical Activity Recognition

6.1 Introduction

6.1.1 Overview of Wearable Sensor-Based Activity Recognition

Human activity recognition through wearable sensors has emerged as a cornerstone technology for smart aging applications, enabling continuous health monitoring, fall detection, and behavior analysis that support independent living. With the proliferation of Internet of Things (IoT) devices and advances in sensor miniaturization, wearable sensing systems offer unprecedented opportunities for understanding human activities in real-world environments.

The ability to automatically recognize physical activities from sensor data collected by smartphones, smartwatches, and other wearable devices holds immense potential for eldercare applications [21]. These systems can monitor daily routines, detect anomalies in behavior patterns, track rehabilitation progress, and provide timely assistance when needed. However, developing robust and accurate activity recognition systems faces several fundamental challenges that must be addressed to realize this potential.

In this chapter, we present three complementary approaches that tackle the most pressing challenges in wearable sensor-based activity recognition. Our work addresses the critical issues of limited labeled training data, distribution shifts across different users, and intelligent sensor selection in multi-modal environments. These challenges are particularly relevant in the context of smart aging, where personalized and adaptive systems are essential for accommodating the diverse needs and capabilities of older adults.

Q. Z. Sheng et al., *Harnessing Artificial Intelligence and Pervasive Internet of Things for an Empowered Aging*, https://doi.org/10.1007/978-3-032-16502-2_6

6.1.2 Challenges and Opportunities

Despite significant advances in sensor technologies and machine learning, several fundamental challenges continue to limit the effectiveness of wearable activity recognition systems:

- *Insufficient Labeled Data*: One of the most significant barriers to deploying activity recognition systems is the scarcity of properly labeled training data. Obtaining ground-truth activity labels is tedious, time-consuming, and error-prone, especially when working with older adults who may have cognitive limitations or difficulty in providing consistent annotations. This challenge is compounded by the need for personalized models that can adapt to individual behavior patterns and physical capabilities.
- *Intra-class Variability*: The same activity may be performed differently by different individuals, or even by the same individual under different conditions. Factors such as age, physical condition, fatigue, and environmental context can significantly affect how activities are performed. This variability is particularly pronounced in aging populations, where mobility limitations and health conditions can alter typical movement patterns.
- *Distribution Shift Across Users*: Human-generated sensor data inherently suffer from distribution shifts due to diverse biological conditions, behavior patterns, and sensor placement variations. When training data from one set of users is applied to different users, the performance often degrades significantly due to person-specific differences in movement patterns, sensor positioning, and physiological characteristics.
- *Multi-modal Sensor Fusion*: Modern wearable devices incorporate multiple sensors (accelerometers, gyroscopes, magnetometers) across different body positions. However, not all sensor modalities are equally informative for recognizing specific activities, and their relative importance varies both spatially and temporally. Effectively selecting and combining information from multiple sensors remains a complex challenge.

These challenges present significant opportunities for advancing the field through innovative machine learning approaches that can handle uncertainty, adapt to individual differences, and intelligently process multi-modal sensor data.

6.1.3 Contributions

This chapter presents three novel methodological contributions that address the fundamental challenges in wearable sensor-based activity recognition for smart aging applications:

First, we propose a robust semi-supervised activity recognition approach that extracts intrinsic shared structures from activities to handle intra-class variability while utilizing both labeled and unlabeled data. Our Robust Semi-supervised Activity Recognition (RSAR) method uses $\ell_{2,1}$ minimization to effectively resist outliers in noisy sensor data and improve recognition accuracy by discerning underlying commonalities from activities. The approach integrates shared structure discovery with graph-based manifold regularization, enabling effective learning even when labeled training data is scarce.

Second, we develop a distributionally robust semi-supervised learning model that addresses distribution shifts between labeled and unlabeled data in people-centric sensing applications. Our method reduces person-specific discrepancy while preserving task-specific consistency, enabling effective knowledge transfer across different users. The approach recognizes that distribution shifts in human activity data can be decomposed into person-specific variations that should be minimized and task-specific patterns that should be preserved across different user populations.

Third, we introduce a multi-agent spatial-temporal attention model that considers the spatially-temporally varying salience of sensor features and the relationships between activities and corresponding body part motions. The multi-agent framework treats activity recognition as a collaborative decision-making problem, deploying multiple intelligent agents that independently select informative sensor modalities while sharing information to coordinate their selection policies for optimal recognition strategies. The model provides explainable insights through attention visualization that enhance system interpretability for practical deployments.

6.1.4 Chapter Organization

The remainder of this chapter is organized as follows: Sect. 6.2 reviews key research in wearable sensor-based activity recognition, semi-supervised learning, and attention mechanisms, establishing the theoretical foundations and current approaches in these fields. Section 6.3 presents our semi-supervised learning framework with shared structure discovery for handling insufficient labeled data, addressing the fundamental challenge of limited annotations in wearable activity recognition systems. Section 6.4 introduces the distributionally robust learning approach for managing distribution shifts across different users, enabling effective knowledge transfer in people-centric sensing applications. Section 6.5 describes the multi-agent attention method for intelligent sensor selection in multi-modal environments, providing advanced solutions for complex activity recognition scenarios. Finally, Sect. 6.6 explores broader implications of these technologies for smart aging applications, including implementation challenges, methodological synergies, and future research directions.

6.2 Background and Related Work

6.2.1 *Wearable Sensor-Based Activity Recognition*

Wearable sensor-based activity recognition has evolved significantly with advances in sensor technologies and machine learning techniques. Early approaches relied on handcrafted features extracted from accelerometer and gyroscope data, using traditional machine learning methods such as decision trees, support vector machines, and naive Bayes classifiers [3, 18, 20, 22, 25, 29].

The proliferation of smartphones and wearable devices has enabled the collection of rich multi-modal sensor data, including acceleration, angular velocity, and magnetic field measurements from multiple body positions. This has led to more sophisticated recognition systems that can handle complex activities and adapt to individual differences [11, 22].

Recent advances in deep learning have further transformed the field, enabling end-to-end learning from raw sensor data without the need for manual feature engineering [15, 23]. However, these approaches often require large amounts of labeled training data, which remains a significant challenge in practical deployments.

6.2.2 *Semi-Supervised Learning for Activity Recognition*

Semi-supervised learning has emerged as a promising approach to address the challenge of limited labeled data in activity recognition. These methods leverage both labeled and unlabeled data to improve recognition performance while reducing annotation requirements.

Graph-based semi-supervised learning methods construct similarity graphs connecting labeled and unlabeled samples, then propagate labels based on manifold assumptions [28, 35]. Other approaches include co-training methods that use multiple classifiers trained on different feature sets [27], and sparse coding frameworks that exploit unlabeled data to handle annotation burden [5].

However, most existing semi-supervised approaches assume that labeled and unlabeled data follow the same distribution, which is often violated in real-world scenarios due to person-specific differences and changing environmental conditions.

6.2.3 *Attention Mechanisms in Sensor Data Analysis*

Attention mechanisms have gained significant attention in various domains for their ability to focus on relevant information while suppressing irrelevant details. In the context of sensor-based activity recognition, attention mechanisms can help identify which sensors, time periods, or spatial locations are most informative for recognizing specific activities.

Recent work has explored spatial attention for selecting relevant sensor modalities [8, 34] and temporal attention for identifying important time segments. However, most existing approaches treat attention as a post-processing step rather than integrating it into a unified learning framework that considers the collaborative nature of multi-modal sensing.

6.2.4 Distribution Shift and Domain Adaptation

Distribution shift represents a fundamental challenge in real-world deployments of activity recognition systems. When training data from one set of users is applied to different users, performance often degrades significantly due to person-specific differences in movement patterns, sensor positioning, and physiological characteristics.

Domain adaptation techniques have been developed to address this challenge, including adversarial training methods that learn domain-invariant features [12], and cycle-consistent approaches that maintain task-relevant information while reducing domain-specific variations [16]. However, most existing methods do not specifically address the unique characteristics of people-centric sensing data.

6.2.5 Research Gaps and Opportunities in Smart Aging

While significant progress has been made in activity recognition, several gaps remain particularly relevant to smart aging applications:

- *Personalization and Adaptation*: Existing systems often assume a one-size-fits-all approach, but aging populations exhibit significant heterogeneity in physical capabilities, cognitive function, and technology adoption. Developing personalized models that can adapt to individual needs while maintaining robustness remains an open challenge.
- *Long-term Deployment*: Most research focuses on controlled experimental settings with limited duration. Long-term deployment in real-world environments introduces challenges related to sensor drift, changing user behavior, and system maintenance that require novel approaches for continuous adaptation and self-calibration.
- *Multi-user Environments*: Smart aging applications often involve multiple occupants or caregivers in the same environment. Developing systems that can distinguish between different users and handle complex social interactions while preserving privacy represents an important research direction.

These gaps motivate our work on developing more robust, adaptive, and intelligent activity recognition systems that can better serve the needs of aging populations.

6.3 Semi-supervised Learning with Shared Structure Discovery

6.3.1 Motivation

The scarcity of labeled training data represents one of the most significant barriers to deploying robust activity recognition systems in real-world environments. This challenge is particularly acute in smart aging applications, where obtaining ground-truth activity labels from older adults can be challenging due to cognitive limitations, privacy concerns, or the difficulty of continuous annotation over extended periods.

Traditional supervised learning approaches require substantial amounts of labeled data to achieve good performance, but acquiring such data is tedious, time-consuming, and often impractical. This is especially problematic when dealing with intra-class variability, where the same activity may be performed differently by different individuals or even by the same individual under varying conditions. For example, walking patterns can vary significantly based on factors such as age, physical condition, fatigue level, or emotional state.

Our motivation stems from two key observations: (1) there exists underlying commonalities or shared structures across different variations of the same activity that can be leveraged to improve recognition robustness, and (2) large amounts of unlabeled sensor data are typically available and can be utilized to enhance learning when properly integrated with limited labeled samples.

We propose a novel approach that integrates shared structure analysis into a semi-supervised learning framework [31]. Our method aims to extract intrinsic shared structures from activities to handle intra-class variability while simultaneously utilizing correlations from both labeled and easily-obtained unlabeled data. By using $\ell_{2,1}$ minimization on both loss function and regularizations, our approach effectively resists outliers in noisy sensor data and improves recognition accuracy by discerning underlying commonalities from activities.

6.3.2 RSAR: A Semi-supervised Framework with Shared Structure Discovery

In this section, we present the core methodology of our Robust Semi-supervised Activity Recognition (RSAR) framework that integrates shared structure discovery with graph-based semi-supervised learning to address both intra-class variability and limited labeled data challenges in wearable sensing.

Figure 6.1 illustrates the main workflow of our proposed framework. Our approach consists of three main components: (1) shared structure learning to capture common patterns across activities, (2) semi-supervised manifold learning to leverage unlabeled data, and (3) a unified optimization framework combining both techniques. First, we segment raw sensing data using a sliding window technique and extract

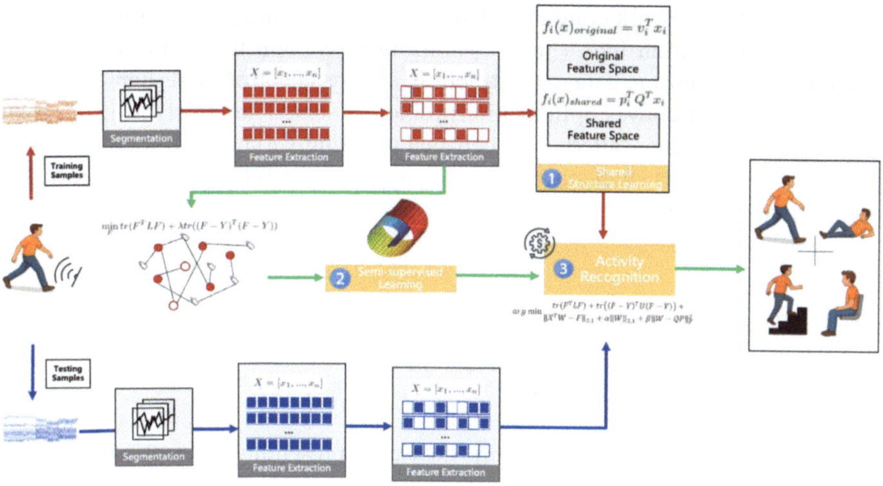

Fig. 6.1 The workflow of our proposed human activity recognition model (3), which is combined with (1) shared structure learning and (2) graph-based semi-supervised learning framework

features from each segment using Canonical Correlation Analysis (CCA) [17] based forward searching. The model then develops $\ell_{2,1}$ based shared structured learning [1] to decode underlying commonalities among features, constructs an adjacency graph using cosine similarity for label propagation via manifold learning [35], and combines both components into a joint optimization framework where model parameters are learned iteratively during training.

Shared Structure Learning. We model activity recognition as learning discriminant functions $f_j(x_i)$ for each activity class $j \in [1, c]$ from feature vectors $x_i \in \mathbb{R}^d$. Our key insight is that activities share underlying structural patterns that can be captured through a shared subspace representation. We formulate each prediction function as $f_j(x_i) = w_j^\top x_i$ where $w_j = v_j + Qp_j$, combining class-specific weights v_j with shared structure weights p_j projected through transformation matrix $Q \in \mathbb{R}^{d \times sd}$.

The shared structure learning objective combines data fitting loss with regularization terms to achieve robustness and feature selection. We employ $\ell_{2,1}$ norms for robustness against sensor noise and outliers commonly present in wearable sensing data. The $\ell_{2,1}$ norm based loss function is robust to outliers while the regularization enables feature selection with joint sparsity.

Semi-supervised Learning Integration. To leverage both labeled and unlabeled data, we incorporate graph-based semi-supervised learning that constructs a similarity graph connecting data points and propagates labels through manifold regularization. The semi-supervised component uses graph Laplacian regularization and label fitting terms, where the graph Laplacian is constructed using cosine similarity with k-nearest neighbors, and a diagonal selection matrix distinguishes labeled from unlabeled samples.

The unified framework combines shared structure learning with semi-supervised manifold regularization into a joint optimization problem that balances manifold smoothness, label fitting, data reconstruction, feature selection, and shared structure discovery. This non-convex optimization problem is solved iteratively using standard optimization techniques, alternating between updating variables until convergence. The solution leverages efficient matrix operations to ensure computational feasibility for real-time applications.

6.3.3 Experimental Validation and Performance Analysis

Experimental Setup and Datasets

We evaluate our approach on four public datasets representing diverse sensor modalities and user populations:

- **USC-HAD** [33]: The dataset is collected in an open environment with 14 participants (7 males, 7 females) with diversity in age, height, and weight. Each participant performs 12 activities including walking forward, walking left, walking right, walking upstairs, going downstairs, jumping up, running, standing, sitting, sleeping, elevator up, and elevator down.
- **Actitracker** [19]: The dataset is collected with 29 subjects performing six activities. All subjects carry Android smartphones in their front pant pockets and perform walk, jog, ascend stairs, descend stairs, sit, and stand for a period of time.
- **UCI HAR** [2]: A group of 30 volunteers with ages ranging from 19 to 48 years old are selected. Each person wears a waist-mounted Samsung Galaxy S II smartphone and performs six activities: standing, sitting, lying down, walking, walking downstairs and walking upstairs.
- **Freedom RFID** [32]: The data includes 12 activities performed by 6 subjects. Each subject stands between RFID signal receiver and transmitter, and the corresponding signal streaming variations are recorded while performing different activities.

Feature Extraction and Validation. For fair comparison, we extract the same types of lightweight statistical features from these four datasets. We divide the continuous sensor data stream into fixed-length segments using a sliding window of $\Delta t = 10$ seconds, which is long enough to be discriminative yet short enough for accurate labeling. From each segment, we extract 12 lightweight statistical features that are widely used in the activity recognition community, as listed in Table 6.1. All features are normalized by standard deviation to account for different scales and units.

We employ person-independent cross-validation, where data from the first to the $(n-1)$th subjects serve as training examples, and data from the left-out nth subject are used for testing. This process iterates for every subject over each dataset, and the final result is the averaged value over all subjects.

Table 6.1 Lightweight statistical features extracted from sensor data

No.	Feature	Description
1	Min	Minimum of signal over the segment
2	Max	Maximum of signal over the segment
3	Mean	Average value of signal over the segment
4	Root Mean Square	Quadratic mean value of signal over the segment
5	Variance	Square of standard deviation
6	Standard Deviation	Mean deviation of the signal compared to the average
7	Kurtosis	Degree of peakedness of the sensor signal distribution
8	Skewness	Degree of asymmetry of the sensor signal distribution
9	Entropy	Measure of the distribution of frequency components
10	Median	Median signal value
11	Zero Crossing Rate	Total number of times the signal changes from positive to negative or back, normalized by the segment length
12	Mean Cross Rate	Total number of times the signal changes from below average to above average, normalized by the segment length

Our method (RSAR) demonstrates superior performance across all datasets compared to supervised baselines (k-NN, SVM, Random Forest, Naive Bayes) and semi-supervised approaches (LapSVM, TSVM, Co-training). Key findings include: (1) consistent improvement over baselines, particularly when labeled data is scarce (2–5 labeled samples per activity), achieving 71.34% accuracy on the Actitracker dataset with minimal training data; (2) robustness to parameter variations, with shared subspace dimension $sd = 5$ and regularization parameters $\alpha = 0.1$, $\beta = 1$ providing optimal performance; and (3) computational efficiency suitable for real-time deployment.

The results validate our hypothesis that shared structure discovery combined with semi-supervised learning effectively addresses both intra-class variability and limited annotation challenges in wearable activity recognition. The $\ell_{2,1}$ norm formulation proves particularly effective for handling sensor noise and outliers common in real-world deployments.

Baseline Methods and Comparative Analysis

To evaluate the performance of our proposed RSAR approach, we conduct extensive experiments comparing with state-of-the-art supervised and semi-supervised methods. We use settings $\alpha = 0.1$, $\beta = 1$, $k = 5$, $sd = 5$ and $\mu = 0.001$ for our method. The training dataset contains both labeled and unlabeled data, while the testing dataset is not available during training. We randomly select m labeled samples ($m = 1, 2, 3, 4, 5, 8, 10, 12, 15$) per activity in the training dataset, resulting in $m \times c$ labeled sensor samples where c is the number of activities per subject in each dataset.

Supervised Baseline Methods:

- ***k*-Nearest Neighbor (*k*NN)**: A common classifier that predicts the class of a sample by majority voting of the class labels of the k nearest training instances. We set $k = 3$ in this work.
- **Linear Support Vector Machine (LSVM)**: Aims at finding the best separation of binary-labeled instances by determining a hyperplane which maximizes the margin between support vectors of different classes. We set $C = 1$ with linear kernel.
- **Random Forest (RF)**: Builds a forest of decision trees with the same distribution but independent output classes, based on random feature selection for each tree. The number of trees is set to 500.
- **Naive Bayes (NB)**: Finds the most posterior probability for a given testing sample based on Bayes' theorem. We model the conditional probability using Gaussian mixture distribution, with the number of Gaussian clusters adaptively determined via Dirichlet Process Gaussian Mixture Model (DPGMM) [6].

Semi-supervised Baseline Methods:

- **Co-training** [7, 27]: Uses two classifier strategies (logistic regression and naive Bayes) trained on different feature subsets (features 1–6 and features 7–12). Each classifier predicts labels for unlabeled data with confidence scores, and high-confidence predictions are iteratively added to the labeled training set to augment both classifiers.
- **GLSVM** [28]: A graph-based semi-supervised framework that constructs similarity graphs to estimate data structure using both labeled and unlabeled data. Labels are propagated on this graph via manifold learning, then both initial labeled data and propagated labels are used to train an SVM classifier.

Comparative Results. Figure 6.2 shows the recognition results on the four datasets with respect to different numbers of labeled training samples. Our method consistently achieves superior performance compared to all baseline methods, particularly when labeled data is scarce. When only one labeled training sample from each activity is used, our method achieves 71.34% accuracy on the Actitracker dataset, significantly outperforming other approaches. The recognition accuracy of most methods improves as the amount of labeled training samples increases, but our algorithm maintains robust performance by learning correlations between features through shared structure analysis.

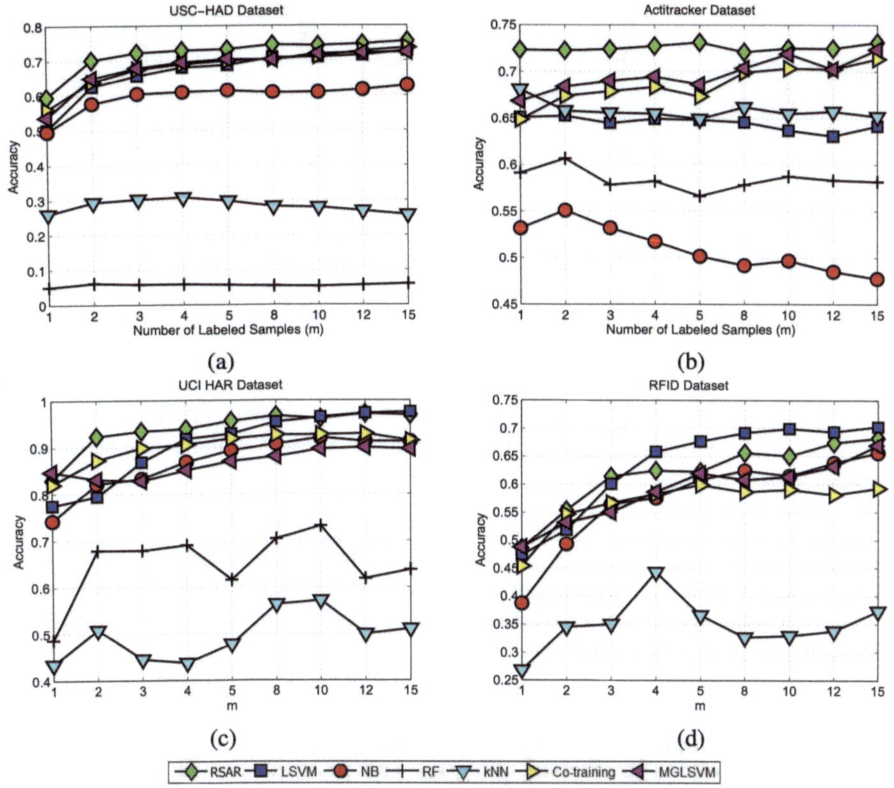

Fig. 6.2 Overall recognition performance comparison using **a** the USC-HAD dataset, **b** the Actitracker dataset, **c** the UCI HAR dataset, and **d** the RFID dataset. Our RSAR approach consistently outperforms baseline methods, especially with limited labeled training data

Parameter Study and Sensitivity Analysis

To understand the impact of key parameters on recognition performance, we conduct comprehensive parameter studies using the Actitracker dataset. Figure 6.3 presents three important analyses.

Shared Subspace Dimension. Figure 6.3a shows performance variations with different dimensions of shared subspace (sd) from 1 to 10, across different numbers of labeled training samples. We observe that recognition accuracy consistently decreases with larger shared subspace dimensions. While a bigger shared subspace may capture more discriminant information, it can also cause over-fitting problems leading to performance deterioration. Based on these results, we set $sd = 5$ as the default value, which provides a good balance between capturing shared structure and avoiding over-fitting.

Regularization Parameters. Figure 6.3b illustrates performance variations with different combinations of α and β tuned on sets $\{10^i | i = -3, -2, -1, 0, 1, 2, 3\}$. The performance is not quite sensitive to β variations but is more affected by α. The opti-

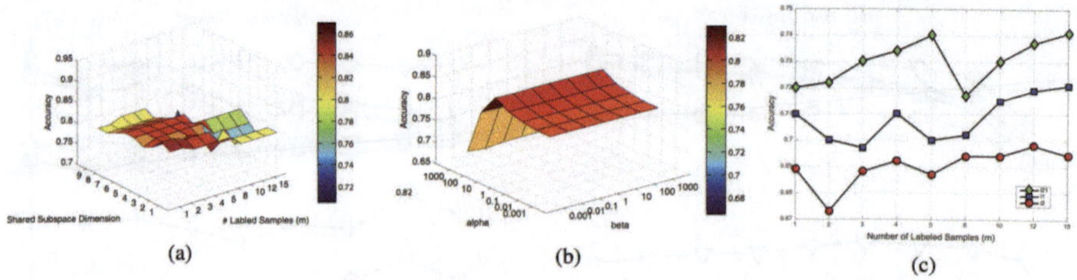

Fig. 6.3 Performance variations with **a** different dimension (sd) of shared subspace and different number of labeled training samples (m); **b** different α and β parameters; **c** comparison of different minimization norms for shared structure analysis over Actitracker dataset

mal combination is $\alpha = 0.1$ and $\beta = 1$ for the Actitracker dataset. We also explore the effects of μ and k, finding that both parameters show relatively low sensitivity to variations.

Norm Comparison. Figure 6.3c compares $\ell_{2,1}$ minimization with ℓ_2 and ℓ_1 norms on shared structure analysis. The $\ell_{2,1}$ minimization consistently outperforms the other methods across different amounts of labeled training data, confirming its effectiveness for handling sensor noise and outliers while performing feature selection with joint sparsity.

Performance Results and Activity-Specific Analysis

Our experimental evaluation demonstrates the effectiveness of the RSAR framework across multiple datasets and scenarios. The method consistently achieves superior performance compared to baseline approaches, particularly in scenarios with limited labeled training data. The results indicate that our approach effectively leverages both labeled and unlabeled data during training, enabling it to outperform supervised learning methods when only small amounts of labeled data are available.

Activity-Specific Recognition. To examine the detailed recognition performance, we analyze the confusion matrices for all four datasets with $m = 2$ labeled training samples per activity, as shown in Fig. 6.4. For the USC-HAD dataset (Fig. 6.4a), our approach works well for most activities such as Sleeping, Sitting, and Jumping. Only for similar activities like Walking Forward, Walking Left, and Walking Downstairs do we observe some misclassification, which is expected given their similar motion patterns. Similar results are observed on the other three datasets (Fig. 6.4b–d), where confusion mainly occurs between activities with similar characteristics.

Performance Analysis. The superior performance of our proposed model can be attributed to several factors: First, our approach takes advantage of both labeled and unlabeled data during the training stage, which enables it to outperform supervised learning methods when only small amounts of labeled data are available. Second, the unified model simultaneously learns from feature correlations through shared struc-

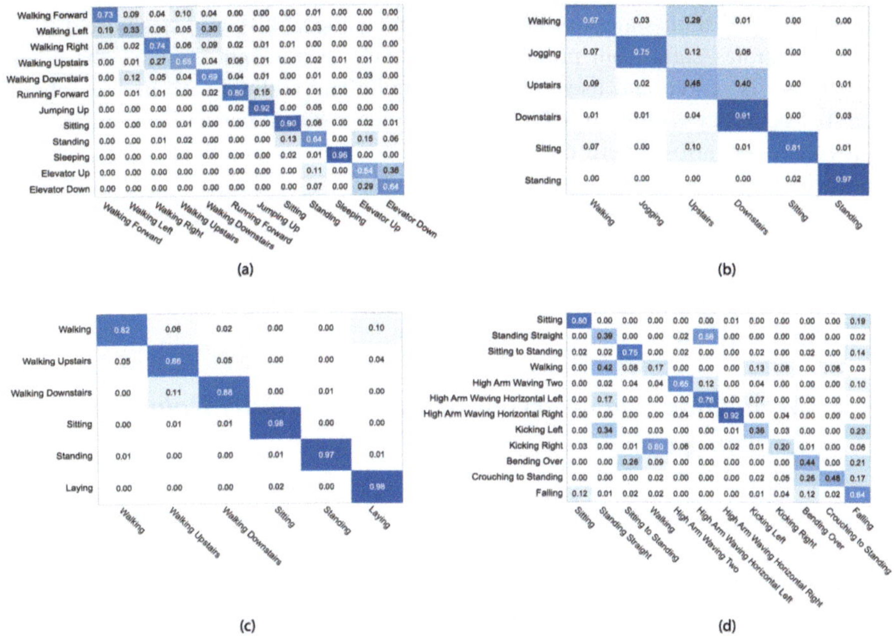

Fig. 6.4 The confusion matrix of our proposed RSAR approach for activity recognition on **a** the USC-HAD dataset, **b** the Actitracker dataset, **c** UCI HAR dataset, and **d** RFID dataset. Each matrix shows the average accuracy per activity with $m = 2$ labeled training samples per activity

ture discovery. Specifically, compared with traditional graph-based semi-supervised methods, we adopt $\ell_{2,1}$ minimization on both loss function and regularization. The $\ell_{2,1}$ norm-based loss function is robust to data outliers, and the $\ell_{2,1}$ norm regularization enables feature selection across all data points with joint sparsity.

6.3.4 Summary of RSAR

In this section, we proposed an approach to recognize human activities via discerning commonalities between multi-type features. First, our approach can simultaneously uncover the intrinsic and invariant low-dimensional subspace to improve overall activity recognition performance against intra-class variability. Second, we adopt the $\ell_{2,1}$ minimization to make our approach more robust to sensor reading outliers. Third, we unify both solutions into a semi-supervised learning framework for reducing the tedious efforts on manual labeling. We conduct extensive experiments to compare our approach with the state-of-the-art methods including supervised and semi-supervised methods. The experimental results on four public datasets show the promising performance of our proposed approach. Our approach outperforms all of these methods, especially when the size of labeled data is small.

The proposed semi-supervised learning framework with shared structure discovery demonstrates significant potential for activity recognition applications where labeled data is scarce and user diversity is high. The method's ability to achieve over 70% accuracy with minimal training samples makes it particularly suitable for deployment scenarios where continuous annotation is impractical, with potential applications in smart aging systems.

6.4 Distributionally Robust Learning for Cross-User Adaptation

6.4.1 Motivation and Overview of Distributionally Robust Learning

While semi-supervised learning offers a promising solution to the labeled data scarcity problem, it faces a fundamental challenge in real-world people-centric sensing applications: distribution shift between labeled and unlabeled data. Human-generated sensor data inherently suffer from significant variability due to diverse biological conditions, behavior patterns, and individual differences in how activities are performed.

In traditional semi-supervised learning, it is commonly assumed that labeled and unlabeled data follow the same underlying distribution. However, this assumption is frequently violated in practice, particularly in activity recognition scenarios where data may be collected from different users, in different environments, or under different conditions. For instance, when training data is collected from one group of users and the system is deployed to serve different users, the performance often degrades significantly due to person-specific differences in movement patterns, sensor positioning, and physiological characteristics.

This challenge is especially relevant in smart aging contexts, where the target population may exhibit different activity patterns compared to younger users who might have provided the initial labeled training data. Older adults may have different mobility patterns, use assistive devices, or perform activities at different paces, leading to significant distribution shifts that can compromise system performance.

Our motivation for developing a distributionally robust approach stems from the need to handle these inherent distribution shifts while still leveraging the benefits of semi-supervised learning. We propose a novel method that explicitly models and addresses the discrepancy between labeled and unlabeled data distributions while preserving task-relevant information that is consistent across different user populations [9].

Our approach focuses on two key objectives: (1) reducing person-specific discrepancy by learning features that are invariant to individual differences, and (2) preserving task-specific consistency to ensure that the learned representations maintain discriminative power for activity recognition across different user groups.

The key insight driving our approach is that we can decompose the distribution shift into two components: person-specific variations that should be minimized, and task-specific patterns that should be preserved. By explicitly modeling and addressing these two aspects, we can create more robust and generalizable activity recognition systems.

6.4.2 *Distributionally Robust Framework and Methodology*

Model Architecture and Components

We address this challenge by learning representations that reduce person-specific discrepancy while preserving task-specific consistency. Our approach recognizes that distribution shifts in human activity data can be decomposed into two components: person-specific variations (which should be minimized) and task-specific patterns (which should be preserved across different user populations).

Our method defines person-specific discrepancy as the distribution divergence between data from different individuals, while task-specific consistency represents the inherent similarity of data from subjects performing the same activities. As illustrated in Fig. 6.5, we employ adversarial training to reduce distribution divergence between labeled and unlabeled data features, while preserving task-specific information through consistency constraints.

We propose a distributionally robust model for semi-supervised learning that handles distribution shifts between labeled and unlabeled data. Our approach addresses scenarios where training data (x^L, y, s) from the labeled set L and unlabeled data (x^U, s) from set U are drawn from different distributions $\mathcal{L}(x)$ and $\mathcal{U}(x)$. To mitigate person-specific discrepancies while preserving task-specific consistency, we learn latent features z such that $P_L(y|z) = P_U(y|z)$.

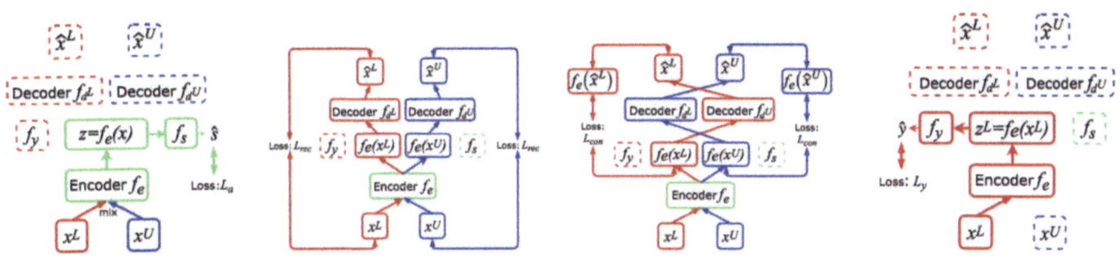

Fig. 6.5 The overview of the proposed model. We define three components of the training procedure: (1) person-specific discrepancy, (2) task-specific consistency, (3) prediction. Four losses are proposed for the objective: the adversarial loss L_a to reduce person-specific discrepancy, the reconstruction loss L_{rec} and the latent consistency loss L_{con} to preserve task-specific consistency and the prediction loss L_y. When minimizing the losses, only the activated parts are trained (indicated as solid lines) while the rest remain fixed (indicated as dashed lines). Red, blue and green denote the training procedures that are associated with the labeled samples, unlabeled samples, and a mixture of all the training samples, respectively

The model consists of five components: an encoder f_e that maps input to latent features z, a label predictor f_y, a distribution predictor f_s, and two decoders f_{dL} and f_{dU} for reconstructing inputs from labeled and unlabeled sets respectively. The training objective combines four loss components:

$$L_{total} = L_a + L_{rec} + L_{con} + L_y \tag{6.1}$$

where the adversarial loss reduces distribution divergence, the reconstruction loss trains domain-specific decoders, the consistency loss preserves task-specific consistency, and the prediction loss ensures discriminative feature learning.

The adversarial loss minimizes distribution divergence by training the encoder to produce features that are indistinguishable by the distribution classifier, effectively aligning the feature distributions of labeled and unlabeled data. The reconstruction loss trains separate decoders for labeled and unlabeled domains, ensuring that domain-specific characteristics are preserved while learning shared representations.

Task-specific consistency is preserved by ensuring that features from cross-domain reconstructions remain consistent, maintaining the semantic meaning of activities across different user populations. The prediction loss ensures discriminative feature learning using standard cross-entropy loss on labeled data, maintaining the model's ability to accurately classify activities.

Training Procedure and Optimization

The training procedure requires careful balancing of the four loss components to achieve optimal performance. Through experimental analysis, we find that a very strong classifier f_s may minimize the feature distribution discrepancy of L and U, but it will also distract the encoder from learning discriminative features for prediction. Therefore, we set a threshold $thre_a$ to seek a balance for the min-max game between person-specific discrepancy and discriminativeness. On the other hand, we require rather strong decoders for reconstruction, so a threshold $thre_{rec}$ is set to guarantee the reconstruction performance.

The training procedure follows an iterative optimization strategy that alternates between updating different model components while respecting these threshold constraints. Specifically, we first train the encoder and decoders until the reconstruction loss reaches the specified threshold, then alternate between training the distribution classifier (until adversarial loss reaches the appropriate threshold) and the encoder (to fool the distribution classifier), while continuously updating the label predictor to maintain discriminative capability throughout the process.

The model demonstrates appropriate sensitivity to key hyperparameters. The adversarial threshold controls the strength of the distribution alignment classifier, and experimental analysis shows that optimal performance is achieved when this threshold balances distribution alignment with discriminative feature learning. Too strong alignment may minimize distribution discrepancy but can distract from learning discriminative features for prediction, while too weak alignment provides limited benefit. The reconstruction threshold affects reconstruction performance, and experimental results indicate that powerful reconstruction ability is significant for the proposed model's effectiveness.

6.4.3 Experimental Validation and Performance Analysis

Experimental Setup and Datasets

We evaluate our distributionally robust model on four people-centric sensing tasks to validate its effectiveness under distribution shift scenarios:

- **EEG-based Intention Recognition**: 108 subjects performing cognitive tasks, with EEG signals recorded for intention classification.
- **EMG-based Muscular Movement Recognition**: 11 subjects performing hand gestures, with EMG sensors capturing muscular activity patterns.
- **MHEALTH Activity Recognition**: 10 participants performing daily activities, with IMU sensors placed at multiple body locations.
- **OPPORTUNITY Gesture Recognition**: 4 subjects performing 17 gesture classes in a smart home environment with multiple sensor modalities.

To simulate realistic distribution shift scenarios, we draw labeled and unlabeled training sets from different subjects. This setup reflects real-world deployment conditions where training data may come from one user population while the system is deployed to serve different users, which is particularly relevant for smart aging applications where training and deployment populations may differ significantly.

Baseline Comparison and Performance Analysis

We compare our model against both traditional semi-supervised methods and state-of-the-art domain adaptation approaches. The baseline methods include:

Semi-supervised Methods:

- **CNN**: A supervised baseline trained with labeled data only.
- **MSS**: Multi-view self-supervised learning approach.
- **DP**: Deep co-training with pseudo-labeling.
- **Tri-Net**: Tri-training approach with three neural networks.

Domain Adaptation Methods:

- **DANN** [12]: Domain-adversarial neural network that learns domain-invariant features.
- **CYCADA** [16]: Cycle-consistent adversarial domain adaptation.
- **ADDA**: Adversarial discriminative domain adaptation.

- **CoGAN**: Coupled generative adversarial networks for cross-domain learning.
- **CycleGAN**: Cycle-consistent generative adversarial network for domain translation.

Table 6.2 presents comprehensive performance comparison across all four datasets. Our model significantly outperforms both traditional semi-supervised methods and domain adaptation approaches across all evaluation metrics. Specifically, we achieve 77.01% accuracy on EEG, 77.83% on EMG, 95.22% on MHEALTH, and 62.27% on OPPORTUNITY datasets, representing substantial improvements over the best baseline methods (3–7% over CYCADA and CycleGAN).

Table 6.2 Performance comparison with state-of-the-art methods. CNN is a supervised baseline trained with labeled data only. * denotes domain adaptation methods. The best performance is indicated in bold

Dataset	Metric	Semi-supervised				Domain adaptation*
		CNN	MSS	DP	Tri-Net	DANN*
EEG	Accuracy	66.62	63.22	67.90	67.69	70.79
	Precision	65.46	58.38	63.27	62.36	69.34
	Recall	67.47	64.54	68.61	68.45	71.87
EMG	Accuracy	64.56	64.74	64.78	66.78	69.55
	Precision	62.11	63.57	63.71	64.23	66.28
	Recall	66.29	66.97	67.61	68.94	72.15
MHEALTH	Accuracy	86.67	87.83	88.82	87.07	89.85
	Precision	85.68	85.53	86.38	84.21	87.56
	Recall	87.06	85.22	85.14	86.30	90.62
OPPORTUNITY	Accuracy	48.56	44.15	47.47	46.57	54.82
	Precision	49.64	45.37	46.88	45.18	55.86
	Recall	48.98	44.16	44.84	43.92	55.90
Dataset	Metric	Domain adaptation methods*				
		CYCADA*	ADDA*	CoGAN*	CycleGAN*	**Ours***
EEG	Accuracy	73.29	67.18	71.02	72.69	**77.01**
	Precision	73.28	62.11	63.83	63.43	**73.85**
	Recall	73.58	68.10	71.94	73.36	**75.77**
EMG	Accuracy	74.03	66.55	72.37	74.46	**77.83**
	Precision	71.18	65.83	70.79	70.88	**73.35**
	Recall	75.93	68.10	73.19	73.32	**76.11**
MHEALTH	Accuracy	92.08	88.93	90.35	91.08	**95.22**
	Precision	90.61	83.72	86.75	87.29	**94.28**
	Recall	92.32	90.53	90.48	91.25	**96.32**
OPPORTUNITY	Accuracy	58.83	52.81	58.38	59.23	**62.27**
	Precision	58.06	47.13	57.30	53.51	**60.39**
	Recall	58.06	52.15	58.31	60.92	**62.47**

Performance Analysis. The results demonstrate that our model effectively handles distribution shifts in people-centric sensing scenarios. Traditional semi-supervised methods (MSS, DP, Tri-Net) perform poorly as they assume labeled and unlabeled data follow the same distribution, which is violated in our experimental setup. Domain adaptation methods (DANN, CYCADA, ADDA, CoGAN, CycleGAN) perform better by learning domain-invariant features, but they do not explicitly preserve task-specific consistency. Our model achieves the best performance by simultaneously reducing person-specific discrepancy through adversarial training while preserving task-specific consistency through reconstruction and latent consistency constraints.

Ablation Study

To understand the contribution of each component in our model, we conduct comprehensive ablation studies. Table 6.3 presents four configurations: (1) L_y only: a regular CNN trained with prediction loss on labeled data; (2) L_y+L_a: adding adversarial loss to reduce person-specific discrepancy; (3) L_y+L_{rec}+L_{con}: adding reconstruction and consistency losses to preserve task-specific consistency; (4) Our full model: combining all components.

The ablation results reveal several important insights: (1) Adding adversarial loss (L_a) provides significant improvement (3–6%) over the supervised baseline, confirming the importance of reducing person-specific discrepancy. (2) Adding reconstruction and consistency losses without adversarial training provides modest improvement (2–3%), indicating that task-specific consistency preservation alone is insufficient. (3) The full model combining all components achieves the best performance

Table 6.3 Ablation Study. L_y denotes a regular CNN trained with prediction loss only; L_y+L_a adds person-specific discrepancy reduction; L_y+L_{rec}+L_{con} adds task-specific consistency preservation; Our Model combines all components

Configuration	EEG			EMG		
	Accuracy	Precision	Recall	Accuracy	Precision	Recall
L_y	66.62	65.46	67.47	64.56	62.11	66.29
L_y+L_a	70.79	69.34	71.88	69.55	66.28	72.15
L_y+L_{rec}+L_{con}	68.85	67.83	69.35	67.40	65.16	69.57
Our Model	**77.01**	**73.85**	**75.77**	**77.83**	**73.35**	**76.11**
Configuration	MHEALTH			OPPORTUNITY		
	Accuracy	Precision	Recall	Accuracy	Precision	Recall
L_y	86.67	85.68	87.06	48.56	49.64	48.98
L_y+L_a	89.85	87.56	90.62	54.82	55.86	55.90
L_y+L_{rec}+L_{con}	87.41	86.13	88.38	51.85	52.23	54.23
Our Model	**95.22**	**94.28**	**96.32**	**62.27**	**60.39**	**62.47**

with 6–8% improvement over partial configurations, demonstrating that both person-specific discrepancy reduction and task-specific consistency preservation are necessary and complementary.

Visualization and Sensitivity Analysis

Through visualization analysis, we observe that our model effectively reduces the distribution discrepancy between labeled and unlabeled data in the learned feature space. The adversarial training component successfully aligns the feature distributions from different user populations, while the reconstruction and consistency components ensure that task-relevant discriminative information is preserved.

The model demonstrates appropriate sensitivity to key hyperparameters. The adversarial threshold ($thre_a$) controls the strength of distribution alignment, and our experiments show that balancing this threshold is crucial: too strong alignment may sacrifice discriminative power, while too weak alignment provides limited benefit. The reconstruction threshold ($thre_{rec}$) ensures powerful reconstruction capability, which is significant for the model's effectiveness in preserving task-specific information.

The model scales well to multi-subject scenarios and shows robust performance across diverse user populations, making it particularly suitable for practical deployment in smart aging applications where training data from younger adults may need to generalize to older adult populations with different movement patterns and physical capabilities.

6.4.4 *Summary of Distributionally Robust Learning*

We proposed a novel distributionally-robust semi-supervised method for handling shifted distributions of the labeled and the unlabeled data. The model first reduces person-specific discrepancy by aligning the distributions of the labeled data and unlabeled data. Task-specific consistency is further proposed for extracting label-related features. We experimentally validate our model on a variety of people-centric sensing tasks. The results demonstrate the outperformance of the proposed model compared with the state-of-the-art. Our model is generic and can be applied to various people-centric sensing applications where distribution shift is a concern.

This distributionally robust approach addresses a critical gap in activity recognition systems where training data from one population may not generalize well to different target populations. By explicitly modeling and reducing person-specific variations while preserving task-relevant information, the method enables more reliable deployment of activity recognition systems across diverse user groups, with particular relevance for smart aging applications where training and deployment populations may differ significantly.

6.5 Multi-agent Attention for Intelligent Sensor Selection

6.5.1 Motivation

Multi-modal wearable sensors generate rich data streams, but effective utilization requires addressing two key challenges: spatially-temporally varying feature salience and the collective nature of human activities involving coordinated motions across multiple body parts. Traditional approaches fail to capture these complex interrelationships and global connections.

Our multi-agent attentional approach treats activity recognition as a collaborative decision-making problem [10]. We deploy multiple intelligent agents, each responsible for selecting informative sensor modalities associated with specific body motions. These agents work independently while sharing information and coordinating their selection policies to learn optimal recognition strategies. This approach is particularly relevant for smart aging applications where movement patterns may differ due to mobility limitations or compensatory strategies.

6.5.2 Multi-agent Framework and Methodology

Architecture and Agent Coordination. We formulate activity recognition on multi-modal sensor data where each input sample $(\mathbf{x}, y)$ consists of a 2D matrix $\mathbf{x} \in R^{K \times P}$ representing sensor readings over time window K with P features, and activity label $y \in [1, ..., C]$. The sensor matrix combines multi-modal data from different body positions.

The model employs three agents that collaborate to recognize activities by decomposing them into sub-motions, as illustrated in Fig. 6.6. The framework operates through three key phases: (1) independent sensor selection by each agent, (2) shared observation processing and encoding, and (3) collaborative decision-making for final activity classification. At each step, agents select active time periods and individual modality locations, observe small patches extracted from the sensor matrix, and encode them into higher-level representations through linear transformations and concatenation operations.

Agents share observations to create collaborative representations and maintain hidden states for sequential decision-making. The selection policies for next locations are determined through policy networks that take shared observations and hidden states as input. After multiple steps, final predictions are made using softmax classification. Agents receive delayed rewards based on classification accuracy and are trained using REINFORCE with Monte Carlo sampling to optimize their collaborative selection policies.

Optimization Framework. The overall training objective combines classification loss with reinforcement learning for policy optimization. The classification loss uses

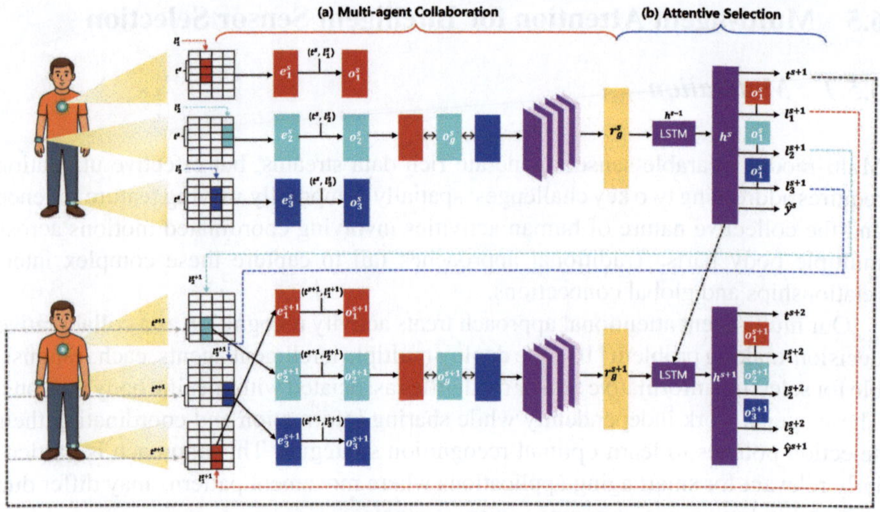

Fig. 6.6 Multi-agent attentional activity recognition framework overview. The architecture consists of three main components: (1) Multi-agent collaboration module where three agents independently select informative sensor modalities and time periods from the input sensor matrix; (2) Attention mechanism that processes selected sensor patches and generates higher-level representations through shared observation encoding; (3) Collaborative decision-making process where agents coordinate their selection policies using shared information to optimize joint recognition performance. Each agent focuses on specific body motions while sharing observations to achieve comprehensive activity understanding

standard cross-entropy loss to measure prediction accuracy, while the reinforcement learning component optimizes agent selection policies. However, selection policies involve non-differentiable parameters for choosing sequences of locations. We deploy a Partially Observable Markov Decision Process (POMDP) framework to solve the optimization problem. Each episode is modeled as a trajectory representing the sequence of observations, locations, and predictions made by the agents.

The training objective is to learn the optimal selection policy that maximizes the expected reward using the REINFORCE algorithm. The gradient computation uses policy gradients to update the selection strategies based on classification performance feedback. Monte Carlo sampling is employed to handle the stochastic nature of the policy learning, providing gradient approximations that enable effective training of the multi-agent selection policies. The overall optimization maximizes the expected reward while minimizing the classification loss through iterative training with Monte Carlo sampling.

6.5.3 Experimental Validation and Performance Analysis

Experimental Setup

We evaluate our multi-agent attentional model on four real-world datasets using Leave-One-Subject-Out (LOSO) cross-validation to ensure fairness and generalizability. The datasets include: MHEALTH [4] (10 subjects), PAMAP2 [26] (9 subjects), UCI HAR [2] (30 subjects), and MARS (8 subjects).

The experimental settings are configured as follows: The time window of inputs is 20 with 50% overlap. The size of each observation patch is set to $\frac{K}{5} \times \frac{P}{5}$, where $K \times P$ is the size of the inputs. In the partial observation module, the sizes of θ_e, θ_{li}, and θ_o are 128, 128, and 220, respectively. The convolutional layer in the shared observation module uses a filter size of $1 \times M$ with 40 feature maps, where M denotes the width of o_g^s. The LSTM cell size is 220, the episode length is 40, and the Gaussian distribution defining the selection policies has a variance of 0.22.

Comparison with State-of-the-Art Methods

To verify the overall performance of our proposed model, we compare it with several state-of-the-art methods: a convolutional model on multichannel time series for HAR (MC-CNN) [30], a CNN-based multi-modal fusion model (C-Fusion) [24], a deep multi-modal HAR model with classifier ensemble (MARCEL) [14], an ensemble of deep LSTM learners (E-LSTM) [13], a parallel recurrent model with convolutional attentions (PRCA) [8], and a weighted average spatial LSTM with selective attention (WAS-LSTM) [34].

Table 6.4 presents the comprehensive performance comparison across four evaluation metrics (Accuracy, Precision, Recall, and F1-score) on all four datasets. Our model consistently outperforms all compared methods across all datasets and metrics. Specifically, we achieve 96.12% accuracy on MHEALTH, 90.33% on PAMAP2, 85.72% on UCI HAR, and 88.29% on MARS, representing significant improvements over the best baseline methods.

Performance Analysis Across Datasets. The results reveal interesting patterns across different datasets. For MHEALTH and PAMAP2, models with higher variance such as MARCEL, E-LSTM, PRCA, WAS-LSTM and our model perform better than MC-CNN and C-Fusion, as these datasets contain numerous features and complex patterns. For UCI HAR and MARS with fewer features, MARCEL, E-LSTM, PRCA and our model still perform well, while WAS-LSTM's performance deteriorates due to its complex structure requiring more input features. Our model eliminates the instability of regular selective attentions through coordinated multi-agent collaboration, achieving consistent superior performance across all datasets.

Table 6.4 The prediction performance of the proposed approach and other state-of-the-art methods. * denotes attention-based state-of-the-art. The best performance is indicated in bold. MH=MHEALTH, PMP=PAMAP2, HAR=UCI HAR

	Method	MC-CNN	C-Fusion	MARCEL	E-LSTM	PRCA*	WAS-LSTM*	Ours*
MH	Accuracy	87.19±0.77	88.66±0.62	92.35±0.46	91.58±0.38	93.32±0.75	91.42±1.25	**96.12±0.37**
	Precision	86.50±0.61	86.36±0.72	93.17±0.84	90.50±0.68	92.11±0.96	91.35±0.70	**95.46±0.33**
	Recall	87.28±0.62	89.68±0.74	92.81±0.93	91.58±0.59	92.25±0.94	91.99±1.14	**96.76±0.30**
	F1	86.89±0.66	87.98±0.79	92.98±0.74	91.03±0.68	92.17±1.06	91.66±1.21	**96.10±0.47**
PMP	Accuracy	81.16±1.32	81.86±0.74	82.87±0.81	83.21±0.68	82.39±1.04	84.89±2.18	**90.33±0.62**
	Precision	81.57±0.89	81.63±0.53	83.51±0.71	84.01±0.54	82.44±0.99	84.44±1.54	**89.25±0.78**
	Recall	81.43±0.64	81.96±0.89	81.12±0.79	83.88±0.74	82.86±0.90	84.20±1.33	**90.49±0.94**
	F1	81.50±0.72	81.79±0.71	82.29±0.76	83.94±0.95	82.64±1.19	84.81±1.06	**89.86±0.81**
HAR	Accuracy	75.86±0.59	74.64±0.78	80.16±0.72	80.78±0.94	81.29±1.22	71.29±1.08	**85.72±0.83**
	Precision	76.93±0.78	73.30±0.75	81.63±0.50	81.34±0.43	80.55±1.26	70.76±0.93	**85.61±0.53**
	Recall	75.81±0.39	74.07±0.48	80.81±0.63	80.63±0.54	81.66±1.03	71.10±1.71	**85.08±0.72**
	F1	76.36±1.11	73.68±0.83	81.21±0.85	80.98±0.64	81.11±1.02	70.92±1.16	**85.34±0.58**
MARS	Accuracy	81.34±0.59	81.48±0.56	81.68±0.87	81.59±0.77	85.38±0.82	74.82±1.42	**88.29±0.87**
	Precision	81.68±0.62	81.84±0.68	81.23±0.84	81.79±0.85	85.99±1.07	75.89±1.54	**88.75±0.81**
	Recall	81.06±0.90	82.15±0.82	82.44±0.54	81.65±0.93	84.95±0.95	74.80±1.63	**87.20±0.67**
	F1	81.32±0.42	81.99±0.71	81.85±0.97	81.71±0.81	85.46±1.02	75.34±1.27	**87.96±0.74**

Ablation Study

To examine the contributions of individual components, we perform a detailed ablation study with six configurations, as shown in Table 6.5. We systematically remove five components: (a) the selection module, (b) the transformation from e_i^s to o_i^s ($i \in \{1, 2, 3\}$), (c) the convolutional network for higher-level representations, (d) the temporal attentive selection, and (e) the multi-agent collaboration.

The ablation results reveal that: (1) S1 provides a baseline CNN performance without any attention; (2) S2 shows that attention without proper observation encoding performs worse, as the model cannot incorporate selection history; (3) S3 improves by 5–7% over S2 by adding observation transformation that feeds back selection history; (4) S4 further improves by convolutional merging of partial observations; (5) S5 adds temporal attention, achieving 3–5% improvement; (6) S6, our full model with all components, achieves the best performance with 5–7% improvement over S5, demonstrating that multi-agent collaboration provides significant benefits.

Attention Visualization and Interpretability

Our proposed method decomposes activities into participating motions, with agents independently deciding the most salient modalities from each motion, making the

Table 6.5 Ablation Study. S1-S6 are six structures created by systematically removing components: (a) selection module, (b) partial observation processing, (c) convolutional merge, (d) temporal attention, (e) multi-agent. S1 is a baseline CNN without any attention mechanism. S6 is our full model

	MHEALTH				PAMAP2			
	Accuracy	Precision	Recall	F1	Accuracy	Precision	Recall	F1
S1	85.75	84.67	85.83	84.34	79.60	79.86	79.68	79.57
S2	80.59	80.37	80.95	80.00	71.49	71.62	71.38	71.49
S3	86.08	85.67	84.62	85.14	77.68	77.35	77.74	77.04
S4	88.32	87.11	87.25	87.17	78.39	78.44	78.86	78.64
S5	91.93	90.85	91.38	91.88	85.53	83.66	83.38	83.51
S6	**96.12**	**95.46**	**96.76**	**96.10**	**90.33**	**89.25**	**90.49**	**89.86**
	UCI HAR				MARS			
	Accuracy	Precision	Recall	F1	Accuracy	Precision	Recall	F1
S1	73.68	73.79	73.98	73.38	79.78	79.37	79.49	79.31
S2	68.95	67.41	67.92	67.66	71.15	71.23	71.99	71.15
S3	75.45	75.54	75.49	75.88	78.34	78.42	78.48	78.40
S4	76.29	76.55	77.66	77.11	81.38	81.99	81.95	81.46
S5	80.71	80.95	80.44	80.11	85.51	84.94	85.73	84.81
S6	**85.72**	**85.61**	**85.08**	**85.34**	**88.29**	**88.75**	**87.20**	**87.96**

Table 6.6 The active modalities for activities selected by the agents. *X*, *Y*, *Z* denote the axis of data. Acc, Ang and Magn denote acceleration, angular velocity and magnetism, respectively. The most frequently selected locations are indicated in bold

Activity	Agent	Most selected modalities
Standing	1	**Y, Z-Magn-Ankle**, X, Y-Acc-Arm
	2	**Y-Acc-Ankle**, ECG1,2-Chest
	3	**X, Y-Ang-Ankle**
Going upstairs	1	**Y,Z-Acc-Ankle**, X, Y-Ang-Ankle
	2	**X,Y, Z-Acc-Ankle**, X, Y-Ang-Ankle
	3	**Y, Z-Acc-Arm**, X, Y, Z-Ang-Arm
Running	1	**Y, Z-Acc-Chest**, ECG1,2-Chest
	2	**X, Y, Z-Acc-Ankle**
	3	X, Y, Z-Acc-Arm, **X,Y-Ang-Arm**
Lying	1	**Y, Z-Acc-Arm**, X, Y, Z-Ang-Arm
	2	**Y, Z-Magn-Ankle**
	3	**X, Y, Z-Magn-Arm**

model explainable. We visualize the recognition process for standing, going upstairs, running, and lying on the MHEALTH dataset. Table 6.6 lists the most frequently selected modalities by different agents for these activities.

The visualization results demonstrate intuitive and explainable attention patterns: (1) For standing and lying, magnetism (orientation) sensors are selected as the most active features, which makes sense as these activities are easily distinguished by body orientation. (2) For going upstairs, Z-axis acceleration is specifically selected, reflecting the characteristic "upward" motion. (3) For running, agents select acceleration, ECG signals, and arm swing features, which align with the high-intensity nature of this activity. Each agent focuses on a subset of modalities during specific time periods, avoiding information loss while capturing the most discriminative features. This explainability enhances system interpretability and facilitates debugging for practical deployments.

6.5.4 *Summary of Multi-agent Attentional Activity Recognition*

We proposed a multi-agent spatial-temporal attention model that addresses the inherent characteristics of human activities: spatially-temporally varying feature salience and collective motions across body parts. The multi-agent framework enables intelligent sensor selection while the attention mechanism focuses on informative modalities during their active periods. Experimental results on four real-world datasets demonstrate superior performance compared to state-of-the-art methods.

The multi-agent attentional approach represents an advanced solution for activity recognition, showing how intelligent sensor selection and collaborative decision-making can significantly improve performance. The method's ability to decompose complex activities into manageable sub-motions and coordinate recognition across multiple body parts makes it particularly suitable for smart aging applications where activity patterns may be complex and varied. The explainable nature of the attention mechanism provides valuable insights for system optimization and user understanding.

6.6 Discussion and Future Directions

This chapter has presented three complementary methodological approaches to address fundamental challenges in wearable sensor-based physical activity recognition. The methods collectively advance the state-of-the-art in handling limited labeled data, cross-user distribution shifts, and intelligent sensor selection in multi-modal environments–challenges that are particularly relevant for practical deployment in diverse application domains including smart aging systems.

6.6.1 *Methodological Synergies and Implications*

The three presented approaches form a methodological progression that addresses interconnected challenges in activity recognition:

- *Semi-supervised Learning Foundation*: The RSAR framework establishes a robust foundation by demonstrating that shared structure discovery can effectively utilize unlabeled data while maintaining robustness to sensor noise through $\ell_{2,1}$ minimization. This capability is essential for scenarios where continuous data annotation is impractical, making the approach suitable for long-term monitoring applications.
- *Cross-user Generalization*: The distributionally robust approach extends this foundation by explicitly addressing the reality that training and deployment populations often differ. By decomposing distribution shifts into person-specific variations (to be minimized) and task-specific patterns (to be preserved), this method enables more reliable cross-population deployment–a critical consideration when developing systems that must work across diverse user groups with varying physical capabilities and movement patterns.
- *Intelligent Sensor Selection*: The multi-agent attention framework represents the most advanced solution, providing both performance improvements and interpretability through collaborative sensor selection. The explainable nature of the attention mechanism offers valuable insights into which sensors contribute most to recognition decisions, facilitating system optimization and user understanding.

6.6.2 Practical Deployment Considerations

The experimental validation demonstrates the practical viability of these approaches across diverse datasets and sensing modalities. Key considerations for real-world deployment include:

- *Computational Efficiency*: All three methods are designed with computational feasibility in mind, using efficient matrix operations and iterative optimization strategies that can accommodate resource-constrained wearable devices. The intelligent sensor selection capability of the multi-agent approach can further enhance efficiency by focusing computational resources on the most informative data streams.
- *Adaptability and Personalization*: The combination of semi-supervised learning with distribution adaptation provides natural mechanisms for system adaptation without requiring extensive retraining. This adaptability is valuable for accommodating individual differences and changing conditions over time.
- *System Interpretability*: The attention mechanisms and shared structure discovery provide interpretable insights into the recognition process, which can be valuable for system debugging, optimization, and user confidence in diverse application contexts.

6.6.3 Future Research Directions

While the presented approaches demonstrate significant advances, several areas warrant further investigation:

- *Temporal Dynamics and Long-term Adaptation*: Current methods focus primarily on cross-sectional performance but could benefit from enhanced mechanisms to handle gradual changes in user behavior, physical capabilities, or environmental conditions that occur over extended deployment periods.
- *Multi-modal Integration*: Future work could explore deeper integration of diverse sensor modalities beyond traditional inertial sensors, potentially incorporating physiological signals, environmental sensors, or contextual information to enhance recognition accuracy and provide richer activity understanding.
- *Privacy-preserving Learning*: As activity recognition systems become more prevalent, developing federated or privacy-preserving learning approaches that can leverage distributed data while protecting user privacy represents an important research direction.
- *Edge Computing Optimization*: Further optimization for edge computing environments, including model compression techniques and adaptive computation strategies, could enhance the practical deployment potential of these methods on resource-constrained devices.

The comprehensive framework presented in this chapter provides a solid methodological foundation for next-generation activity recognition systems that can effectively handle the challenges of real-world deployment across diverse user populations and application contexts.

References

1. Ando, R.K., Zhang, T.: A framework for learning predictive structures from multiple tasks and unlabeled data. J. Mach. Learn. Res. **6**, 1817–1853 (2005)
2. Anguita, D., Ghio, A., Oneto, L., Parra, X., Reyes-Ortiz, J.L.: A public domain dataset for human activity recognition using smartphones. In: 21st European Symposium on Artificial Neural Networks, Computational Intelligence and Machine Learning (ESANN), pp. 437–442. i6doc.com publ./ESANN, Bruges, Belgium (2013)
3. Bao, L., Intille, S.S.: Activity recognition from user-annotated acceleration data. In: Ferscha, A., Mattern, F. (eds.) Pervasive Computing, Pervasive 2004. Lecture Notes in Computer Science, vol. 3001, pp. 1–17. Springer, Berlin (2004)
4. Baños, O., García, R., Holgado-Terriza, J.A., Damas, M., Pomares, H., Rojas, I., Sáez, A., Villalonga, C.: mhealthdroid: a novel framework for agile development of mobile health applications. In: International Workshop on Ambient Assisted Living, pp. 91–98. Springer, Berlin (2014)
5. Bhattacharya, S., Nurmi, P., Hammerla, N., Plötz, T.: Using unlabeled data in a sparse-coding framework for human activity recognition. Pervasive Mob. Comput. **15**, 242–262 (2014)
6. Blei, D.M., Jordan, M.I.: Variational inference for dirichlet process mixtures. Bayesian Anal. **1**(1), 121–143 (2006)
7. Blum, A., Mitchell, T.: Combining labeled and unlabeled data with co-training. In: Proceedings of the Eleventh Annual Conference on Computational Learning Theory (COLT), pp. 92–100. ACM (1998)
8. Chen, K., Yao, L., Wang, X., Zhang, D., Gu, T., Yu, Z., Yang, Z.: Interpretable parallel recurrent neural networks with convolutional attentions for multi-modality activity modeling. In: 2018 International Joint Conference on Neural Networks (IJCNN), pp. 3016–3021. IEEE (2018)
9. Chen, K., Yao, L., Zhang, D., Chang, X., Long, G., Wang, S.: Distributionally robust semi-supervised learning for people-centric sensing. In: Proceedings of the Thirty-Third AAAI Conference on Artificial Intelligence (AAAI-19). AAAI Press (2019)
10. Chen, K., Yao, L., Zhang, D., Guo, B., Yu, Z.: Multi-agent attentional activity recognition. In: Proceedings of the Twenty-Eighth International Joint Conference on Artificial Intelligence (IJCAI-19). IJCAI (2019)
11. Clarkson, B., Pentland, A.: Unsupervised clustering of ambulatory audio and video. In: Proceedings of the 1999 IEEE International Conference on Acoustics, Speech, and Signal Processing (ICASSP), vol. 6, pp. 3037–3040. IEEE (1999)
12. Ganin, Y., Ustinova, E., Ajakan, H., Germain, P., Larochelle, H., Laviolette, F., Marchand, M., Lempitsky, V.: Domain-adversarial training of neural networks. J. Mach. Learn. Res. **17**(1), 2096–2103 (2016)
13. Guan, Y., Plötz, T.: Ensembles of deep lstm learners for activity recognition using wearables. Proc. ACM Interactive, Mobile, Wearable Ubiquitous Technol. (IMWUT) **1**(2), 11 (2017)
14. Guo, H., Chen, L., Peng, L., Chen, G.: Wearable sensor based multimodal human activity recognition exploiting the diversity of classifier ensemble. In: Proceedings of the 2016 ACM International Joint Conference on Pervasive and Ubiquitous Computing (UbiComp), pp. 1112–1123 (2016)

15. Hammerla, N.Y., Halloran, S., Plötz, T.: Deep, convolutional, and recurrent models for human activity recognition using wearables. In: Proceedings of the Twenty-Fifth International Joint Conference on Artificial Intelligence (IJCAI), pp. 1533–1540 (2016)
16. Hoffman, J., Tzeng, E., Park, T., Zhu, J.Y., Isola, P., Saenko, K., Efros, A.A., Darrell, T.: Cycada: cycle-consistent adversarial domain adaptation. In: Proceedings of the 35th International Conference on Machine Learning (ICML), pp. 1994–2003 (2018)
17. Hotelling, H.: Relations between two sets of variates. In: Biometrika, pp. 321–377 (1936)
18. Hunh, T., Blanke, U., Schiele, B.: Scalable recognition of daily activities with wearable sensors. In: Location- and Context-awareness. Lecture Notes in Computer Science, pp. 50–67. Springer, Berlin (2007)
19. Kwapisz, J.R., Weiss, G.M., Moore, S.A.: Activity recognition using cell phone accelerometers. ACM SIGKDD Explor. Newsl **12**(2), 74–82 (2011)
20. Logan, B., Healey, J., Philipose, M., Tapia, E.M., Intille, S.S.: A long-term evaluation of sensing modalities for activity recognition. Springer, Berlin (2007)
21. Lu, J., Zheng, X., Sheng, M., Jin, J., Yu, S.: Efficient human activity recognition using a single wearable sensor. IEEE Internet Things J. **7**(11), 11137–11146 (2020)
22. Maurer, U., Smailagic, A., Siewiorek, D.P., Deisher, M.: Activity recognition and monitoring using multiple sensors on different body positions. In: Proceedings of the International Workshop on Wearable and Implantable Body Sensor Networks (BSN 2006), p. 4. IEEE (2006)
23. Pouyanfar, S., Sadiq, S., Yan, Y., Tian, H., Tao, Y., Reyes, M.P., Shyu, M., Chen, S., Iyengar, S.S.: A survey on deep learning: algorithms, techniques, and applications. ACM Comput. Surv. (CSUR) **51**(5), 92 (2018)
24. Radu, V., Tong, C., Bhattacharya, S., Lane, N.D., Mascolo, C., Marina, M.K., Kawsar, F.: Multimodal deep learning for activity and context recognition. Proc. ACM Interactive, Mobile, Wearable Ubiquitous Technol. (IMWUT) **1**(4), 157 (2018)
25. Ravi, N., Dandekar, N., Mysore, P., Littman, M.L.: Activity recognition from accelerometer data. In: Proceedings of the AAAI 2005 Spring Symposium Series, pp. 1541–1546 (2005)
26. Reiss, A., Stricker, D.: Introducing a new benchmarked dataset for activity monitoring. In: Wearable Computers (ISWC), pp. 108–109. IEEE (2012)
27. Stikic, M., Laerhoven, K.V., Schiele, B.: Exploring semi-supervised and active learning for activity recognition. In: Proceedings of the 2008 IEEE International Symposium on Wearable Computers (ISWC'08), pp. 81–88. IEEE (2008)
28. Stikic, M., Larlus, D., Schiele, B.: Multi-graph based semi-supervised learning for activity recognition. In: Proceedings of the 2009 IEEE International Symposium on Wearable Computers (ISWC'09), pp. 85–92. IEEE (2009)
29. Tapia, E.M., Intille, S.S., Larson, K.: Activity recognition in the home using simple and ubiquitous sensors. In: Pervasive Computing. Lecture Notes in Computer Science. Springer, Berlin (2004)
30. Yang, J., Nguyen, M.N., San, P.P., Li, X., Krishnaswamy, S.: Deep convolutional neural networks on multichannel time series for human activity recognition. In: Proceedings of the IJCAI, pp. 3995–4001 (2015)
31. Yao, L., Nie, F., Sheng, Q.Z., Gu, T., Li, X., Wang, S.: Learning from less for better: Semi-supervised activity recognition via shared structure discovery. In: Proceedings of the 2016 ACM International Joint Conference on Pervasive and Ubiquitous Computing (UbiComp '16), pp. 13–24. ACM, Heidelberg, Germany (2016)
32. Yao, L., Sheng, Q.Z., Li, X., Wang, S., Gu, T., Ruan, W., Zou, W.: Freedom: Online activity recognition via dictionary-based sparse representation of rfid sensing data. In: Proceedings of the IEEE International Conference on Data Mining (ICDM). IEEE (2015a)

33. Zhang, M., Sawchuk, A.A.: Usc-had: A daily activity dataset for ubiquitous activity recognition using wearable sensors. In: Proceedings of the 2012 ACM Conference on Ubiquitous Computing (Ubicomp'12), pp. 1036–1043. ACM (2012)
34. Zhang, X., Yao, L., Huang, C., Wang, S., Tan, M., Long, G., Wang, C.: Multi-modality sensor data classification with selective attention. In: Proceedings of the Twenty-Seventh International Joint Conference on Artificial Intelligence (IJCAI), pp. 3111–3117 (2018)
35. Zhou, D., Bousquet, O., Lal, T.N., Weston, J., Schölkopf, B.: Learning with local and global consistency. Adv. Neural. Inf. Process. Syst. **16**, 321–328 (2004)

Chapter 7
EEG-Based Cognitive Activity Recognition

7.1 Introduction

7.1.1 Overview of Cognitive Activity Recognition

Cognitive activity recognition represents a critical frontier in artificial intelligence and IoT applications for smart aging. As the global population ages, there is an increasing need for intelligent systems that can understand, monitor, and assist with cognitive processes. The ability to accurately recognize and interpret cognitive activities through brain signals, behavioral patterns, and multi-modal data fusion opens new possibilities for personalized healthcare, assistive technologies, and quality-of-life improvements for aging populations.

This chapter presents three advanced artificial intelligence (AI) approaches that collectively address the challenges of cognitive activity recognition. These methods leverage the power of deep learning [23], graph neural networks, and cross-modal learning to create more robust and effective cognitive monitoring systems that can be integrated into smart aging environments.

7.1.2 Challenges and Opportunities

The field of cognitive activity recognition faces several interconnected challenges that are particularly relevant for smart aging applications:

Signal Processing and Data Limitations: Electroencephalography (EEG) signals are inherently noisy, containing artifacts from physiological activities and exhibiting low signal-to-noise ratios. The correlations between brain signals and cognitive intentions are often ambiguous, especially in aging populations where neural patterns may change over time. Additionally, obtaining labeled data in healthcare settings is

Q. Z. Sheng et al., *Harnessing Artificial Intelligence and Pervasive Internet of Things for an Empowered Aging*, https://doi.org/10.1007/978-3-032-16502-2_7

expensive and requires expert knowledge, creating scarcity that limits the development of robust cognitive recognition systems.

Multi-Modal Integration and Real-Time Processing: Understanding cognitive activities requires integrating information from multiple modalities such as brain signals and visual stimuli. Traditional approaches struggle with cross-modal alignment and generalization to unseen scenarios. Furthermore, smart aging applications demand real-time processing capabilities, creating tension between model complexity and computational efficiency requirements.

These challenges present significant opportunities for innovation. More specifically, advanced AI techniques can enable personalized cognitive monitoring that adapts to individual patterns, provides early detection of cognitive decline, and supports aging individuals through brain-computer interfaces and assistive technologies. Semi-supervised learning approaches can maximize the utility of limited labeled data while leveraging abundant unlabeled observations for more robust and comprehensive cognitive assessment systems.

7.1.3 Contributions

This chapter makes several significant contributions to the field of cognitive activity recognition for smart aging:

- *EEG-Based Intention Recognition*: We introduce both cascade and parallel convolutional recurrent neural network models for precisely identifying human intended movements and instructions by effectively learning the compositional spatio-temporal representations of raw EEG streams. Our approach achieves high accuracy near 98.3% and outperforms existing methods with a significant accuracy increase of 18% in cross-subject validation scenarios. The models demonstrate robust capabilities across different BCI systems and can generalize to various human intentions.
- *Adversarial Variational Embedding Framework*: We present a novel semi-supervised Adversarial Variational Embedding (AVAE) approach that harnesses deep generative models and generative adversarial networks collectively under a unified framework. The proposed VAE++ produces exclusive latent codes for accurate classification while providing meaningful prior distributions for GAN generators. This approach addresses the limitation of traditional VAEs where learned representations are not exclusive for specific input samples.
- *Self-Supervised Cross-Modal Learning*: We develop a self-supervised cross-modal learning paradigm for retrieving exact visual matching for EEG clips evoked by visual stimuli. Our EEGVis-CMR model maximizes mutual information between correct EEG-image pairs and demonstrates superior performance in both instance-level retrieval and semantic-level classification tasks. The approach overcomes limitations of supervised reconstruction methods and shows potential for handling open-set scenarios.

- *Unified Framework for Smart Aging*: These three approaches collectively provide a comprehensive framework for cognitive activity recognition that can be integrated into smart aging systems, offering multiple levels of cognitive monitoring and assistance capabilities.

7.1.4 Chapter Organization

The remainder of this chapter is organized as follows. Section 7.2 provides the background and related work on EEG-based brain-computer interfaces (BCIs), variational autoencoders and generative adversarial networks for semi-supervised learning, and cross-modal learning approaches. We also identify research gaps and opportunities specifically relevant to smart aging applications. Section 7.3 presents our EEG-based intention recognition approach, including the motivation and overview, detailed methodology for cascade and parallel convolutional recurrent networks, experimental evaluation on large-scale datasets, and comprehensive analysis of results in both laboratory and real-world BCI scenarios. Section 7.4 describes the adversarial variational embedding framework for robust semi-supervised learning, covering the motivation behind VAE++, the integration with semi-supervised GANs, experimental validation across multiple real-world applications, and performance comparisons with state-of-the-art methods. Section 7.5 introduces the self-supervised cross-modal visual retrieval approach, explaining the motivation for moving beyond reconstruction-based methods, the technical details of the EEGVis-CMR model, comprehensive empirical studies on EEG-visual datasets, and analysis of both quantitative and qualitative results. Finally, Sect. 7.6 provides an overall discussion of the three approaches, their complementary nature, implications for smart aging applications, and future research directions.

7.2 Background and Related Work

7.2.1 EEG-Based Brain-Computer Interfaces

The brain-computer interface (BCI) technology enables direct communication between the brain and external devices, offering tremendous potential for smart aging applications [1]. EEG-based BCIs are particularly promising due to their non-invasive nature and portability [46]. Traditional approaches to EEG-based intention recognition have relied heavily on handcrafted features and domain-specific preprocessing steps [42], which often require extensive expert knowledge and may miss critical information in the raw signals.

Recent advances in deep learning have shown promise for improving EEG signal analysis [23]. However, most existing deep learning approaches either focus on complex preprocessing steps, such as converting raw EEG signals to images [3], or neglect the subtle spatial and temporal information contained within EEG signals. The challenge of handling cross-subject and multi-class scenarios remains largely unaddressed, despite being crucial for real-world applications in smart aging environments.

7.2.2 *Semi-supervised Learning with Deep Generative Models*

Semi-supervised learning has gained significant attention in healthcare and aging-related applications where labeled data is scarce but unlabeled data are abundant. Variational Autoencoders (VAEs) have emerged as powerful tools for learning latent representations that can be used for both generation and classification tasks [21]. However, traditional VAEs suffer from the limitation that learned latent representations are stochastically sampled from prior distributions, making them non-exclusive for specific input samples.

Generative Adversarial Networks (GANs) have also shown promise in semi-supervised settings [30], but they typically generate samples from pre-defined distributions that are independent of input data distributions. This can obstruct convergence and makes it difficult to control the distribution of generated data. The combination of VAEs and GANs for semi-supervised learning remains an active area of research with significant potential for healthcare applications.

7.2.3 *Cross-Modal Learning and Neural Activity Decoding*

Cross-modal learning aims to understand relationships between different modalities of data, such as brain signals and visual stimuli. Traditional approaches to neural activity decoding have followed classification-then-generation procedures under supervised learning, which leads to several limitations. First, generative models cannot guarantee cross-modal alignment at the instance level. Second, the scope of generation is limited to fixed sets of visual classes, making novel classes challenging to handle.

Recent advances in contrastive learning, particularly inspired by models like CLIP, have shown promise for cross-modal tasks. However, the success of such approaches typically depends on large-scale datasets, which are often not available for human-centered EEG recognition tasks. The development of effective cross-modal learning approaches for brain-computer interfaces in low-data regimes remains an open challenge.

7.2.4 Research Gaps and Opportunities in Smart Aging

Despite significant progress in individual areas, several research gaps remain in applying cognitive activity recognition to smart aging:

- *Integration Challenges*: Current approaches often focus on single modalities or isolated techniques. There is a need for integrated frameworks that can combine EEG-based intention recognition, robust representation learning, and cross-modal understanding for comprehensive cognitive monitoring.
- *Adaptation to Aging Populations*: Most existing methods are developed and tested on young, healthy populations. The unique characteristics of aging brains, including changes in neural patterns and increased variability, require specialized approaches and validation.
- *Real-World Deployment*: Laboratory-based cognitive recognition systems often fail to translate to real-world smart aging environments due to environmental noise, user variability, and system integration challenges.
- *Personalization and Adaptability*: Smart aging systems need to adapt to individual users over time, accounting for progressive changes in cognitive abilities and personal preferences.

These gaps present significant opportunities for developing next-generation cognitive activity recognition systems that can truly benefit aging populations through improved monitoring, assistance, and quality of life enhancement.

7.3 EEG-Based Intention Recognition

7.3.1 Motivation

Brain-computer interface (BCI) technology enables direct communication between the brain and external devices, providing alternative pathways for individuals with motor disabilities or communication difficulties [46]. EEG-based BCIs are particularly promising due to their non-invasive nature and portability, making them suitable for practical deployment in smart aging environments [4, 34]. However, EEG-based systems face significant challenges including noise from physiological activities [17], ambiguous correlations between signals and intentions, and reliance on complex preprocessing [42, 49]. Most existing approaches either neglect spatial-temporal dependencies or require extensive domain expertise for feature engineering.

Our approach addresses these limitations by converting 1D EEG sequences to 2D spatial meshes that preserve correlations between brain regions, and employing unified end-to-end trainable models with cascade and parallel architectures. Experimental validation demonstrates 98.3% accuracy on large-scale datasets and 93% accuracy in real-world BCI scenarios, with significant improvements in cross-subject generalization.

7.3.2 *Spatio-Temporal Neural Network Architecture for EEG Processing*

Our approach addresses the challenges of intention recognition from EEG signals by converting traditional 1D EEG sequences to 2D spatial meshes and employing specialized neural network architectures to capture both spatial and temporal patterns [51]. This methodology is particularly relevant for smart aging applications where robust, real-time intention recognition can enable intuitive brain-computer interfaces for assistive technologies.

Converting 1D EEG Sequences to 2D EEG Meshes

The overall EEG data acquisition and preprocessing flowchart of our proposed method is shown in Fig. 7.1. The EEG based BCI system uses a wearable headset with multiple electrodes to capture the EEG signals. When a subject *imagines* performing a certain instruction, the electrodes of the headset acquire the fluctuations of the voltages from the scalp. The EEG electrode map in Fig. 7.1 depicts the electrodes placement of an example BCI headset. The electrode map varies from different BCI systems according to the different number of recording channels. The sensory readings from the EEG acquisition system represent time series data at the acquiring frequency. Typically, the raw data from EEG signal acquisition system at time index t is a one-dimensional (1D) data vector $\mathbf{r}_t = [s_t^1, s_t^2, s_t^i, \ldots, s_t^n]^T$, where s_t^i is the reading data of the ith electrode channel at time stamp t. The acquisition system totally contains n channels. For the observation period $[t, t+N]$, there are $(N+1)$ 1D data vectors, each of which contains n elements corresponding to n electrodes of the acquisition headset.

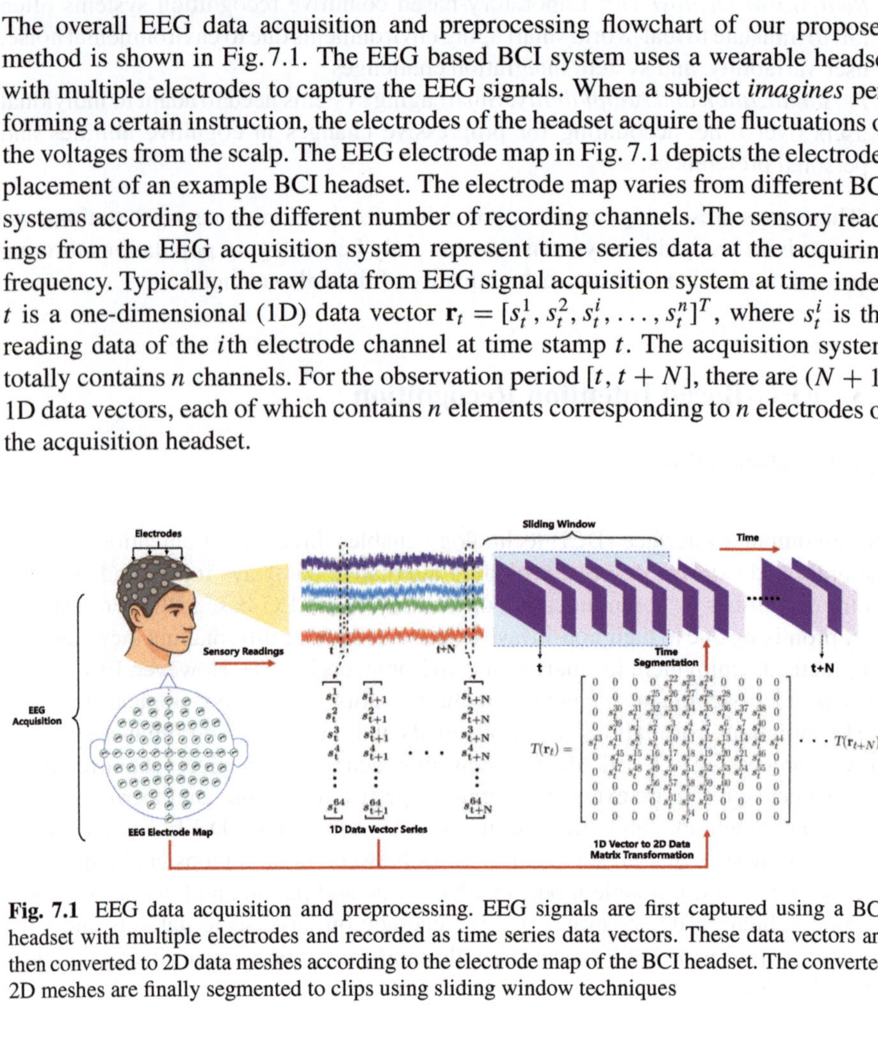

Fig. 7.1 EEG data acquisition and preprocessing. EEG signals are first captured using a BCI headset with multiple electrodes and recorded as time series data vectors. These data vectors are then converted to 2D data meshes according to the electrode map of the BCI headset. The converted 2D meshes are finally segmented to clips using sliding window techniques

The key innovation lies in converting these 1D vectors to 2D meshes according to the spatial electrode distribution. This transformation preserves the spatial relationships between brain regions, as different areas correspond to different cognitive activities. The transformation maps each electrode reading to its corresponding spatial position in a 2D mesh structure, with non-electrode positions padded with zeros.

After 2D mesh transformation, we apply sliding window segmentation to create clips with 50% overlap between consecutive segments. Each segment $\mathbf{S}_j = [\mathbf{m}_t, \mathbf{m}_{t+1}, \ldots, \mathbf{m}_{t+S-1}]$ contains S data meshes, where our goal is to recognize human intentions from these windowed segments.

Neural Network Architectures

We propose two complementary architectures: cascade and parallel convolutional recurrent networks, each designed to extract spatial and temporal features from EEG data.

Cascade Architecture: As illustrated in Fig. 7.2, this approach first extracts spatial features from each 2D mesh using a deep CNN, then processes the temporal sequence of spatial features through LSTM layers. The CNN applies three convolutional layers with kernel size 3×3, starting with 32 feature maps and doubling in each subsequent layer. A fully connected layer converts the final feature maps to spatial representations $\mathbf{f}_k$. The sequence of spatial features is then processed by two stacked LSTM layers to capture temporal dependencies, with only the final time step output used for classification.

Parallel Architecture: As shown in Fig. 7.3, this approach extracts spatial and temporal features concurrently. The CNN part processes 2D mesh segments similarly to the cascade model, while the RNN part processes the original 1D sequences. Spatial features from each time step are aggregated through summation, while temporal features come from the final LSTM output. The extracted features are fused through concatenation before final classification.

Both architectures employ dropout regularization and softmax classification to predict intention categories. The parallel approach offers computational advantages while the cascade approach provides more structured feature extraction, making them suitable for different deployment scenarios in smart aging applications.

7.3.3 *Experimental Evaluation and Implementation Results*

We evaluated our proposed models on both public datasets and real-world BCI data to demonstrate their effectiveness for intention recognition across different scenarios relevant to smart aging applications.

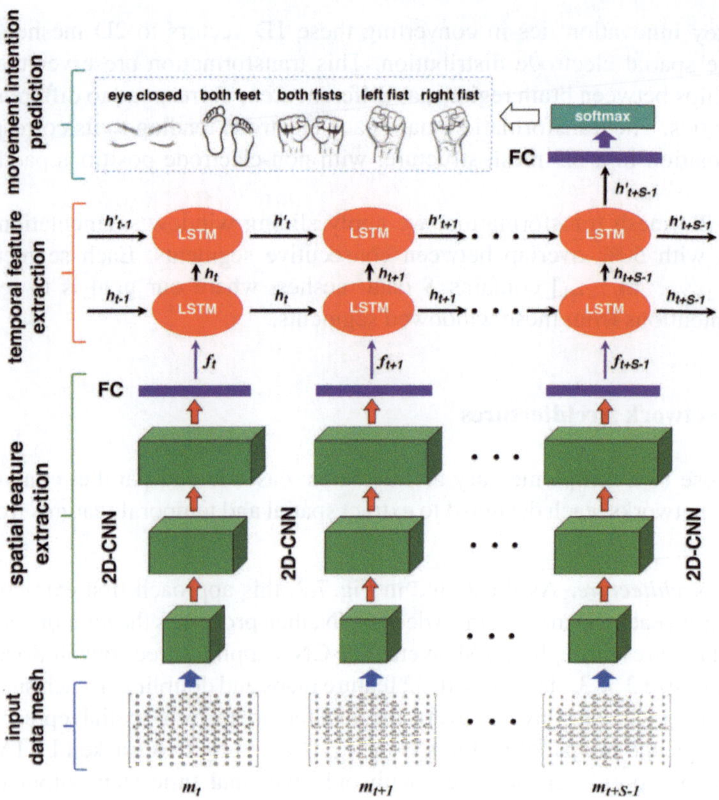

Fig. 7.2 Cascade convolutional recurrent neural network architecture. The 2D-CNN extracts spatial features from each EEG mesh, then LSTM processes the temporal sequence of spatial features for final intention classification

Dataset and Experimental Setup. Our evaluation utilized the PhysioNet EEG Motor Movement/Imagery Dataset [10], which contains EEG recordings from 109 subjects performing motor movement and imagery tasks. The dataset includes recordings with 64 electrode channels 160 Hz sampling rate [37], covering five brain activities: eye closed baseline, imagining moving both feet, both fists, left fist, and right fist. We focused on cross-subject multi-class scenarios to ensure robust generalization, which is crucial for practical BCI applications in smart aging contexts where individual variability is high.

All neural networks were implemented using TensorFlow and trained on GPU from scratch. We used stochastic gradient descent with Adam optimizer [20], learning rate of 10^{-4}, and dropout probability of 0.5. The 2D data meshes were transformed to size 10×11, with window size set to 10 for temporal segmentation.

Comparison with State-of-the-Art Methods. We compared our approaches against established methods including Support Vector Machines with Common Spatial Patterns [39], Filter Bank CSP approaches, Random Forest classifiers [19], and recent

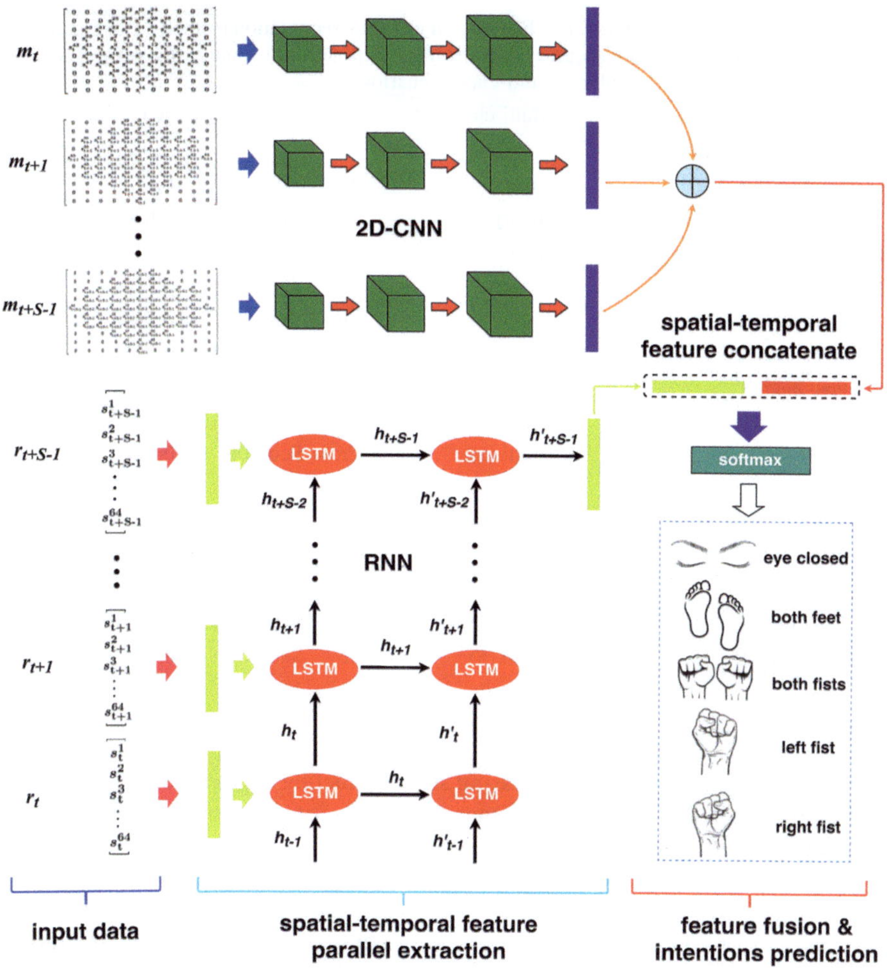

Fig. 7.3 Parallel recurrent convolutional neural network architecture. CNN and RNN extract spatial and temporal features concurrently, which are then fused for final classification. The concatenation operation is shown as an example fusion strategy

deep learning methods [44]. Table 7.1 summarizes the overall performance of our proposed models and comparison models. Both our cascade and parallel models achieve high accuracy near 98.3%, consistently outperforming state-of-the-art methods and baseline models across all evaluation metrics.

Notably, when compared with Bashivan et al.'s CNN-RNN approach [3], our method demonstrated approximately 18–30% improvement (from 69.68% to 98.35% for cascade and 98.28% for parallel models). This significant performance gain is likely due to our direct use of raw EEG data without lossy spectral feature extraction that can miss critical information in short-duration brain activities. Bashivan's

Table 7.1 Performance comparison of EEG-based intention recognition methods. Our cascade and parallel models achieve 98.3% accuracy, significantly outperforming state-of-the-art methods and baseline approaches in cross-subject multi-class scenarios

Method	Multi-class	Validation	Accuracy
State-of-the-art methods			
Major and Conrad 2017 [6]	Binary	Intra-Sub	0.72
Shenoy et al. 2015 [39]	Binary	Intra-Sub	0.8206
Pinheiro et al. 2016 [17]	Binary	Cross-Sub (10)	0.8505
Kim et al. 2016 [19]	Binary	Cross-Sub (105)	0.805
Zhang et al. 2017 [44]	Multi (5)	Cross-Sub (20)	0.794
Bashivan et al. 2016 [3]	Multi (5)	Cross-Sub (108)	0.6731
Baseline models			
1D-CNN	Multi (5)	Cross-Sub(108)	0.8622
2D-CNN	Multi (5)	Cross-Sub(108)	0.8841
3D-CNN	Multi (5)	Cross-Sub(108)	0.9238
RNN (64)	Multi (5)	Cross-Sub(108)	0.8493
RNN (16)	Multi (5)	Cross-Sub(108)	0.7468
Proposed methods			
Cascade model	Multi (5)	Cross-Sub (108)	**0.9831**
Parallel model	Multi (5)	Cross-Sub (108)	**0.9828**

method employs complex preprocessing steps extracting spectral features and converting them to 2D images, which may introduce compression artifacts and lose informative messages within raw signals.

Furthermore, our 3D-CNN baseline model also achieves competitive results (89.32% accuracy) compared to state-of-the-art approaches, demonstrating the effectiveness of incorporating spatial-temporal information. However, the 3D-CNN model only captures local temporal patterns through 3D convolutions, whereas our cascade and parallel models leverage global temporal dependencies through LSTM layers, resulting in superior performance.

Analysis of Spatial and Temporal Information. Systematic analysis using 1D-CNN, 2D-CNN, and 3D-CNN baseline models revealed that incorporating both spatial and temporal information is crucial for effective intention recognition. Our 2D mesh representation significantly outperformed traditional 1D approaches, while the combination of spatial CNN features with temporal RNN processing provided superior results compared to either modality alone. The results confirm that global temporal information captured by RNN components is more effective than local temporal patterns from 3D convolutions.

Architectural Variants and Ablation Studies. Investigation of different architectural configurations showed that three CNN layers and two RNN layers provide the optimal trade-off between performance and computational efficiency. Table 7.2 presents detailed performance comparisons of cascade model variants, demonstrating that: (1) Deeper CNN architectures (3-layer) consistently outperform shallower ones, improv-

Table 7.2 Performance comparison of cascade model architectural variants. The optimal configuration (3-layer CNN + FC + 2-layer RNN + FC) achieves 98.31% accuracy, demonstrating the importance of architectural depth and intermediate fully-connected layers

Architecture configuration	Accuracy	F1 score
1-layer CNN + FC + 2-layer RNN + FC	0.9310	0.9207
2-layer CNN + FC + 2-layer RNN + FC	0.9712	0.9676
3-layer CNN + FC + 2-layer RNN + FC	**0.9831**	**0.9804**
3-layer CNN + 2-layer RNN + FC (no FC between)	0.9217	0.9117
3-layer CNN + FC + 2-layer RNN (no final FC)	0.9801	0.9783
3-layer CNN + FC + 1-layer RNN + FC	0.9813	0.9791

Table 7.3 Performance comparison of parallel model fusion strategies. Simple concatenation of 3-layer CNN outputs achieves 98.28% accuracy, outperforming more complex fusion methods with additional processing layers

Architecture configuration	Fusion method	Accuracy	F1 score
1-layer CNN + FC + RNN	Concatenation	0.9487	0.9432
2-layer CNN + FC + RNN	Concatenation	0.9727	0.9697
3-layer CNN + FC + RNN	**Concatenation**	**0.9828**	**0.9810**
3-layer CNN + FC + RNN	Summation	0.9813	0.9792
3-layer CNN + FC + RNN	Concatenation + FC	0.9696	0.9661
3-layer CNN + FC + RNN	Concatenation + Conv	0.9666	0.9626

ing accuracy from 93.10 to 98.31%; (2) The fully-connected layer between CNN and RNN components is essential - removing it causes performance to drop to 92.17%; (3) Two-layer RNN provides optimal temporal modeling capacity.

For the parallel model, we examined different fusion strategies including concatenation, summation, and additional processing layers after fusion. Table 7.3 shows that basic fusion methods (concatenation and summation) achieve excellent results with accuracy higher than 98%, demonstrating that simple fusion approaches are sufficient when individual spatial and temporal components are well-designed. The best parallel model uses 3-layer CNN branches with direct concatenation, achieving 98.28% accuracy without requiring complex fusion mechanisms.

The experimental results confirm that our spatio-temporal approach effectively handles the inherent challenges of EEG-based intention recognition, including cross-subject variability and environmental noise, making it well-suited for deployment in real-world assistive technologies for aging populations.

7.3.4 Summary of EEG-Based Intention Recognition

The spatio-temporal representation approach demonstrates significant advantages for EEG-based intention recognition in practical cross-subject and multi-class scenarios.

The two unified end-to-end trainable deep learning models effectively handle both movement intention and instruction intention recognition tasks. Experimental validation on both public datasets and real-world BCI data confirms the effectiveness and feasibility of these models across diverse human intentions and various EEG recording resolutions.

The systematic investigation of model variants and the influence of spatio-temporal information provides valuable insights for practical BCI system development. This approach represents an important step toward accurate human intention recognition for smart aging applications, offering robust performance under realistic conditions with reduced electrode counts and environmental noise.

7.4 Adversarial Variational Embedding

7.4.1 Motivation

Semi-supervised learning is crucial for smart aging applications where labeled data is often scarce and expensive to acquire [9]. Traditional approaches using Variational Autoencoders (VAEs) and semi-supervised Generative Adversarial Networks (GANs) face critical limitations: VAE-learned latent codes are non-exclusive due to stochastic sampling [28], creating consistency issues for classification tasks, while GAN models generate data from pre-defined distributions independent of input data [30], leading to convergence difficulties.

To address these challenges, we propose the Adversarial Variational Embedding (AVAE) framework that combines VAE++ with semi-supervised GANs [53]. The key innovation is VAE++, which produces exclusive latent codes for reliable classification while providing meaningful prior distributions for GAN generators. This approach is particularly suitable for cognitive activity recognition in smart aging contexts where consistent and reliable assessments are essential.

Experimental validation across four real-world applications demonstrates superior performance over state-of-the-art methods, confirming the effectiveness of combining exclusive latent representations with adversarial training for semi-supervised learning scenarios.

7.4.2 AVAE Framework: Integrating VAE++ with Semi-supervised GANs

The AVAE framework addresses the challenge of learning exclusive latent representations for semi-supervised classification by combining a modified VAE (VAE++) with a semi-supervised GAN in a unified framework.

Problem Formulation. Consider a dataset with labeled samples and unlabeled samples, where our goal is to learn effective latent representations that enable accurate classification even with limited labeled data.

VAE++ Architecture. Traditional VAE learns latent representations through stochastic sampling, creating non-exclusive representations that vary across different runs for the same input. VAE++ addresses this limitation by introducing an exclusive latent code that is deterministically computed from input data through an encoder network. As illustrated in Fig. 7.4, while standard VAE relies solely on stochastically sampled representations that are non-repeatable, VAE++ generates both exclusive and stochastic representations, enabling reliable classification performance.

The exclusive code is used to generate the traditional stochastic representation, which is then processed by the decoder for reconstruction. The VAE++ loss combines reconstruction error and KL divergence to maintain the generative properties while ensuring exclusive latent codes.

Adversarial Training. The semi-supervised GAN component treats the exclusive latent code as "real" and the generated representation as "fake". The discriminator performs both adversarial classification (real vs. fake) and semantic classification using both labeled and unlabeled data. For labeled inputs, the supervised loss encourages correct class prediction, while for unlabeled inputs, the unsupervised loss focuses on real/fake discrimination.

This dual training objective encourages the VAE++ to learn more robust and informative latent codes, as illustrated in the complete AVAE architecture shown in Fig. 7.5. The framework enables effective semi-supervised learning by leveraging both generative modeling capabilities and adversarial training dynamics, making it particularly suitable for smart aging applications with limited labeled data.

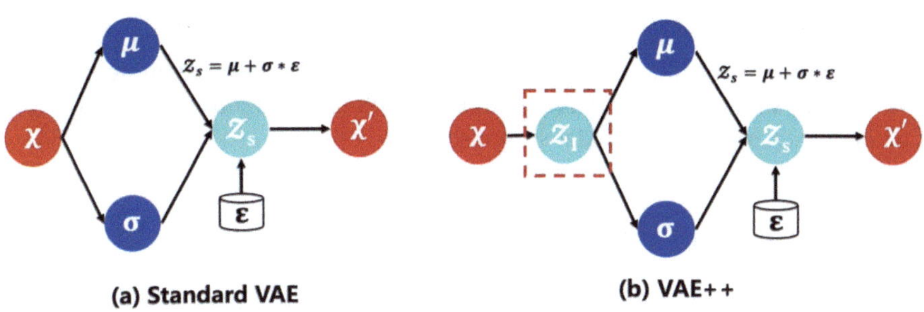

Fig. 7.4 Comparison of the standard VAE and the proposed VAE++. **x** and **x**′ denote the input and the reconstructed data. μ and σ denote the learned expectation and standard deviation, z_s denotes the stochastically sampled latent representation which is composed by μ, σ, and ε, where ε is randomly sampled from $\mathcal{N}(0, 1)$. In standard VAE, z_s is regarded as the learned representation while, in VAE++, z_I denotes the proposed exclusive latent representation which can be used for classification

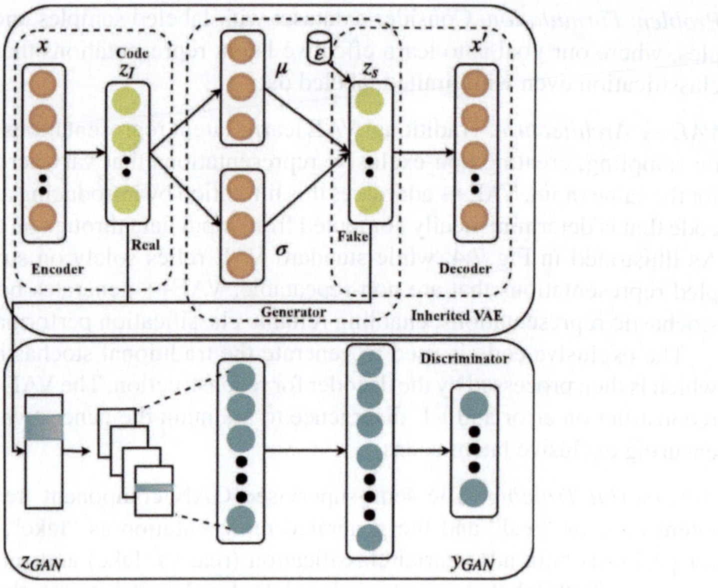

Fig. 7.5 The detailed architecture of the proposed Adversarial Variational Embedding (AVAE) framework. The framework integrates VAE++ with a semi-supervised GAN, where the encoder generates exclusive latent codes for classification and stochastic representations for reconstruction. The discriminator performs both adversarial training (distinguishing real from generated representations) and semantic classification, enabling effective semi-supervised learning with limited labeled data

7.4.3 Experimental Evaluation Results

We evaluated the AVAE framework across four different application domains to demonstrate its versatility and effectiveness in semi-supervised learning scenarios relevant to smart aging: activity recognition, neurological diagnosis [33], image classification [11], and recommender systems.

Experimental Setup

Our evaluation employed standardized datasets including PAMAP2 for activity recognition (containing IMU sensor data from 9 participants performing 5 common activities), TUH for neurological diagnosis (EEG data for epileptic seizure detection from 18 subjects), MNIST for image classification (handwritten digits), and Yelp for recommender systems (restaurant rating predictions). All experiments used a Leave-One-Subject-Out strategy where applicable, with supervision rates varying from 20 to 100% to evaluate semi-supervised performance.

Baseline Comparisons

We compared AVAE against two categories of state-of-the-art methods: (1) algorithm-related approaches including M2 [21], Adversarial Autoencoders (AAE) [25], Ladder Variational Autoencoders (LVAE) [43], Auxiliary Deep Generative Models (ADGM) [24], semi-supervised GAN (SGAN) [30], CatGAN [41], kernel-based methods [47], and virtual adversarial training [27]; and (2) application-specific state-of-the-art methods for each domain. Additionally, we conducted ablation studies comparing the standard VAE, VAE++, with our complete AVAE framework.

Key Results and Analysis

Table 7.4 presents the comprehensive performance comparison on the PAMAP2 activity recognition dataset. The experimental results demonstrate consistent superior performance of AVAE across all supervision rates. At 60% supervision rate, AVAE achieved 84.91% accuracy, outperforming all algorithm-related state-of-the-art methods (M2, AAE, LVAE, ADGM) and application-specific state-of-the-art approaches (achieving 79.63–82.49% accuracy). This represents approximately 5% improvement over standard VAE (79.63%) and 3% over VAE++ (81.94%).

The ablation studies confirmed that each component, particularly the adversarial training mechanism (GAN), contributes significantly to performance enhancement. The proposed latent layer z_I and adversarial training between the discriminator and VAE++ effectively encourages the model to learn and refine informative latent representations. Notably, VAE using only the stochastic mean (μ) performs significantly worse (67.85% at 60% supervision), confirming the necessity of the exclusive latent code design. The performance progressively improves from standard VAE to VAE++ to the complete AVAE framework, demonstrating the value of each architectural innovation.

To further understand the learned representations, Fig. 7.6 visualizes the latent features using t-SNE dimensionality reduction on the PAMAP2 dataset. The visualization clearly demonstrates the progressive improvement in feature quality: standard VAE produces overlapping clusters with poor class separation, VAE++ achieves moderate separability, while the complete AVAE framework generates highly discriminative features with distinct class boundaries. This visual evidence corroborates the quantitative performance improvements and validates the effectiveness of the exclusive latent code design combined with adversarial training.

Table 7.4 Overall comparison of semi-supervised classification accuracy (%) on activity recognition. All the baselines and our approach are working on the same dataset and sharing the same experiment settings for each specific application

Dataset	Rate (%)	Algorithm-related State-of-the-art				Application-related State-of-the-art				Ablation Study			Ours AVAE
		M2	AAE	LVAE	ADGM	[5]	[22]	[13]	[52]	VAE (μ)	VAE	VAE++	
Activity Recognition (PAMAP2)	20	64.83±0.16	63.67±0.23	69.82±0.69	67.31±0.45	72.31±0.16	70.95±0.08	67.31±0.14	76.68±0.31	58.43±0.13	76.51±0.53	78.12±0.55	78.63±0.38
	40	68.55±0.23	76.83±0.25	76.43±0.19	75.21±0.38	80.51±0.24	75.38±0.12	77.28±0.21	80.15±0.16	62.74±0.15	76.78±0.22	80.88±0.58	81.37±0.29
	60	72.35±0.21	77.39±0.19	78.69±0.27	79.34±0.29	80.29±0.21	76.89±0.05	79.69±0.15	82.49±0.33	67.85±0.08	79.63±0.29	81.94±0.19	84.91±0.17
	80	75.88±0.35	78.28±0.11	81.44±0.23	80.38±0.16	82.12±0.16	79.59±0.18	81.65±0.09	83.56±0.11	73.43±0.06	81.75±0.17	82.08±0.26	85.36±0.21
	100	77.59±0.17	80.79±0.14	84.39±0.18	83.66±0.16	83.64±0.17	81.96±0.11	82.38±0.13	84.59±0.24	76.85±0.06	82.37±0.25	83.29±0.18	86.41±0.06

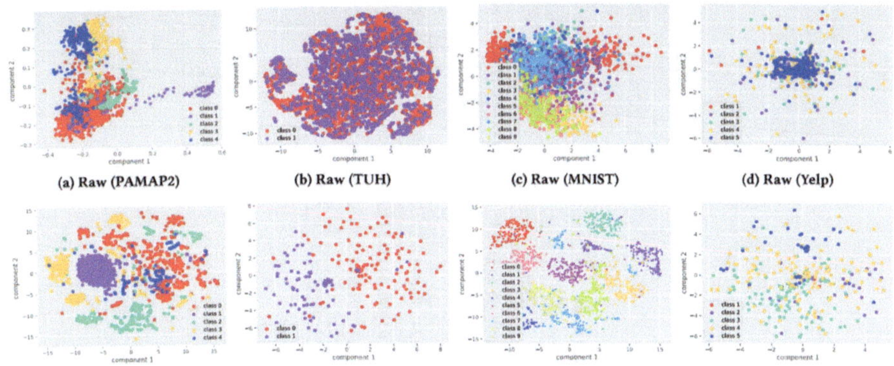

(a) Raw (PAMAP2) (b) Raw (TUH) (c) Raw (MNIST) (d) Raw (Yelp)

(e) Learned feature (PAMAP2) (f) Learned feature (TUH) (g) Learned feature (MNIST) (h) Learned feature (Yelp)

Fig. 7.6 t-SNE visualization of learned feature representations on the PAMAP2 dataset at 60% supervision rate. **a** Features learned by standard VAE show significant overlap between activity classes, indicating poor discriminability. **b** VAE++ produces more separable clusters with reduced inter-class confusion. **c** Complete AVAE framework generates highly discriminative and well-separated feature spaces, with clear boundaries between different activity classes. Each color represents one of five activity classes (lying, sitting, standing, walking, running), demonstrating AVAE's superior ability to learn exclusive latent representations for classification

Application Domain Evaluations

We further evaluated AVAE across four diverse application domains to demonstrate its versatility:

- *Neurological Diagnosis*: Table 7.5 presents the comprehensive comparison on the TUH dataset [29] for epileptic seizure detection (18 subjects, 22 channels, 250 Hz). Our AVAE approach outperforms all competitive baselines across all supervision rates. At 60% supervision level, AVAE achieves the highest accuracy of 95.21%, which represents approximately 4% improvement over algorithm-related state-of-the-art methods (76.32–87.65%) and application-specific approaches including hybrid deep learning [54] (91.28%), filter bank-based methods [15] (92.58%), deep ConvNets [38] (85.36%), and statistical models [12] (90.38%). The approach effectively distinguishes between normal and seizure states, with some misclassification occurring at seizure onset/termination phases where symptoms resemble normal activity.
- *Image Classification*: On the MNIST dataset (handwritten digits), AVAE demonstrated superior performance across all supervision rates, achieving accuracies from 95.12% at 20% supervision to 99.85% at 100% supervision. The results confirm the framework's ability to learn discriminative features through joint training of VAE++ and semi-supervised GAN.
- *Recommender Systems*: Applied to restaurant rating prediction using the Yelp dataset (192,609 businesses, 1,637,138 users), AVAE showed consistent improvements with accuracies from 70.19% to 79.98% across different supervision levels,

Table 7.5 Overall comparison of semi-supervised classification accuracy (%) on neurological diagnosis

Dataset	Rate (%)	Algorithm-related State-of-the-art				Application-related state-of-the-art				Ablation study			Ours ΛVAE
		M2	AAE	LVAE	ADGM	[54]	[15]	[38]	[12]	VAE (μ)	VAE	VAE++	
Neurological Diagnosis (TUH)	20	71.28±0.16	80.13±0.95	82.51±0.19	86.32±0.12	87.66±0.23	86.58±0.36	82.19±0.24	86.33±0.21	80.58±0.69	86.37±0.24	86.86±0.53	93.69±0.18
	40	75.52±0.16	82.95±0.26	84.58±0.16	86.99±0.05	89.25±0.19	91.58±0.35	84.21±0.08	89.23±0.34	81.55±0.24	89.69±0.27	91.28±0.25	94.32±0.28
	60	76.32±0.29	86.21±0.32	87.51±0.26	87.65±0.16	91.28±0.37	92.58±0.26	85.36±0.32	90.38±0.24	82.59±0.03	90.84±0.27	92.87±0.31	95.21±0.21
	80	79.65±0.37	88.53±0.28	89.56±0.25	88.05±0.12	92.59±0.26	93.25±0.31	85.16±0.24	91.59±0.16	83.21±0.21	91.69±0.25	93.96±0.28	97.86±0.26
	100	82.59±0.31	89.58±0.25	90.25±0.21	88.65±0.26	93.52±0.18	94.29±0.25	86.42±0.26	92.44±0.25	84.21±0.65	92.38±0.41	94.65±0.24	98.13±0.32

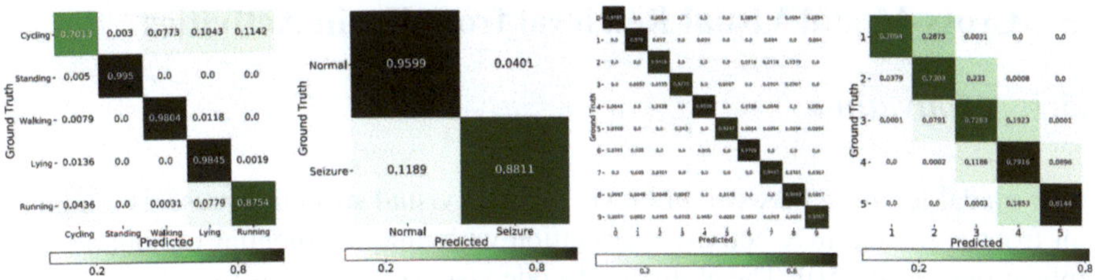

(a) Confusion matrix of PAMAP2 (b) Confusion matrix of TUH (c) Confusion matrix of MNIST (d) Confusion matrix of Yelp

Fig. 7.7 Confusion matrices of AVAE performance across four application domains at 60% supervision rate. **a** Activity Recognition (PAMAP2): 5 activities with high inter-class discrimination, primary confusion between standing and sitting. **b** Neurological Diagnosis (TUH): Binary classification achieving 95.21% accuracy with minimal confusion. **c** Image Classification (MNIST): 10 digit classes showing strong diagonal patterns with minor confusions between visually similar digits (e.g., 4–9, 3–5). **d** Recommender Systems (Yelp): 5-level rating prediction demonstrating consistent performance across rating categories

outperforming both semi-supervised algorithms and content-based recommendation methods including cosine similarity-based approaches [32], factorization machines [35], and deep neural network enhanced FM methods [16].

- *Activity Recognition*: On the PAMAP2 dataset (IMU sensor data from 9 participants), AVAE achieved 84.91% accuracy at 60% supervision rate, representing approximately 5% improvement over standard VAE and 3% over VAE++.

As visualized in Fig. 7.7, the confusion matrices across all four domains demonstrate AVAE's strong classification performance and generalization capability across diverse semi-supervised learning scenarios.

7.4.4 Summary of Adversarial Variational Embedding

We presented an effective and robust semi-supervised latent representation framework, AVAE, by proposing a modified VAE model and integration with generative adversarial networks. The VAE++ and GAN share the same generator. In order to automatically learn the exclusive latent code, in the VAE++, we explore the latent code's posterior distribution and then stochastically generate a latent representation based on the posterior distribution. The discrepancy between the learned exclusive latent code and the generated latent representation is constrained by semi-supervised GAN. The latent code of AVAE is finally served as the learned feature for classification. The proposed approach is evaluated on four real-world applications and the results demonstrate the effectiveness and robustness of it.

7.5 Cross-Modal Visual Retrieval from Brain Activities

7.5.1 *Motivation*

Cross-modal learning between brain signals and visual stimuli represents a significant frontier in cognitive activity recognition with unique potential for smart aging applications [7, 40, 50]. The ability to decode visual experiences from brain signals could revolutionize assistive technologies for aging populations with communication difficulties or motor impairments.

Traditional approaches follow supervised classification-then-generation frameworks [18, 31, 45], using EEG signals to reconstruct visual stimuli. However, these reconstruction-based methods learn mappings between modality distributions but fail to reproduce exact visual stimuli that evoked the brain activity. This limitation is problematic for applications requiring precise understanding of cognitive states and visual experiences.

The fundamental problem is that image generation relies on semantic classes rather than actual visual content [26, 36], as illustrated in Fig. 7.8a. For instance, if

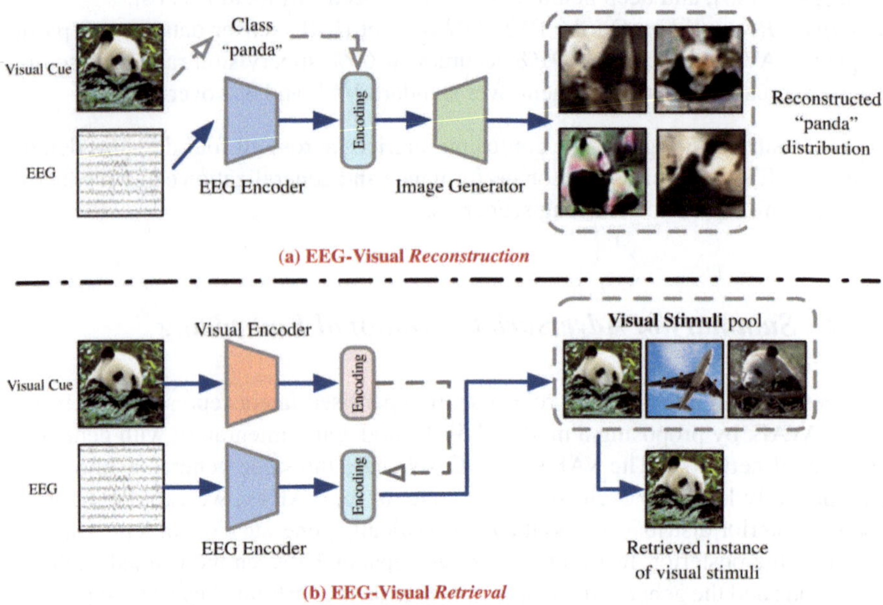

Fig. 7.8 Conceptual comparison between reconstruction-based and retrieval-based approaches for EEG-visual correspondence. **a** Traditional reconstruction methods generate category-level images based on semantic classes, producing generic representations that may differ significantly from the actual viewed stimulus. **b** Our proposed retrieval approach directly identifies and returns the exact visual stimulus from a candidate set by maximizing mutual information between EEG encodings and visual features, enabling instance-level correspondence without requiring class labels

a subject views a specific image while EEG is recorded, existing models can only generate generic category images, not the exact viewed stimulus.

To address these limitations, we propose a self-supervised cross-modal retrieval paradigm that seeks instance-level alignment by maximizing mutual information between EEG encodings and visual stimuli [48]. Our EEGVis-CMR model offers three key advantages: (1) exact visual stimulus retrieval without class information access, (2) higher-quality outputs through direct retrieval rather than generation [2], and (3) enhanced open-set recognition capabilities crucial for real-world applications where novel visual experiences are common.

7.5.2 EEGVis-CMR: Self-supervised Cross-Modal Learning Framework

Our EEGVis-CMR approach addresses the limitations of reconstruction-based methods by formulating EEG-visual correspondence as a self-supervised retrieval problem. Instead of generating images from EEG signals, we maximize mutual information between EEG encodings and their corresponding visual stimuli through contrastive learning. The framework comprises three key components: dual-modal encoding, self-supervised contrastive learning, and instance-level retrieval optimization.

Framework Architecture and Processing Pipeline

Given N paired EEG-image tuples as input, EEGVis-CMR employs a dual-encoder architecture to extract modality-specific features. The framework operates through four sequential stages: (1) feature extraction using domain-specific encoders for both EEG signals and visual stimuli, (2) transformation into joint multi-modal representations via learned projection matrices, (3) optimization of a shared latent space where paired EEG-visual encodings are drawn together while non-paired encodings are pushed apart, and (4) instance-level retrieval through similarity comparison in the learned representation space.

The core innovation lies in creating a shared latent representation space optimized with respect to an instance-level discriminative objective. This enables direct comparison between any EEG encoding and visual encoding to derive model predictions, as illustrated in Fig. 7.9. Unlike reconstruction-based approaches that require complex generative models, our retrieval paradigm achieves superior performance through simplified training objectives and direct instance matching.

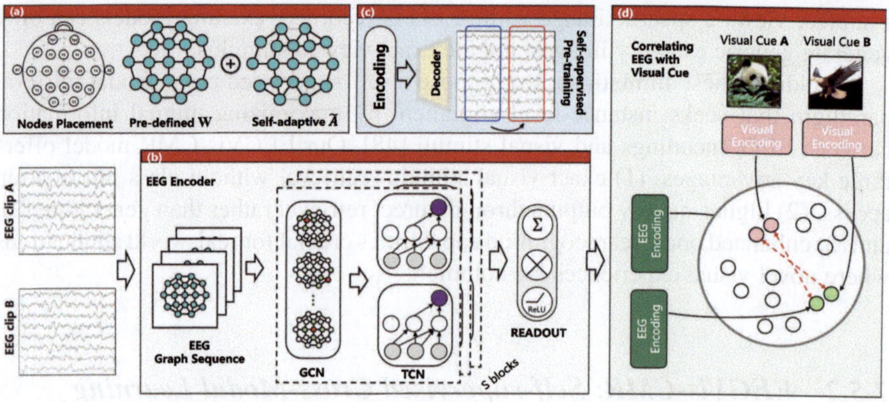

Fig. 7.9 EEGVis-CMR framework architecture. **a** EEG sensor placement following the 10–20 international system with pre-defined adjacency matrix W and self-adaptive adjacency $\tilde{\mathbf{A}}$. **b** Temporal Graph Convolution Network for EEG encoding that processes signal clips and generates corresponding EEG representations. **c** Self-supervised pre-training module that predicts future T' timesteps from historical T signal measurements. **d** Contrastive learning mechanism that correlates EEG and visual encodings by maximizing mutual information between correct EEG-image pairs

Dual-Modal Encoding Architecture

Visual Feature Encoder. We employ pre-trained convolutional neural networks (AlexNet, ResNet, or Vision Transformer) to extract hierarchical visual representations, leveraging transfer learning from large-scale image datasets [36]. The CNN features are projected into the joint representation space via learned linear transformations.

EEG Signal Encoder. The EEG encoder utilizes Temporal Graph Convolution Networks (TGCN) to capture both spatial correlations among electrode channels and temporal dependencies across time sequences. The TGCN models EEG signals as an undirected weighted graph where nodes represent electrode channels and edges encode spatial relationships.

We incorporate both pre-defined adjacency matrices based on physical electrode placement following the 10–20 system and self-adaptive adjacency matrices that learn dynamic brain connectivity patterns from data. The spatial graph features are processed through gated temporal convolution layers to capture long-range temporal dependencies while maintaining computational efficiency. Channel-wise attention mechanisms enable selective emphasis on relevant electrode contributions during different cognitive states.

Contrastive Learning Optimization

To establish correspondence between EEG and visual modalities, we employ a contrastive learning objective that maximizes mutual information between correctly paired EEG-image tuples. Both EEG and visual encodings are projected into a shared multi-modal representation space using learned projection matrices. The contrastive loss function encourages high similarity for positive pairs while minimizing similarity with negative samples within each training batch.

The framework incorporates a mixup-based augmentation strategy specifically designed for EEG signals to improve robustness in low-data regimes typical of neuroimaging studies. This augmentation combines each EEG clip with both ground-truth data from other clips and predicted future timesteps from a self-supervised pre-trained EEG autoencoder, enhancing model generalization across diverse cognitive patterns.

Self-supervised Pre-training

To enhance EEG representation learning, we implement a self-supervised pre-training strategy where the EEG encoder learns to predict future signal timesteps from historical measurements. This temporal prediction task provides task-agnostic supervision that helps the encoder develop robust EEG representations transferable to downstream cross-modal retrieval objectives. The pre-training phase operates independently of visual modality, enabling the EEG encoder to capture intrinsic temporal patterns and brain dynamics before fine-tuning on the cross-modal correspondence task.

7.5.3 Experimental Evaluation and Implementation Results

We conducted comprehensive experiments to evaluate the effectiveness of our EEGVis-CMR approach across different scenarios and compared it with state-of-the-art reconstruction-based methods. Our evaluation focuses on both instance-level retrieval accuracy and semantic-level classification performance.

Datasets: We used the largest publicly-accessible single-subject EEG dataset measuring brain activity evoked by visual stimuli, containing 40,000 images and corresponding EEG segments. The visual cues from ImageNet belong to 40 classes (1000 images each), with EEG recorded using 96 channels 4096 Hz for two seconds per stimulus.

Evaluation Protocols: We examined EEGVis-CMR with two protocols: (1) instance-level EEG-visual retrieval measuring exact image retrieval capability, and (2) semantic-level classification. Performance metrics included mean Reciprocal Rank (MRR) and mean Average Precision (mAP) for retrieval tasks.

Table 7.6 Quantitative results of EEGVis-CMR and comparison methods [8, 14] on EEG-visual retrieval. For visual encoder variants, AN and RN indicate AlexNet and ResNet-50, respectively. We report the performance difference obtained with pre-training the EEG encoder. Mean and std are from 5-fold cross-validation with the same random seed. The best results are **bolded**. The subscripts indicate the p-value from pairwise Welch's t-test for statistical significance ($p \leq 0.05$)

Metric	AN	RN	RNN	CNN	w/o pre	[8]	[14]	Ours (w/o mixup)	Ours (Full)
MRR ($\times 10^2$)	25.82 ± 0.82	31.26 ± 1.25	27.55 ± 0.77	28.86 ± 0.83	32.79 $\pm 1.65_{(0.02)}$	23.29 $\pm 0.83_{(0.00)}$	17.83 $\pm 2.01_{(0.00)}$	35.59 $\pm 0.87_{(0.01)}$	**38.13 ± 1.87**
mAP ($\times 10^2$)	11.93 ± 0.26	14.54 ± 0.39	12.52 ± 0.23	13.15 ± 0.33	15.68 $\pm 0.58_{(0.00)}$	11.25 $\pm 0.31_{(0.00)}$	8.96 $\pm 0.27_{(0.00)}$	16.49 $\pm 0.37_{(0.00)}$	**17.58 ± 0.25**

Instance-Level Retrieval Performance: Table 7.6 presents comprehensive quantitative comparisons of EEGVis-CMR and state-of-the-art contrastive learning approaches on EEG-visual retrieval. Our full EEGVis-CMR framework achieved the best performance with MRR of 38.13% and mAP of 17.58%, significantly outperforming existing contrastive learning methods (MRR: 23.29 and 17.83%) and demonstrating superior retrieval capability. The model showed consistent trends across variants—configurations achieving higher MRR also produced higher mAP values, confirming the effectiveness of the contrastive self-supervised framework for EEG-vision cross-modality learning.

Pre-training of EEG encoders proved empirically effective, as shown in the performance comparison with and without pre-training steps in Table 7.6. The full EEGVis-CMR model with mixup augmentation outperformed the variant without mixup (MRR: 35.59% vs. 38.13%), demonstrating the benefit of data augmentation strategies for this task.

Encoder Impact Analysis: The results in Table 7.6 reveal that more powerful visual encoders led to improved performance. ResNet-50 (RN) achieved MRR of 31.26% and mAP of 14.54%, significantly outperforming AlexNet (AN) with 25.82 and 11.93% respectively, given they share the same EEG encoder. This confirms that visual encodings play a crucial role as factual supervision to EEG encodings—more discriminative visual representations enable better cross-modal learning despite introducing more noise than ground truth semantic labels.

For EEG encoders, the GNN-based TGCN approach (28.86% MRR) proved more effective than RNN (27.55%) and CNN (included in variants) architectures. The TGCN encoder successfully incorporates non-Euclidean structures, dynamic connectivity, and long-range temporal dependencies, demonstrating superior capability for EEG signal modeling in this cross-modal learning task.

The comprehensive ablation studies visualized in Fig. 7.10 systematically validate the contribution of each component in the EEGVis-CMR framework, confirming the design choices for both encoder architectures and training strategies.

Semantic-Level Classification: Table 7.7 presents semantic-level EEG-visual classification results across 40 visual classes (39 closed-set + 1 open-set). EEGVis-CMR

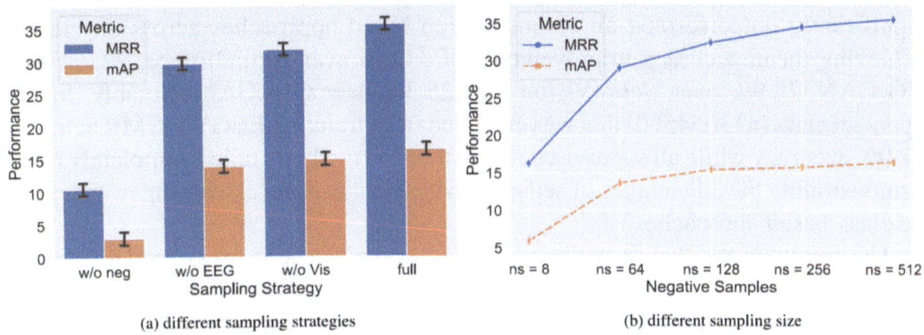

Fig. 7.10 Ablation studies of EEGVis-CMR components on EEG-visual retrieval performance. **a** Impact of different visual encoder architectures: ResNet-50 significantly outperforms AlexNet in both MRR and mAP metrics, demonstrating the importance of discriminative visual features. **b** Impact of different EEG encoder architectures: TGCN (GNN-based) achieves superior performance compared to RNN and CNN encoders by effectively modeling spatial-temporal EEG patterns. **c** Effect of pre-training: Models with EEG encoder pre-training show consistent improvements over non-pretrained variants. **d** Effect of data augmentation: Full model with mixup augmentation achieves the highest performance, validating the effectiveness of data augmentation strategies for cross-modal learning

Table 7.7 The EEG-visual classification results on representative visual classes. The first 9 classes are evaluated under a closed-set setting, whereas the last class (n13054560) is left for open-set recognition. Results are from 5 different evaluation splits. EEGVis-CMR significantly outperforms reconstruction-based approaches, especially demonstrating superior open-set recognition capability

Visual Class	Brain2Image	VG-GAN	NeuroVision	CapsGAN	EEGVis-CMR
n02106662	0.029 ± 0.018	0.163 ± 0.025	0.058 ± 0.034	0.099 ± 0.024	$\mathbf{0.395 \pm 0.124}$
n02124075	0.091 ± 0.012	0.220 ± 0.032	0.162 ± 0.104	0.203 ± 0.025	$\mathbf{0.617 \pm 0.211}$
n02510455	0.181 ± 0.067	0.238 ± 0.119	0.274 ± 0.033	0.283 ± 0.062	$\mathbf{0.565 \pm 0.137}$
n02690373	0.227 ± 0.052	0.433 ± 0.052	0.327 ± 0.126	0.358 ± 0.078	$\mathbf{0.606 \pm 0.086}$
n03590841	0.773 ± 0.041	0.907 ± 0.069	0.775 ± 0.066	0.836 ± 0.067	$\mathbf{0.597 \pm 0.104}$
n03773504	0.152 ± 0.024	0.203 ± 0.056	0.228 ± 0.031	0.257 ± 0.031	$\mathbf{0.616 \pm 0.093}$
n07753592	0.775 ± 0.056	0.554 ± 0.069	0.763 ± 0.080	0.613 ± 0.041	$\mathbf{0.894 \pm 0.049}$
n07873807	0.371 ± 0.026	0.347 ± 0.040	0.316 ± 0.099	0.375 ± 0.056	$\mathbf{0.631 \pm 0.095}$
n11939491	0.206 ± 0.059	0.348 ± 0.092	0.285 ± 0.044	0.302 ± 0.083	$\mathbf{0.606 \pm 0.203}$
Open-set Recognition (unseen during training)					
n13054560	0.000 ± 0.000	0.000 ± 0.000	0.000 ± 0.000	0.000 ± 0.000	$\mathbf{0.179 \pm 0.096}$

significantly outperformed all reconstruction-based approaches across all classes, achieving mean accuracy improvements of 34.6% over Brain2Image, 22.7% over VG-GAN, 28.9% over NeuroVision, and 25.3% over CapsGAN. Notably, for the open-set class (n13054560) that was excluded from training, EEGVis-CMR achieved 17.9% accuracy while all supervised reconstruction methods failed completely (0%), demonstrating the advantages of self-supervised instance-level learning over semantic class-based approaches.

The results reveal that visual features play a crucial role in cross-modal learning. Approaches incorporating visual features (VG-GAN, CapsGAN) outperformed those relying solely on class supervision (Brain2Image, NeuroVision) by 6.2–11.2%. However, EEGVis-CMR's self-supervised instance-level learning approach proved most effective, retrieving true visual cues instead of synthesizing approximate images.

Qualitative Assessment: Comparison with reconstruction-based approaches (Brain2Image, VG-GAN, NeuroVision) demonstrated that while reconstruction methods synthesize distinguishable images belonging to correct visual classes, none produce images identical to actual stimuli. EEGVis-CMR directly retrieves exact paired images without requiring complex image generator training. The open-set recognition capability is particularly noteworthy—supervised reconstruction methods cannot generate images outside training classes, while EEGVis-CMR's contrastive learning framework creates a multi-modal representation space enabling retrieval based on instance-level similarity rather than predefined semantic classes.

As illustrated in Fig. 7.11, the qualitative comparison visually demonstrates the fundamental advantage of retrieval over reconstruction: while generation-based approaches produce class-consistent but instance-different outputs, our retrieval approach successfully identifies and returns the exact visual stimuli that evoked the recorded brain activity.

7.5.4 *Summary of Cross-Modal Visual Retrieval*

The self-supervised cross-modal visual retrieval approach offers significant advantages over traditional reconstruction-based methods for EEG-visual tasks. Our EEGVis-CMR framework demonstrates that retrieval paradigms can achieve superior performance through simpler training objectives, higher-quality outputs, and enhanced generalization capabilities.

Key Advantages: The retrieval approach provides three main benefits: (1) simplified training objectives that avoid the instability and complexity of adversarial generation; (2) high-quality outputs through direct retrieval of real visual instances rather than synthesized approximations; and (3) enhanced open-set recognition capabilities that enable handling of unseen visual classes without explicit semantic supervision.

Limitations and Future Directions: The primary limitation is the requirement for visual stimulus databases during inference, which may restrict deployment in

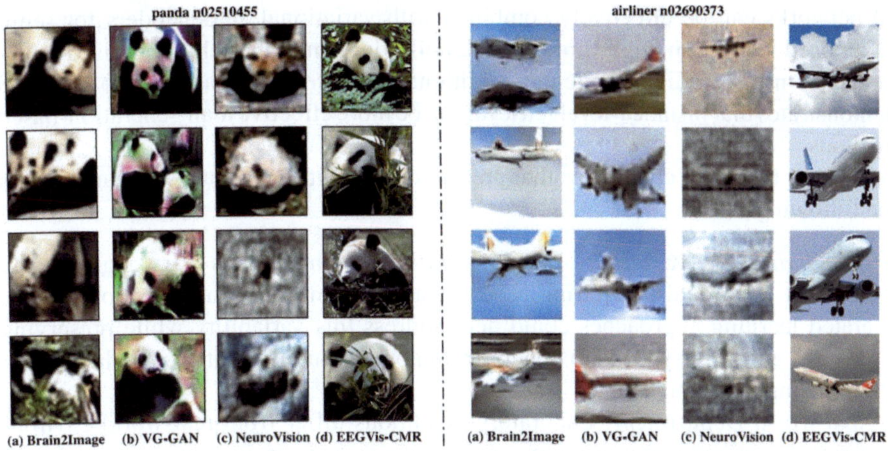

Fig. 7.11 Qualitative comparison of EEG-to-visual results between reconstruction-based and retrieval-based approaches. Each row shows: (left) the ground truth visual stimulus viewed by the subject during EEG recording, followed by outputs from four reconstruction methods (Brain2Image, VG-GAN, NeuroVision, CapsGAN), and (right) the top-3 retrieval results from EEGVis-CMR. Reconstruction methods generate semantically relevant but visually distinct images from the actual stimuli, while EEGVis-CMR successfully retrieves the exact original image (highlighted with green border) within top-ranked candidates. The last row demonstrates open-set recognition: reconstruction methods fail to generate unseen class instances, while EEGVis-CMR can still retrieve semantically similar images from the candidate database

resource-constrained environments. Future work should explore combining the complementary merits of retrieval and reconstruction approaches, potentially enabling exact reconstruction once instance-level correlations are successfully modeled. Extension to multi-modal scenarios involving additional modalities like text could lead to more comprehensive brain-computer interface systems.

7.6 Discussion and Future Directions

This chapter has presented three complementary approaches to cognitive activity recognition: *EEG-based intention recognition*, *adversarial variational embedding*, and *self-supervised cross-modal visual retrieval*. While these methods were developed for general cognitive recognition tasks, they demonstrate potential applications in IoT-enabled environments.

The three approaches collectively address fundamental challenges in cognitive activity recognition through distinct methodological innovations. The novel EEG mesh representation and hybrid neural network architectures demonstrate effective integration of spatial and temporal information for robust brain signal processing. The adversarial variational embedding framework shows how generative adversarial networks can be effectively combined with variational autoencoders for semi-supervised learning in high-dimensional, noisy domains. The self-supervised cross-modal learning paradigm challenges traditional reconstruction-based approaches and demonstrates that instance-level retrieval can be more effective than generation-based methods.

Several technical challenges that present opportunities for future research are as the following:

- *Inter-individual Variability and Adaptation*: Brain signals vary significantly between individuals, requiring robust adaptation mechanisms. Developing federated learning approaches could help address this variability while preserving privacy, enabling systems to benefit from population-level patterns without compromising individual data.
- *Real-world Deployment*: Laboratory conditions differ from real-world environments due to ambient noise, movement artifacts, and varying environmental conditions. Optimizing cognitive recognition algorithms for edge computing platforms could enable real-time processing in IoT environments while reducing communication overhead.
- *Multi-modal Integration*: Combining brain signals with other sensor modalities (accelerometers, ambient sensors, wearable devices) could provide more comprehensive and robust cognitive state estimation. This integration is particularly relevant for developing systems that can adapt to changes in cognitive patterns over time.
- *Privacy and Ethics*: Brain-computer interfaces raise important questions about mental privacy and data protection that must be addressed in any practical deployment.

The cognitive activity recognition approaches presented in this chapter advance the state-of-the-art in brain-computer interfaces, semi-supervised learning, and cross-modal learning. The emphasis on non-invasive methods, robustness to real-world conditions, and data-efficient learning addresses key requirements for practical cognitive monitoring systems. One important future work should focus on translating these research advances into deployable systems that can operate effectively in realistic environments while addressing privacy and ethical considerations.

References

1. Ahn, M., Lee, M., Choi, J., Jun, S.C.: A review of brain-computer interface games and an opinion survey from researchers, developers and users. Sensors **14**(8), 14601–14633 (2014)
2. Arjovsky, M., Chintala, S., Bottou, L.: Wasserstein generative adversarial networks. In: Proceedings of the 34th International Conference on Machine Learning (ICML), pp. 214–223. PMLR (2017)
3. Bashivan, P., Rish, I., Yeasin, M., Codella, N.: Learning representations from eeg with deep recurrent-convolutional neural networks. In: International Conference on Learning Representations (ICLR) (2016)

4. Bright, D., Nair, A., Salvekar, D., Bhisikar, S.: Eeg-based brain controlled prosthetic arm. In: Proceedings of the Conference on Advances in Signal Processing (CASP), pp. 479–483. IEEE (2016)
5. Chen, K., Yao, L., Wang, X., Zhang, D., Gu, T., Yu, Z., Yang, Z.: Interpretable parallel recurrent neural networks with convolutional attentions for multi-modality activity modeling. In: Proceedings of the 2018 International Joint Conference on Neural Networks (IJCNN), pp. 3016–3021. IEEE (2018)
6. Chollet, F.: Xception: Deep learning with depthwise separable convolutions. In: Proceedings of the IEEE Conference on Computer Vision and Pattern Recognition (CVPR), pp. 1800–1807. IEEE (2017)
7. Defossez, A., Caucheteux, C., Rapin, J., Kabeli, O., King, J.R.: Decoding speech from non-invasive brain recordings (2022). arXiv:2208.12266
8. Deldari, S., Xue, H., Saeed, A., Smith, D.V., Salim, F.D.: Cocoa: Cross modality contrastive learning for sensor data. Proc. ACM Interactive Mobile Wearable Ubiquitous Technol. (IMWUT) **6**, 1–28 (2022) (ACM)
9. Dizaji, K.G., Wang, X., Huang, H.: Semi-supervised generative adversarial network for gene expression inference. In: Proceedings of the 24th ACM SIGKDD International Conference on Knowledge Discovery and Data Mining, pp. 552–560. ACM (2018)
10. Goldberger, A.L., Amaral, L.A., Glass, L., Hausdorff, J.M., Ivanov, P.C., Mark, R.G., Mietus, J.E., Moody, G.B., Peng, C.K., Stanley, H.E.: Physiobank, physiotoolkit, and physionet: components of a new research resource for complex physiologic signals. Circulation **101**(23), E215–E220 (2000)
11. Gong, C., Tao, D., Maybank, S.J., Liu, W., Kang, G., Yang, J.: Multi-modal curriculum learning for semi-supervised image classification. IEEE Trans. Image Process. **25**(7), 3085–3098 (2016)
12. Goodwin, T.R., Harabagiu, S.M.: Deep learning from eeg reports for inferring underspecified information. In: Proceedings of the 2017 AMIA Joint Summits on Translational Science, pp. 229–238. AMIA (2017)
13. Guo, H., Chen, L., Reng, L., Chen, C.: Wearable sensor based multimodal human activity recognition exploiting the diversity of classifier ensemble. In: Proceedings of the 2010 UbiComp Conference, pp. 102–110. ACM (2010)
14. Han, J., Zhang, S., Men, A., Chen, Q.: Cross-modal contrastive hashing retrieval for infrared video and eeg. Sensors **22**(22), 8804 (2022)
15. Harati, A., Golmohammadi, M., Lopez, S., Obeid, I., Picone, J.: Improved eeg event classification using differential energy. In: Proceedings of the 2015 IEEE Signal Processing in Medicine and Biology Symposium (SPMB), pp. 45–48. IEEE (2015)
16. He, X., Chua, T.: Neural factorization machines for sparse predictive analytics. In: Proceedings of the 2017 ACM SIGIR Conference, pp. 355–364. ACM (2017)
17. Heydari, E., Shahbakhti, M.: Adaptive wavelet technique for eeg de-noising. In: Proceedings of the 8th Biomedical Engineering International Conference (BMEiCON), pp. 1–4. IEEE (2015)
18. Kavasidis, I., Palazzo, S., Spampinato, C., Giordano, D., Shah, M.: Brain2image: Converting brain signals into images. In: Proceedings of the 25th ACM International Conference on Multimedia (MM), pp. 1809–1817. ACM (2017)
19. Kim, Y., Ryu, J., Kim, K., Took, C.C., Mandic, D.P., Park, C.: Motor imagery classification using mu and beta rhythms of eeg with strong uncorrelating transform-based complex common spatial patterns. Comput. Intell. Neurosci. Article ID 123456 (2016)
20. Kingma, D.P., Ba, J.: Adam: A method for stochastic optimization. In: Proceedings of the 3rd International Conference on Learning Representations (ICLR) (2015)
21. Kingma, D.P., Mohamed, S., Rezende, D.J., Welling, M.: Semi-supervised learning with deep generative models. Adv. Neural Inf. Process. Syst. **27**, 3581–3589 (2014) (NeurIPS)
22. Lara, O.D., Perez, A.J., Labrador, M.A., Posada, J.D.: Centinela: a human activity recognition system based on acceleration and vital sign data. Pervasive Mob. Comput. **8**(5), 717–729 (2012)
23. LeCun, Y., Bengio, Y., Hinton, G.: Deep learning. Nature **521**(7553), 436–444 (2015)
24. Maaløe, L., Sønderby, C.K., Sønderby, S.K., Winther, O.: Auxiliary deep generative models (2016). arXiv:1602.05473

25. Makhzani, A., Shlens, J., Jaitly, N., Goodfellow, I., Frey, B.: Adversarial autoencoders (2015). arXiv:1511.05644
26. Mirza, M., Osindero, S.: Conditional generative adversarial nets (2014). arXiv:1411.1784
27. Miyato, T., ichi Maeda, S., Ishii, S., Koyama, M.: Virtual adversarial training: a regularization method for supervised and semi-supervised learning. IEEE Trans. Pattern Anal. Mach. Intell. **41**(8), 1972–1986 (2019)
28. Narayanaswamy, S., Paige, T.B., de Meent, J.V., Desmaison, A., Goodman, N., Kohli, P., Wood, F., Torr, P.: Learning disentangled representations with semi-supervised deep generative models. In: Advances in Neural Information Processing Systems, vol. 30, pp. 99–109. NeurIPS (2017)
29. Obeid, I., Picone, J.: The temple university hospital eeg data corpus. Front. Neurosci. **10**, 196 (2016)
30. Odena, A.: Semi-supervised learning with generative adversarial networks (2016). arXiv:1606.01583
31. Palazzo, S., Spampinato, C., Kavasidis, I., Giordano, D., Schmidt, J., Shah, M.: Decoding brain representations by multimodal learning of neural activity and visual features. IEEE Trans. Pattern Anal. Mach. Intell. **43**(11), 3833–3849 (2021)
32. Pazzani, M.J., Billsus, D.: Content-based recommendation systems. In: The Adaptive Web: Methods and Strategies of Web Personalization. Lecture Notes in Computer Science, vol. 4321, pp. 325–341. Springer, Berlin (2007)
33. Peng, L., Chen, W., Zhou, W., Li, F., Yang, J., Zhang, J.: An immune-inspired semi-supervised algorithm for breast cancer diagnosis. Comput. Methods Programs Biomed. **134**, 259–265 (2016)
34. Qiu, S., Li, Z., He, W., Zhang, L., Yang, C., Su, C.: Brain-machine interface and visual compressive sensing-based teleoperation control of an exoskeleton robot. IEEE Trans. Fuzzy Syst. **25**(1), 58–69 (2017)
35. Rendle, S.: Factorization machines with libfm. ACM Trans. Intell. Syst. Technol. **3**(3), 57:1–57:22 (2012)
36. Russakovsky, O., Deng, J., Su, H., Krause, J., Satheesh, S., Ma, S., Huang, Z., Karpathy, A., Khosla, A., Bernstein, M.S., et al.: Imagenet large scale visual recognition challenge. Int. J. Comput. Vision **115**(3), 211–252 (2015)
37. Schalk, G., McFarland, D.J., Hinterberger, T., Birbaumer, N., Wolpaw, J.R.: Bci 2000: a general-purpose brain-computer interface (bci) system. IEEE Trans. Biomed. Eng. **51**(6), 1034–1043 (2004)
38. Schirrmeister, R.T., Gemein, L., Eggensperger, K., Hutter, F., Ball, T.: Deep learning with convolutional neural networks for decoding and visualization of eeg pathology (2017). arXiv:1708.08012
39. Shenoy, H.V., Vinod, A.P., Guan, C.: Shrinkage estimator based regularization for eeg motor imagery classification. In: Proceedings of the 2015 10th International Conference on Information, Communications and Signal Processing (ICICS), pp. 1–5. IEEE (2015)
40. Spampinato, C., Palazzo, S., Kavasidis, I., Giordano, D., Souly, N., Shah, M.: Deep learning human mind for automated visual classification. In: Proceedings of the IEEE Conference on Computer Vision and Pattern Recognition (CVPR), pp. 6809–6817. IEEE (2017)
41. Springenberg, J.T.: Unsupervised and semi-supervised learning with categorical generative adversarial networks. In: Proceedings of the International Conference on Learning Representations (ICLR) (2016)
42. Sun, S., Zhou, J.: A review of adaptive feature extraction and classification methods for eeg-based brain-computer interfaces. In: Proceedings of the 2014 International Joint Conference on Neural Networks (IJCNN), pp. 1746–1753. IEEE (2014)
43. Sønderby, C.K., Raiko, T., Maaløe, L., Sønderby, S.K., Winther, O.: Ladder variational autoencoders. In: Advances in Neural Information Processing Systems, vol. 29, pp. 3738–3748. NeurIPS (2016)
44. Tabar, Y.R., Halici, U.: A novel deep learning approach for classification of eeg motor imagery signals. J. Neural Eng. **14**(1), 016003 (2017)

45. Tirupattur, P., Rawat, Y.S., Spampinato, C., Shah, M.: Thoughtviz: Visualizing human thoughts using generative adversarial network. In: Proceedings of the 26th ACM International Conference on Multimedia (MM), pp. 950–958. ACM (2018)
46. WAhnang, H., Li, Y., Long, J., Yu, T., Gu, Z.: An asynchronous wheelchair control by hybrid eeg–eog brain-computer interface. Cogn. Neurodynamics **8**(5), 399–409 (2014)
47. Weston, J., Ratle, F., Mobahi, H., Collobert, R.: Deep learning via semi-supervised embedding. In: Neural Networks: Tricks of the Trade. Lecture Notes in Computer Science, vol. 7700, pp. 639–655. Springer, Berlin (2012)
48. Ye, Z., Yao, L., Zhang, Y., Gustin, S.: Self-supervised cross-modal visual retrieval from brain activities. Pattern Recogn. **145**, 109915 (2024)
49. Yin, Z., Wang, Y., Liu, L., Zhang, W., Zhang, J.: Cross-subject eeg feature selection for emotion recognition using transfer recursive feature elimination. Front. Neurorobot. **11**, 19 (2017)
50. Zhang, D., Chen, K., Jian, D., Yao, L.: Motor imagery classification via temporal attention cues of graph embeded eeg signals. IEEE J. Biomed. Health Inform. **24**(9), 2570–2579 (2020)
51. Zhang, D., Yao, L., Zhang, X., Wang, S., Chen, W., Boots, R.: Cascade and parallel convolutional recurrent neural networks on eeg-based intention recognition for brain computer interface. In: Proceedings of the Thirty-Second AAAI Conference on Artificial Intelligence (AAAI-18), pp. 1703–1710. AAAI Press, New Orleans, LA, USA (2018)
52. Zhang, X., Yao, L., Huang, C., Wang, S., Tan, M., Long, G., Wang, C.: Multi-modality sensor data classification with selective attention. In: Proceedings of the 2018 Tianjin Jiao Tong University Conference on Advanced Technologies (TJCAT), pp. 122–130. TJCAT (2018)
53. Zhang, X., Yao, L., Yuan, F.: Adversarial variational embedding for robust semi-supervised learning. In: Proceedings of the 25th ACM SIGKDD International Conference on Knowledge Discovery and Data Mining, KDD '19, pp. 139–147. ACM, Anchorage, AK, USA (2019)
54. Ziyabari, S., Shah, V., Golmohammadi, M., Obeid, I., Picone, J.: Objective evaluation metrics for automatic classification of eeg events (2017). arXiv:1712.10107

Part III
Interactive and Cooperative Ambient Intelligence

This part advances beyond basic sensing and recognition to explore intelligent systems that actively interact with and assist users through sophisticated ambient intelligence technologies. Building upon the foundational capabilities established in Parts I and II, these chapters demonstrate how environmental and wearable sensing can be integrated with interactive technologies to create cooperative intelligent environments that understand, predict, and respond to human needs.

Chapter 8 introducesWeb-based interactive ambient intelligence, presenting a comprehensive IoT management framework that bridges physical and virtual worlds through intuitive web interfaces. The chapter demonstrates a real-world smart home prototype with 121 connected devices, showcasing layered architecture approaches for scalable device management, real-time monitoring, and rule-based automation. This foundation establishes the technological infrastructure necessary for creating responsive intelligent environments.

Chapter 9 presents intent-aware interactive IoT for collaborative ambient intelligence, introducing a novel framework that combines intent recognition, semantic reasoning, and robotic actuation. The chapter demonstrates how systems can understand and predict human intentions through contextual sensing and historical interaction patterns, enabling robots to provide proactive physical assistance. The proposed methodology achieves over 90% success rates in complex manipulation tasks, representing a significant advancement in human-robot collaborative intelligence.

Chapter 10 explores brain-computer interface integration for IoT cognitive interactivity, presenting a unified deep learning framework that enables direct brain-to-device communication. Through innovative techniques including selective attention mechanisms and spatial LSTM architectures, the system achieves 93.6% accuracy in mental task recognition with sub-second response times. This technology opens new possibilities for cognitive control of ambient intelligence systems, particularly valuable for users with mobility limitations.

Collectively, these three chapters establish a comprehensive framework for interactive and cooperative ambient intelligence that seamlessly integrates web-based management, intent-aware robotics, and cognitive interfaces. The resulting systems provide multiple interaction modalities that can adapt to diverse user capabilities and preferences, creating truly accessible and responsive intelligent environments for smart aging applications.

Chapter 8
Web-Based Interactive Ambient Intelligence

8.1 Introduction

8.1.1 Overview of Web-Based IoT

As noted by Tim Berners-Lee, the inventor of the World Wide Web, it's not the documents that are actually interesting, it's the things they're about. The last level of abstraction for the Web is to connect physical things [4, 10]. With recent advances in RFID, wireless sensor networks, and Web services, the Internet of Things (IoT) offers the capability of integrating information from both the physical and virtual worlds, creating intelligent environments that can support daily living activities. With IoT, it becomes possible to infer the status of real-world entities with minimal delay using a standard Web browser [1, 2], an interface modality that is familiar to most users.

IoT represents the evolution from systems linking digital documents to systems relating digital information to real-world physical items. While IoT offers numerous opportunities and benefits, it also presents significant technical challenges in developing applications for real-world environments [1, 9]. Web-based IoT solutions offer a promising approach to creating accessible, intuitive interfaces that can be easily managed by residents and caregivers, with particular potential for smart aging applications where technology accessibility and ease of use are paramount considerations.

8.1.2 Challenges and Opportunities

One of the main challenges is to smoothly and seamlessly integrate the virtual and physical worlds to effectively manage things of interest (TOIs) in IoT [6, 8, 13, 16, 19]. This is critical for a number of important applications, such as

Q. Z. Sheng et al., *Harnessing Artificial Intelligence and Pervasive Internet of Things for an Empowered Aging*, https://doi.org/10.1007/978-3-032-16502-2_8

object discovery (for example, finding a quiet restaurant), recommendation (suggesting a device that can consume a video stream), and mashup (composing device functionalities for a new service). A crucial prerequisite is acknowledging the seamless information access, exchange, and manipulation between the two worlds.

For smart home applications, these challenges are compounded by the need for interfaces that accommodate diverse user capabilities, requirements for reliable operation with minimal maintenance, privacy and security concerns related to home monitoring, and the importance of contextual awareness to support safe and comfortable living environments. However, these challenges also present significant opportunities to develop IoT systems that enhance independence, safety, and quality of life for residents in their homes, with particular benefits for aging-in-place scenarios.

8.1.3 Contributions

In this chapter, we explore a new direction in realizing information integration between the physical and virtual worlds. We design and develop a system that offers an integrated Web-based interface to manage (that is, connect, monitor, control, mashup, and visualize) things in an IoT environment, which helps people be aware of their surroundings and thereby make better decisions.

Our work presents a comprehensive architecture that includes a layered framework for managing information produced by physical things and a rule-based approach to aggregate individual things for building context-aware, personalized value-added services. We demonstrate the practical feasibility of this approach through a functional prototype implementation in a real-world inhabited home environment with 121 connected devices, showing how residents can access, control, and compose physical resources in a variety of daily living contexts.

Additionally, we provide practical insights and future research directions for IoT applications in smart home environments, including applications for independent living, environmental monitoring, and intelligent systems that can enhance quality of life for residents with diverse needs and capabilities. The system's design principles and implementation experiences offer valuable guidance for developing accessible IoT solutions that can support aging-in-place scenarios while maintaining user autonomy and privacy.

8.1.4 Chapter Organization

The remainder of this chapter is organized as follows. Section 8.2 presents background and related work in developing IoT applications, with a focus on approaches relevant to smart home environments and smart aging applications. Section 8.3 details our Web-based management system for the Internet of Things, including system architecture, key components, and experimental validation through a demonstrator application in a smart home setting. Finally, Sect. 8.4 discusses implications for smart aging applications, identifies future research directions, and explores the evolution of smart aging technologies.

8.2 Background and Related Work

8.2.1 IoT System Architectures and Smart Environments

With billions of things interconnected and present over the Web, there are significant software engineering challenges in developing Internet of Things (IoT) applications, due to their unique and inherent characteristics. The SENSEI project[1] proposes an architectural framework that focuses on addressing scalability issues in wireless sensor and actuator networks. SemSorGrid4Env [7] develops a service-oriented architecture and middleware that assists developers in building large-scale, semantic-based sensor network applications. Both projects, however, deal with the connectivity issues of IoT: how to connect heterogeneous things to the Web rather than how to describe and model things.

The recent research and development activities at the Commonwealth Scientific and Industrial Research Organization (CSIRO) [12] offer some interesting experiences in applying IoT in a number of application domains, such as smart farming. They developed an ontology-enabled architecture where the sensor observations are published as linked data cubes for long-term data analysis and sharing at the national scale. However, the system doesn't provide suitable integrated abstractions for things.

University of Washington researchers developed an IoT application, which unfortunately only focuses on managing the collected RFID data [14]. The Paraimpu platform [8] provides a Web-based social platform for people to connect, compose, and share things. To perform mashups of heterogeneous things, Paraimpu exploits several strong abstractions. In the Hyperpipe project, things are represented as Web services and connected using pipes so that users can easily compose things for new services.

8.2.2 Web-Based Integration and Smart Aging Applications

Most things are resource-constrained and the traditional service-oriented architecture (SOA) standards like SOAP and Business Process Execution Language (BPEL) might not be applicable [5]. Many research projects are actively solving these challenges and one notable effort is the IoT6 project [20], which focuses on investigating

[1] https://senseiproject.eu/.

IPv6 and related standards, such as the Constraint Application Protocol (CoAP) [3] and IPv6 over Low-Power Wireless Personal Area Networks (6LoWPAN)[2] to overcome IoT's current fragmentation.

Despite advances in IoT technologies, several research gaps remain in the context of smart aging applications:

- *Usability for Diverse Users*: Many existing IoT systems lack interfaces specifically designed for users who may have limited technological proficiency or physical limitations. Web-based approaches that provide intuitive, accessible interfaces could significantly improve adoption rates across different user groups.
- *Integration with Healthcare Systems*: There is limited research on how to effectively integrate smart home IoT systems with healthcare monitoring and emergency response systems - a critical requirement for supporting aging-in-place.
- *Contextual Awareness*: Current IoT systems often lack sufficient contextual awareness to differentiate between normal and concerning behaviors in home environments. Improved algorithms for detecting and responding to potential emergencies or daily living difficulties are needed.
- *Privacy-Preserving Monitoring*: Finding the right balance between helpful monitoring and privacy invasion remains a significant challenge. Systems that can provide necessary oversight while respecting dignity and autonomy are urgently needed.
- *Adaptive Systems*: IoT environments need to adapt to changing user capabilities and needs over time, requiring systems that can evolve without requiring significant reconfiguration or technical intervention.

8.3 Web-Based IoT Management Framework

8.3.1 Motivation and Overview of Web-Based IoT Management

The Internet of Things (IoT) system presented here seamlessly integrates virtual and physical worlds to efficiently manage things of interest (TOIs), where services and resources offered by things can be monitored, visualized, and aggregated for value-added services by users. Our approach provides a layered architecture that effectively bridges the physical and virtual domains through web-based interfaces and technologies that prioritize accessibility and intuitive interaction. While the system is demonstrated in a general smart home context, the design principles and architectural choices make it particularly suitable for smart aging contexts, as it enables intuitive monitoring and control of everyday objects with minimal technical requirements.

[2] http://tools.ietf.org/wg/6lowpan.

In this section, we describe our approach to addressing the challenges of web-based IoT management in smart environments. Our system aims to provide intuitive interfaces and seamless integration between physical objects and digital representations, enabling effective monitoring and control of smart environments. The approach prioritizes ease of use while maintaining robust functionality, making it suitable for various applications including potential deployment in aging-in-place scenarios. Using practical experience gained from this system, we identify several R&D opportunities for building future IoT applications.

8.3.2 System Architecture and Core Components

Figure 8.1 shows our system's architecture [17]. The architecture is layered, developed using the Microsoft .NET framework and SQL Server 2012. The system maps physical things and their related data to corresponding virtual resources, which it can aggregate and visualize via a range of software components. The system provides two ways to identify physical objects and connect them to the Web. The first is to use RFID technology, where physical objects are attached with RFID tags and interrogated by RFID readers. The second is to combine sensors with objects to transfer the raw data to the network. Then the raw data captured by readers and sensors is processed further. In the following, we describe the key system modules and their implementation details.

Data Access and the Sensor Hive

The data access layer manages RFID tags and sensors associated with physical things; collects raw RFID and sensor data and processes them; and provides a universal API for higher-level programs to retrieve the status of things. Due to inherent characteristics of RFID and sensor data (it's volatile, for example) [2, 11], this layer contains several software components for filtering and cleaning the collected raw data, and adapting such data for high-level applications. The advantage of the data access layer is to allow the system to provide data synchronously. This is important, since some devices work with more than one sensor and the sensor readings may come asynchronously. This layer works in a scalable, plug-and-play fashion, where we can easily plug in new sensors and remove the old sensors.

The sensor hive module in the architecture essentially lets you map physical things to the corresponding virtual resources. To achieve a seamless integration of physical things with an organization's business processes, applications must be able to understand different data semantics. There are several languages, such as Physical

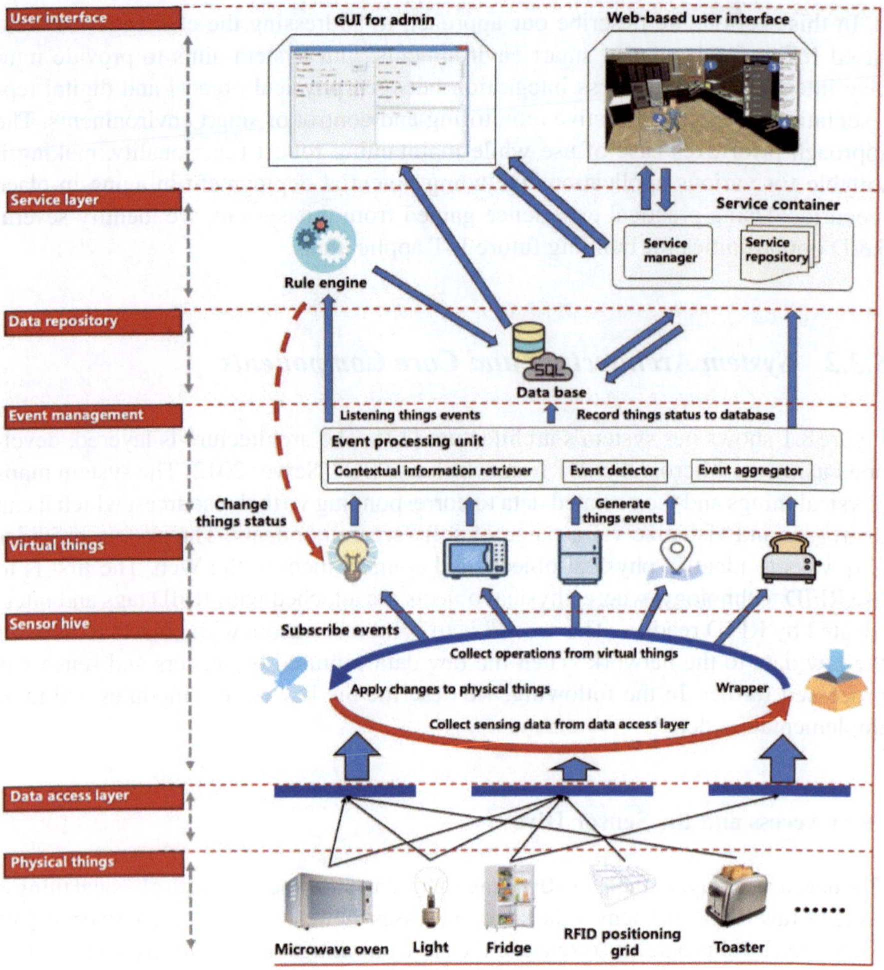

Fig. 8.1 Our system's layered architecture. The system maps physical things and their related data to corresponding virtual resources, which it can aggregate and visualize via a range of software components.

Markup Language,[3] Microformats,[4] and Resource Description Framework (RDF),[5] which we can use to add semantics to the descriptions of things. In our design, we exploit schema.org,[6] an initiative (launched in 2011 by Bing, Google, and Yahoo) that is designed for both human users and machines. The universal RESTful API provided

---

[3] http://web.mit.edu/mecheng/pml.

[4] https://www.microformats.org/.

[5] https://www.w3.org/RDF/.

[6] https://www.schema.org/.

in our design enables higher-level programs to retrieve the status of physical things with specified addresses, without knowing where and how to find the physical sensors associated with the things.

Virtual Things

This module maps a collection of classes (also called *virtual things*, aka *digital twins*) to their corresponding physical things. Each virtual thing communicates with the sensor hive, collects the information, and interprets the current status of the corresponding physical device. For example, the virtual device of a microwave oven can query the sensor values associated with the physical microwave oven from the sensor hive layer, and use this information to decide the oven's current status (idle or in use). A virtual thing is responsible for generating events based on the collected information (such as when the refrigerator door opens), which can be directly used by high-level applications or further processed by other modules (for example, an event-processing unit).

Event Management

This layer focuses on event processing that automatically extracts and aggregates objects' usage events based on the data feeds from the virtual things layer in a pipelined fashion. The pipeline consists of three main phases: event detection, contextual information retrieval, and event aggregation.

The event detector captures and decides whether a physical thing is in use. In our design, there are two ways to detect usage events of things: a sensor-based approach for detecting state changes and RFID-based approach for detecting mobility [16]. In sensor-based detection, an object's usage is reflected by changes of the object's status – for example, the status of a microwave oven moves from idle to busy when it is being used. In the RFID-based detection, an object's movement indicates that the object is being used. For example, if a coffee mug is moving, it is likely that the mug is being used. In this situation, we adopt a generic method based on comparing descriptive statistics of the Received Signal Strength Indication (RSSI) values in consecutive sliding windows [18]. The statistics obtained from two consecutive windows are expected to differ significantly when an object is moved.

The contextual information retriever extracts contextual information contained in things' usage events. In our current design, we focus on three types of contextual information: identity (user), temporality (time stamp) and spatiality (location) [18]. To obtain the identity information, we perform manual labeling, where all participants mark and record their activities. To obtain the temporal information, we split a day into 48 equal intervals of half an hour each. For example, if the time stamp of a usage event is 9:07 am, it will be assigned to the 9:00–9:30 am interval. For the spatial information, we consider two situations. For static objects (perhaps a refrigerator or microwave oven), the spatial information is a prior knowledge. For mobile objects (an RFID-tagged coffee mug, for example), we provide coarse-grain and fine-grain methods for localization. The coarse-grain method uses the RSSI signal received from a tagged object to approximate its proximity to an RFID antenna. Each zone is covered by a mutually exclusive set of RFID antennas. The zone scanned by an antenna with the maximum RSSI signal is regarded as the object's location. The fine-grain method compares the signal descriptors from an object at an unknown location to a previously constructed radio map or fingerprint. We use the weighted k Nearest Neighbors algorithm (w-kNN) to find the most similar fingerprints and compute a weighted average of their 2D positions to estimate the unknown tag location [18].

The event aggregator indexes and stores all the events and services, together with their related information in a database (in the data repository layer), which can be mined for various purposes (for example, finding latent correlations among things, and making recommendations) [18]. A list of elements is constructed, storing the identifiers of objects, their types and values, as well as the calculated contextual information. In this way, applications can focus on the functionalities without worrying about operations, such as connecting to the database, opening connections, querying with specified languages, and handling the results (normally they're raw data and inconvenient to access).

The Service Layer

This layer consists of a rule engine and a service container. The service container converts events and data into corresponding services. In particular, the repository stores the descriptions of services (in the form of RESTful APIs) for things, where applications can easily access the data associated with a particular thing stored in the database (for example, usage history of a device), and manipulate the actuators (such as turning on or off a light). The APIs are represented using JavaScript Object Notation (JSON), which is developed from JavaScript for representing simple data structures and associative objects. The service manager is responsible for abstracting services from the lower level, representing them as services, and storing them into the service repository.

The rule engine allows applications to control a device automatically by establishing a set of rules. A rule consists of two parts: a *condition* and an *action*. A condition is a composition of a set of simple boolean expressions. An action is simply a set of device settings—for example, 'Out-DoorLight.On = true' will turn on the outdoor lighting device. Alternatively, an action can also be a program—for example, 'SendEmail(Microwave,'someone@example.com')' will send an email to the email address. By combining simple Boolean expressions together, the application can setup a complex rule to make devices "smarter".

The rule engine consists of three main components: the *rule composer*, the *rule interpreter*, and the *rule parser*. The rule composer is a Web-based application implementing a user-friendly GUI for rule creation and action setup, in a drag-and-drop fashion. The rule interpreter is software that receives the string expressions of rules from the rule composer. It analyzes and annotates the string statement based on a state machine. The string expression is then translated to a list of annotated objects. The rule parser is implemented based on the shunting-yard algorithm. It first compiles each part of the input sequence into a .NET Expression object. Then, it combines all such objects together into a complex Expression Tree, which will be compiled into a Lambda expression. This Lambda expression object will be stored in memory when the system is running. It can be invoked when a device status changes or time elapses. If the Lambda expression returns true, a corresponding action will be called.

The User Interface Layer

This layer provides access to the management of things (for example, connection, monitoring, control, mashup, and visualization). The Web-based interface offers a 3D scene in a Web browser for users to manage their things of interest. We particularly adopt the Web Graphics Library (WebGL) in HTML5 to enable 3D scene recreation. The 3D models are stored as Digital Asset Exchange (DAE) files, and imported and rendered by using three.js[7] with plugins. Things are visualized and managed by device plugins. Each visualized thing is considered as a device plugin, which contains one or more 3D model or animation settings. For instance, the kettle will show steam when it is boiling water. We can use the ShaderParticleEngine plugin[8] for three.js to create the steam effect for the kettle. Each device plugin also provides a series of APIs, to communicate with the service layer for status changes of the corresponding things, and to reflect such changes on the Web browser. This layer also provides an administrative interface for things management (for example, connecting and disconnecting things, and viewing event logs).

8.3.3 *Experimental Validation and Performance Analysis*

We developed a number of IoT applications based on the proposed system architecture. Here, we particularly focus on introducing a *smart home* application, which has been successfully deployed in a real-world environment (at the first author's home). We attached RFID tags and sensors to 121 physical things (a microwave oven, fridge, coffee mug, laptop, couch, and so on) and Fig. 8.2a shows the statistics of the involved things. Figure 8.2b shows some RFID devices and sensors used in the implementation, and Fig. 8.2c shows part of the kitchen setting, including an IoT-enabled microwave oven and toaster. When users interact with these physical things, events are captured (by RFID readers, for example). The raw data of the events must be processed (through cleaning, transformation, and integration) before storing in the repository. This task greatly benefits from our extensive experience in a recently completed, seven-year RFID research project [15].

[7] https://threejs.org/.

[8] https://github.com/squarefeet/ShaderParticleEngine/.

Category	No. of things
Cooking	48
Entertainment	28
Home office	25
First-aid/medicine	20

(a)

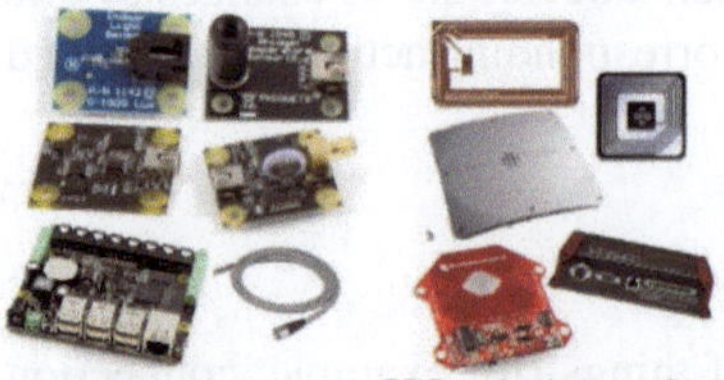

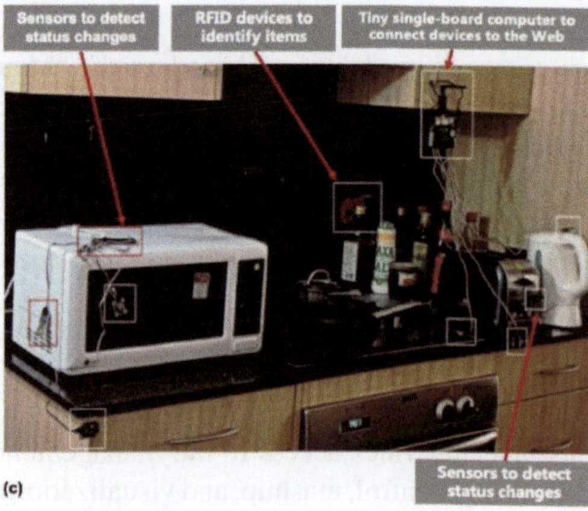

Fig. 8.2 The settings of the smart home Internet of Things (IoT) application. **a** Statistics of the involved physical things, **b** some devices used in the application, and **c** part of the kitchen setting, such as an IoT-enabled microwave oven and toaster

This application offers an integrated Web-based interface where a user can monitor and visualize the status changes of household things of interest in real time. Users can monitor, track, and control the current status of physical things by directly observing the status of their corresponding icons from the Web browser. In addition, this application also augments the physical things with key social network functionality. We developed a real-time notification of things' status by exploiting the Twitter API. Status changes can be sent to Twitter subscribers in real time. Figure 8.3a shows the integrated Web-based user interface.

Real-Time Visualizer and Monitor. This function offers access to, and control of, the physical things, allowing the status of physical things to be visualized in real time. We render the icons with different effects to be consistent with the real status of physical things. For example, if the microwave oven is being used, its corresponding icon in the Web interface will change to a highlighted status (yellow), and otherwise gray (see part 1 of Fig. 8.3a).

The learned position information from the event-processing module (see Fig. 8.1) is used to visualize the locations and traces of TOIs at a coarse-grain level. We divide the testing area into multiple grids in a chessboard style (for example, 3 m * 3 m in the kitchen area). Then, the trace line is generated by connecting the grids' central dots. For example, as part 2 of Fig. 8.3a shows, the trace of a coffee mug held by a subject is displayed in green lines.

Rules Composer. This function provides a graphical interface letting users control the devices by setting up a series of rules via a Web browser without any programming efforts (see part 3 in Fig. 8.3a) with the details shown in Fig. 8.3b. It can create a composite service using the rule-based composition component provided by the

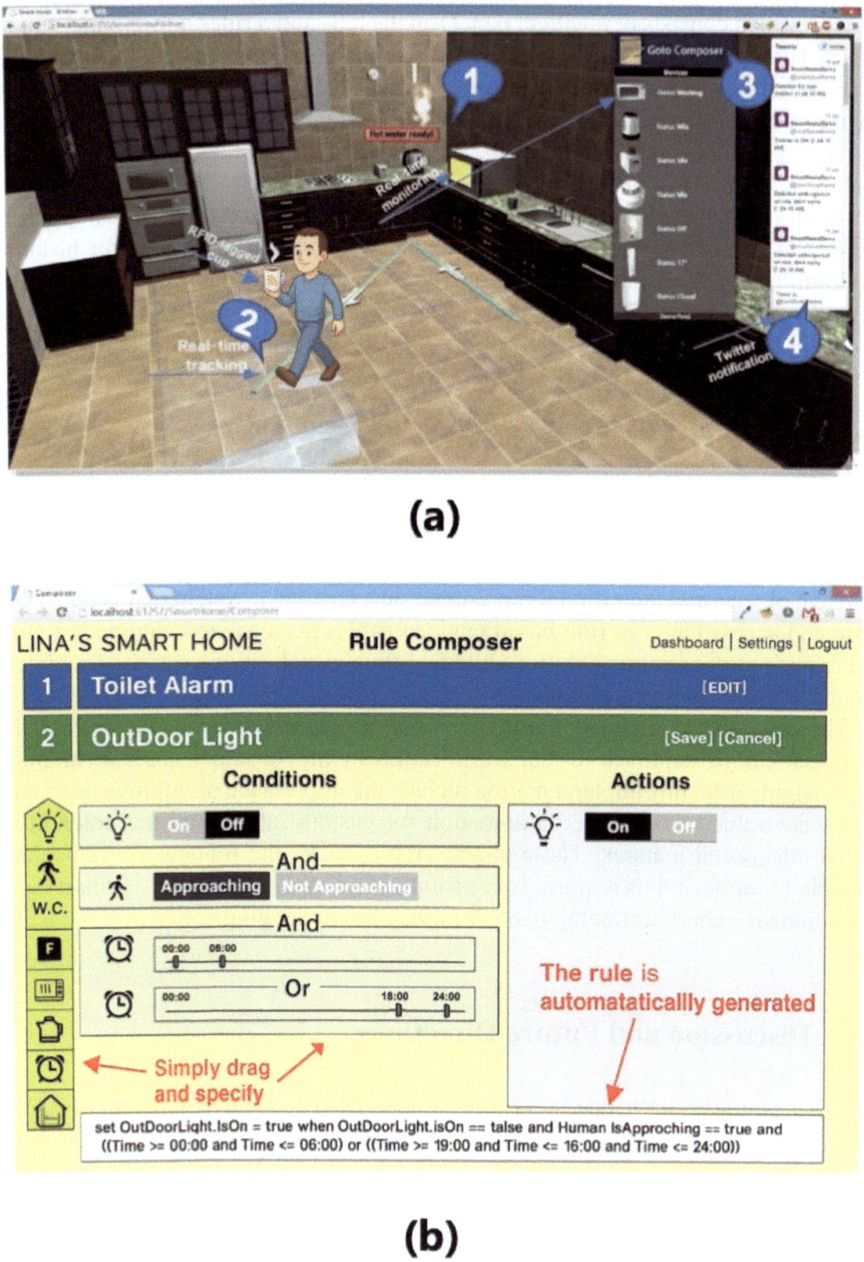

Fig. 8.3 Real-time notification of things' status using Twitter (now X). **a** The 3D Web-based application interface. **b** The rule composer supports users so that they can easily create their own rules. For example, for editing a rule like "turn on the outdoor light when a person is approaching during midnight to 6 am or 6 pm to midnight," a user needs only to drag the person and clock icons to the condition subpanel and the light icon to the action subpanel, and perform some simple adjustments (such as adjusting the clock slider to set the time period)

system, which consists of a widget panel (on the left) and a rules editor panel (on the right). The widget panel shows the virtualized objects (things and people) and each object has a set of actions (the light, for example, is associated with two actions: turn on and turn off). Users simply drag any object's widget to the rules editor panel and start to create a new rule or change the old rules by clicking the "edit" button beside each rule.

An editing panel includes a condition editor and an action editor. The condition editor lets users change or set rules based on contextual information (for instance, environmental information such as temperature, or event information such as a person approaching). Figure 8.3b shows the interface on specifying a rule.

8.3.4 Summary of the Web-Based IoT Framework

Our Web-based IoT management framework demonstrates the feasibility and effectiveness of creating intuitive interfaces for controlling smart environments. Through the layered architecture approach, we have successfully bridged the gap between physical objects and their digital representations, creating a system that is both powerful and accessible. The rule-based engine enables personalized automation without requiring programming skills, while real-time visualization provides immediate feedback on environmental states.

The case study implementation with 121 connected devices proves that this approach can be deployed in real-world settings with consumer-grade technology. Key insights from this implementation include the importance of intuitive user interfaces, the value of rule-based automation for customization, and the potential of social integration features. These characteristics make the framework particularly suitable for applications requiring accessibility and ease of use, such as smart aging environments where technology adoption may be challenging.

8.4 Discussion and Future Directions

The development and deployment of Web-based IoT management frameworks for smart environments present both significant opportunities and ongoing challenges. Our work demonstrates that such frameworks can provide intuitive, accessible interfaces for managing a wide range of connected devices, supporting automation, real-time monitoring, and user-driven customization in everyday settings. While our implementation was validated in a general smart home context, the design principles and technical solutions are broadly applicable to various domains, including—but not limited to—smart aging.

Despite recent advances, several core challenges remain for the broader adoption and evolution of web-based IoT management systems:

- *Scalability and Interoperability*: As the number and diversity of IoT devices continue to grow, scalable architectures and standardized interfaces are essential for seamless integration and management. Future research should focus on robust frameworks that can accommodate heterogeneous devices and protocols, ensuring long-term system flexibility.
- *Data Management and Context Awareness*: Efficient handling of large-scale, continuous, and distributed IoT data streams remains a fundamental issue. Enhancing context awareness—such as inferring user intent, environmental conditions, or device status—will be critical for delivering intelligent and adaptive services.
- *Security and Privacy*: The proliferation of connected devices increases the attack surface for potential security breaches and privacy violations. Balancing robust security mechanisms with user convenience is an ongoing challenge, especially in personal and home environments.
- *User-Centric Design*: Ensuring that interfaces and automation tools remain accessible to users with diverse backgrounds and abilities is vital. This includes not only elderly users, as in smart aging scenarios, but also families, caregivers, and individuals with varying technical skills.

Although our experimental validation was not specifically focused on elderly users, the features of Web-based IoT management—such as intuitive rule-based automation, real-time visualization, and remote monitoring—are well aligned with the needs of smart aging applications. These capabilities can support independent living, safety, and social connectivity for older adults, while also benefiting a broader range of users in smart home and ambient intelligence contexts.

The evolution of Web-based IoT management systems will require ongoing innovation in system architecture, data analytics, and user experience design [10]. Future work should explore deeper integration with healthcare and social support systems, adaptive interfaces that evolve with user needs, and privacy-preserving monitoring solutions. By addressing these challenges, web-based IoT frameworks can play a pivotal role in enabling intelligent, cooperative, and human-centric ambient environments for a wide spectrum of applications.

References

1. Atzori, L., Iera, A., Morabito, G.: The internet of things: a survey. Comput. Netw. **54**(15), 2787–2805 (2010)
2. Barnaghi, P.M., Sheth, A.P., Henson, C.A.: From data to actionable knowledge: big data challenges in the web of things. IEEE Intell. Syst. **28**(6), 6–11 (2013)
3. Bormann, C., Castellani, A.P., Shelby, Z.: Coap: an application protocol for billions of tiny internet nodes. IEEE Internet Comput. **16**(2), 62–67 (2012)
4. Bouguettaya, A., Sheng, Q.Z., Benatallah, B., Neiat, A.G., Mistry, S., Ghose, A., Nepal, S., Yao, L.: An internet of things service roadmap. Commun. ACM **64**(9), 86–95 (2021)

5. Bouguettaya, A., Singh, M.P., Huhns, M.N., Sheng, Q.Z., Dong, H., Yu, Q., Neiat, A.G., Mistry, S., Benatallah, B., Medjahed, B., Ouzzani, M., Casati, F., Liu, X., Wang, H., Georgakopoulos, D., Chen, L., Nepal, S., Malik, Z., Erradi, A., Wang, Y., Blake, M.B., Dustdar, S., Leymann, F., Papazoglou, M.P.: A service computing manifesto: the next 10 years. Commun. ACM **60**(4), 64–72 (2017)
6. Christophe, B., Verdot, V., Toubiana, V.: Searching the 'web of things'. In: Proceedings of the 5th IEEE International Conference on Semantic Computing (ICSC 2011), pp. 308–315. IEEE Computer Society (2011)
7. Gray, A.J.G., Galpin, I., Fernandes, A.A.A., Paton, N.W., Page, K., Sadler, J., Kyzirakos, K., Koubarakis, M., Calbimonte, J.P., Castro, R.G., Corcho, O., Gabaldon, J.E., Aparicio, J.: SemSorGrid4Env Architecture. Project report, University of Southampton (2010). https://eprints.soton.ac.uk/272700/
8. Pintus, A., Carboni, D., Piras, A.: Paraimpu: A platform for a social web of things. In: Mille, A., Gandon, F., Misselis, J., Rabinovich, M., Staab, S. (eds.) Proceedings of the 21st World Wide Web Conference (WWW 2012)—Companion, pp. 401–404. ACM (2012)
9. Qin, Y., Sheng, Q.Z., Falkner, N.J.G., Dustdar, S., Wang, H., Vasilakos, A.V.: When things matter: a data-centric view of the internet of things. CoRR (2014). arxiv:abs/1407.2704
10. Sheng, M., Qin, Y., Yao, L., Benatallah, B. (eds.): Managing the Web of Things: Linking the Real World to the Web. Morgan Kaufmann (2017)
11. Sheng, Q.Z., Li, X., Zeadally, S.: Enabling next-generation rfid applications: solutions and challenges. Computer **41**(9), 21–28 (2008)
12. Taylor, K., Griffith, C., Lefort, L., Gaire, R., Compton, M., Wark, T., Lamb, D.W., Falzon, G., Trotter, M.G.: Farming the web of things. IEEE Intell. Syst. **28**(6), 12–19 (2013)
13. Tran, N.K., Sheng, Q.Z., Babar, M.A., Yao, L.: Searching the Web of Things: State of the Art, Challenges, and Solutions. ACM Comput. Surv. **50**(4), 55:1–55:34 (2017)
14. Welbourne, E., Battle, L., Cole, G., Gould, K., Rector, K., Raymer, S., Balazinska, M., Borriello, G.: Building the internet of things using RFID: the RFID ecosystem experience. IEEE Internet Comput. **13**(3), 48–55 (2009)
15. Wu, Y., Yang, F., Sheng, Q.Z., Falkner, N.J.G., Qin, Y.: Modeling object flows from distributed and federated rfid data streams for efficient tracking and tracing. IEEE Trans. Parallel Distrib. Syst. **24**(10), 2036–2045 (2013)
16. Yao, L., Sheng, Q.Z.: Exploiting latent relevance for relational learning of ubiquitous things. In: X. Chen, G. Lebanon, H. Wang, M.J. Zaki (eds.) 21st ACM International Conference on Information and Knowledge Management (CIKM 2012), pp. 1547–1551. ACM (2012)
17. Yao, L., Sheng, Q.Z., Dustdar, S.: Web-based management of the internet of things. IEEE Internet Comput. **19**(4), 60–67 (2015)
18. Yao, L., Sheng, Q.Z., Gao, B.J., Ngu, A.H.H., Li, X.: A model for discovering correlations of ubiquitous things. In: 2013 IEEE 13th International Conference on Data Mining (ICDM 2013), pp. 1253–1258. IEEE Computer Society (2013)
19. Yao, L., Sheng, Q.Z., Ngu, A.H.H., Li, X.: Things of interest recommendation by leveraging heterogeneous relations in the internet of things. ACM Trans. Internet Technol. **16**(2), 9:1–9:25 (2016)
20. Ziegler, S., Crettaz, C., Ladid, L., Krco, S., Pokric, B., Skarmeta, A.F., Jara, A., Kastner, W., Jung, M.: IoT6—Moving to an IPv6-Based Future IoT. In: Galis, A., Gavras, A. (eds.) The Future Internet, pp. 161–172. Springer, Berlin (2013)

Chapter 9
Intent-Aware Interactive IoT for Collaborative Ambient Intelligence

9.1 Introduction

9.1.1 Overview of Intent-Aware Interactive IoT

The Internet of Things (IoT) represents a paradigm shift in how digital and physical worlds interact, connecting artifacts into networks that can infer the status of real-world entities and enable innovative applications across domains. In the context of elderly care and smart aging, this technology holds particular promise. Ambient intelligence has emerged as a natural evolution of IoT, especially in smart home environments where intelligent systems can assist elderly residents with daily activities, enhancing their independence and quality of life.

Despite the widely recognized potential of IoT for ambient intelligence, few systems demonstrate autonomous execution capabilities in real-world environments. Traditional IoT devices often function in isolation due to incompatible protocols, limiting collaborative potential. The Web of Things (WoT) has advanced by providing standardized descriptions of actions, events, and properties to extend Web protocols, enabling broader interactions between smart objects [17]. However, these connected systems still require human intervention rather than functioning fully autonomously [9].

In smart aging contexts, intelligent environments that proactively assist elderly residents face significant challenges while offering valuable opportunities. The Internet of Robotic Things (IoRT)—the integration of robotics with IoT systems—offers a promising approach to enhance ambient intelligence by enabling physical interactions and assistance with daily tasks.

Intent-aware interactive IoT represents a significant advancement in ambient intelligence for supporting elderly individuals in smart homes. By understanding user intentions through contextual sensing and historical interaction patterns, these systems anticipate needs and provide proactive assistance. For elderly users, intent-aware systems offer four key advantages. These systems reduce cognitive load

Q. Z. Sheng et al., *Harnessing Artificial Intelligence and Pervasive Internet of Things for an Empowered Aging*, https://doi.org/10.1007/978-3-032-16502-2_9

through automatic prediction and facilitation of routine tasks. They enhance safety via anticipatory monitoring of potentially dangerous activities. They increase independence through physical assistance with daily activities. Finally, they improve quality of life through personalized support aligned with individual habits and preferences.

The integration of robotics with intent-aware IoT creates a comprehensive support system bridging digital monitoring and physical assistance—a critical advancement for addressing practical challenges of aging in place.

9.1.2 Challenges and Opportunities

The development of intent-aware interactive IoT systems for smart aging faces several significant challenges. Firstly, accurately interpreting human intentions from sensor data and physical observations remains particularly complex when dealing with elderly users who may have inconsistent interaction patterns. Secondly, creating seamless integration between physical sensing, intention recognition, and robotic actuation in real-world environments presents technical difficulties that extend beyond controlled laboratory settings. Thirdly, ensuring that systems can adapt to individual preferences and habits while maintaining privacy and user autonomy requires careful balance between personalization and protection. The development of reliable and safe robotic assistance that can operate effectively in unstructured home environments adds another layer of complexity to system design.

Despite these challenges, intent-aware IoT presents remarkable opportunities for enhancing elderly care. These systems can enable aging-in-place through intelligent support that predicts and responds to needs, reduce caregiver burden by automating routine assistance tasks, improve quality of life by maintaining independence while providing necessary support, and create preventive health systems that detect early signs of deterioration in daily functioning. The existing research primarily focuses on recommending next actions to take, yet cannot control devices directly to execute those actions. Inspired by multiagent systems, Internet of Robotic Things (IoRT) enables robots to gain awareness of the environment and adapt their actions. However, the limited related research focuses on specialized scenarios [10], such as workplaces and smart cities; it still faces challenges for conducting physical interactions for daily tasks. There remains a significant gap to bring robotics into home applications to support streamlined physical human-machine interactions, particularly for elderly users.

9.1.3 Contributions

In this chapter, we present a novel framework named Intent-aware Interactive Internet of Things that implements ambient intelligence to facilitate seamless collaborations between humans, smart objects, and robots based on a unified IoT platform. Our first key contribution is an end-to-end solution for interactive ambient intelligence, where robots assist humans in physical activities within IoT-enabled smart homes, with specific applications for elderly care through adaptive monitoring and assistance. We further contribute a standardized approach using generic Web-based descriptions to facilitate smart-home device interactions, enabling the system to both decide and execute physical actions in the real world. Additionally, we propose an advanced reinforcement learning methodology for robotic assistants that exploits both successful and failed experiences, implementing policy continuation strategies with Hindsight Experience Replay to expedite learning and demonstrate practical implementation in the OpenAI Gym [2] environment. We evaluate our solution using implementations of public benchmarks on open-source platforms and demonstrate several activities to showcase the effectiveness of the proposed approach in real-life scenarios relevant to elderly care.

9.1.4 Chapter Organization

The remainder of this chapter is organized as follows. Section 9.2 provides background information and reviews the related work in smart home systems, activity recognition, and Internet of Robotic Things, with special attention to applications in smart aging. Section 9.3 presents our Intent-Aware Interactive Internet of Things framework in detail, including its methodology and implementation aspects. Section 9.4 discusses implications for smart aging applications, limitations, challenges, and identifies future research directions in this domain.

9.2 Background and Related Work

9.2.1 Smart Home Systems and Activity Recognition

Smart-home-related studies have attracted enormous attention, thanks to the availability of networked smart devices and improved computing capability. Early studies in the field concern Web management, localization, tracking, or activity recognition. CASAS [3] is one of the earliest smart-home experimental platforms that tracks users with preinstalled devices in apartments. Ruan et al. [14] achieved device-free indoor human localization and tracking. Yao et al. [22, 23] demonstrated a unified management system that integrates and monitors physical devices and finds relevant things according to past human interactions.

In the context of smart aging, activity recognition systems have been utilized to monitor daily activities of elderly residents, detect anomalies in routine behaviors, and provide assistance when needed. These systems typically rely on various sensing technologies, from ambient sensors to wearable devices, to collect data about user activities and environmental conditions.

9.2.2 Internet of Robotic Things and Ambient Intelligence

The concept of Internet of Robotic Things (IoRT) [10] aims to integrate robotics with IoT networks to enhance ambient intelligence capabilities. Mahieu et al. [10] investigated context-aware and personalized interactions on the IoRT. Vermesan et al. [22] reviewed IoRT and clarify some concepts with suggested architectures and applications.

For elderly care applications, IoRT offers the potential to bridge the gap between digital monitoring and physical assistance. Robots integrated with IoT systems can provide tangible help with activities of daily living, from medication reminders to physical assistance with mobility or household tasks. This integration is particularly valuable in the smart aging context, where users may benefit from both environmental intelligence and physical support.

9.2.3 Intent Recognition and Predictive Systems

Intent recognition involves inferring users' goals or desires from observed behaviors, contextual information, and historical patterns. Shemshadi et al. [16] proposed a framework for diversified relevance search in IoT, laying the foundation for IoT search engines [19, 20]. Their follow-up study [5, 24] reveals a real-time multilevel activity monitoring system for a personalized smart home, which continuously tracks daily activities and conducts abnormal activity detection.

For elderly users, intent recognition systems can help anticipate needs and provide timely assistance, potentially compensating for cognitive or physical limitations. By understanding typical behavioral patterns and recognizing deviations, these systems can offer personalized support while promoting independence and safety.

9.2.4 Research Gaps and Opportunities in Smart Aging Applications

Despite significant advances in IoT, activity recognition, and robotics, several research gaps remain in the context of intent-aware systems for smart aging:

- *Adaptive Intent Recognition*: Most existing systems rely on predefined activity patterns and struggle to adapt to the changing capabilities and habits of elderly users as they age.
- *Physical Assistance Integration*: While activity monitoring systems are relatively mature, their integration with physical assistance robots remains limited, particularly in unstructured home environments.

- *Personalization Challenges*: Elderly users have highly individualized needs and preferences, yet many systems lack sophisticated personalization capabilities beyond basic profile configurations.
- *Human-Robot Collaborative Intelligence*: Current systems typically either make recommendations or execute predefined tasks, but rarely engage in true collaborative problem-solving with human users.
- *Ethical Considerations*: The balance between assistance and autonomy, as well as privacy concerns, presents unique challenges in smart aging applications that require thoughtful technical and design approaches.

These research gaps represent significant opportunities for developing more comprehensive intent-aware interactive IoT systems that can truly enhance quality of life for elderly individuals. The studies mentioned previously realize ambient intelligence in certain aspects or applications but are still far from being truly "smart" in the sense of directly assisting human activities, particularly for elderly users with diverse and changing needs.

9.3 Intent-Aware Interactive IoT Framework

9.3.1 Motivation of Intent-Aware Ambient Intelligence

The Internet of Things (IoT) enables the connection of a broad range of artifacts with advanced sensory technologies and produces massive amounts of data to support ambient intelligence. While the potential of IoT systems is widely recognized, little work has demonstrated a system with the ability to execute autonomously in the real world, especially for supporting elderly individuals in their daily activities. Inspired by the success of robotics in specialized IoT environments, we propose an end-to-end solution for a generic, interactive ambient intelligence system where robots can assist humans, particularly elderly users, in conducting activities in IoT-enabled smart homes [6]. Although our experimental framework is designed with general applicability, we focus our discussion on implications and adaptations for elderly care scenarios, aligning with the broader focus of smart aging technologies. We evaluate the solution using implementations of public benchmarks on open-source platforms and use several activities to demonstrate the effectiveness of the proposed solution in real life scenarios that are particularly relevant to elderly assistance.

We envision a scenario (Fig. 9.1) to demonstrate our goal toward ambient intelligence and to motivate this study. Bob is preparing a bowl of cereal as breakfast, and usually, he finishes the meal with a cup of tea. The system detects a series of events in the kitchen at the time, such as movements of a cabinet door, a bowl, the fridge door, cereal containers and such, thereby recognizing that Bob is preparing cereal as breakfast. Based on Bob's daily routine, the system envisages a tea to finish the breakfast and commands a robot with a 3D depth camera to move to the kitchen. The robot then identifies a mug and teaspoon on the bench, confirming the predicted

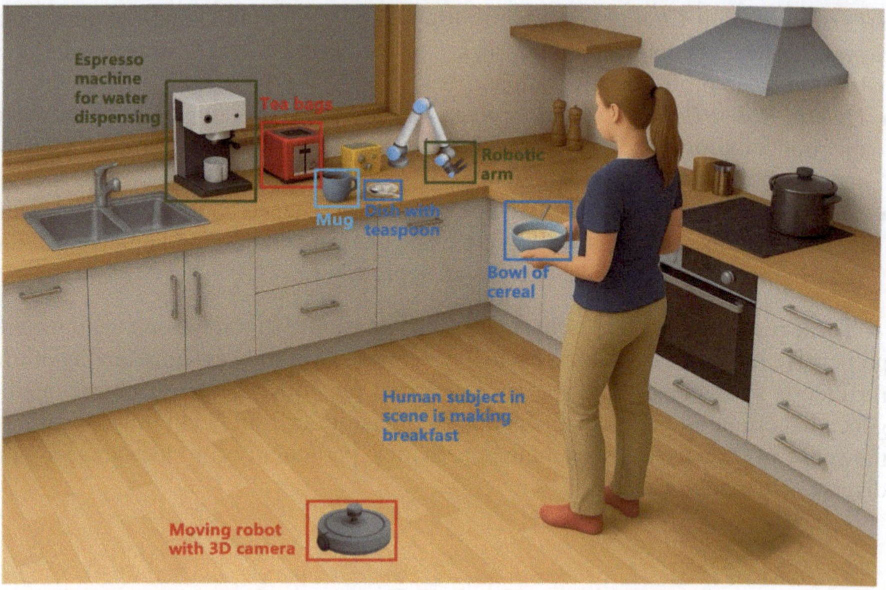

Fig. 9.1 An envisioned scenario of ambient intelligence for smart homes

intent of Bob, followed by the robot coordinating a robotic arm on the bench to make a tea for Bob while the cereal is being consumed. This assistance is particularly valuable as it reduces the physical strain of multiple trips to the kitchen that might be challenging for older adults.

9.3.2 IAIoT: Methodology for Intent-Aware Interactive IoT

Our framework (Fig. 9.2) explores ambient intelligence to enable autonomous robots to collaborate actively with humans in their daily activities in smart homes. The framework can infer human intent, compose actuation for interactions, and finally execute actions via robots.

Problem Setup

We first model human activities and develop a segmentation method for recognizing complex activities with awareness of concurring events and the subject intentions. Then, we finalize conscientious moves and device instructions for the robot assistants. We use the moving robot with a 3D stereo camera as the visual guide for other cooperative robot assistants to collaborate with the human. The 3D camera enables the robot to scan the environment, monitor the subject's activities, and infer the

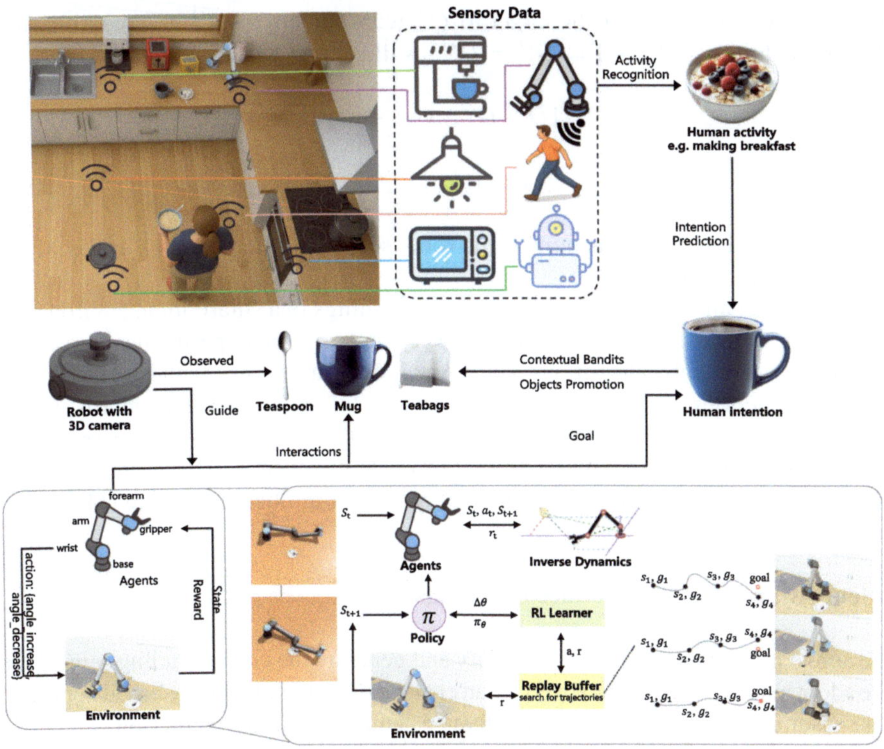

Fig. 9.2 Workflow of the proposed system in our scenario (illustrated in Fig. 9.1). First, the robot observes human activity and infers human's current behavior (i.e., making cereal breakfast) and intent (i.e., having a cup of tea) based on IoT sensory data. Then, the system figures out the objects to interact and works out the procedure for making tea. Finally, the robotic arm is guided to execute the procedure and make the predicted intent a reality (by preparing a cup of tea)

next move of the subject based on the usage history and basic rules preset or learned beforehand. After identifying interactable objects, the robot will receive step-by-step instructions by a smart and adaptive robotic control system.

Let $A \in \mathbb{R}^N$ be a set of activities, where $a_i \in A$ is the ith class of activity in the set. At time t, the system receives sensory input $x_t^A \in \mathbb{R}^d$, along with the predicted activity for this input:

$$x_t^A \rightarrow \widehat{y}_t^A = a_i. \tag{9.1}$$

Suppose $Q_t^A \in R^p$ is the semantic description corresponded to the current input x_t^A. The system matches this description with the semantic keywords $Q_t^O \in R^p$ of the objects detected by the robot R_m. With the contexts and historical usage information (A_H), the system infers the future action of the human at time $t'+1$, $y_{t'+1}^A = \hat{a}_j \in A$; accordingly, the action compositor $\alpha(\cdot)$ produces executable procedure with a series of interactions $I \in R^M$ for the target to Q^A with objects to Q^O assumed that in a short time duration $Q^O_t + 1 = Q^O_t = Q^O$, as illustrated below:

$$\{Q^A_t, Q^O, A_H\} \rightarrow \hat{a}_j \tag{9.2}$$

$$I = \alpha(\hat{a}_j, Q^O). \tag{9.3}$$

Once receiving the interactions I, the robot sees each interaction ι_m as a goal and learns to reach these goals.

We abstract all the connected and interactive things in a smart home environment as Web resources to support dynamic discovery, and perform hypermedia interactions as standardized Web interactions via normal Web protocols, such as HTTP. The device interactions are realized via Web services following WS-* standards, where JSON-based serialization help ease the implementation. Besides, we adapt a semantic description of Web-based Artifacts (based on Ricci et al. [13]) as the first-class abstraction for a clear integration and deployment of multiagent system (MAS).

Intent-Awareness With Connected Things

We aim to predict the next human activity and generate the corresponding semantics. We adopt a workflow inspired by Triboan et al. [21] a semantic theory based approach for sensor event segmentation, to facilitate a semantic activity prediction.

Activity Modeling. The environmental context (EC) consists of human subject (H_n), location (L_m), ambient characteristic (AC_o), sensor characteristics (S_p), and interactable objects (Obj_q) of classes (C_i).

$$EC = \{H_n, L_m, AC_o, S_p, Obj_q\}. \tag{9.4}$$

Sensor Environment (SR) describes the semantic relationship (R_e) between sensor events and objects where $SR = a_n(R_e, EC) \rightarrow R_e \rightarrow SE\ SE = instance(R_e, S_p)$. Since the actual activities performed by human may not match the system's prior knowledge (as noted in [10]), we additionally consider human preferences ($Pref_r$) below:

$$Pref_r = instance(R_e, a_n \cap Preference) \rightarrow R_e. \tag{9.5}$$

Semantic Decision. Based on the above relationships, we recognize activities using ontology-based semantic reasoning methods. Given a set of the streamed sensory events E^s and possible activity candidates A', we construct an activity thread AT_i by conducting Terminology Box ($\mathsf{T-Box}$) reasoning on regular, generic activities, and Assertion Box ($\mathsf{A-Box}$) reasoning for user preferred activities:

$$AT_i = \{tBox[A', E^s], aBox[Pref_r[Pref', E^s]]\}. \tag{9.6}$$

We analyze the metadata of sensor event $e_m \in E^s$ for the corresponding entity (ET_K) to deduce candidate relationships with activities; the concurrent activities can be inferred during this process using the above semantic reasoner.

Sensor Events Segmentation. We generalize the concept of sensory events to contain status and usage information gathered in the IoT networks. Inspired by Mallick et al. [11] we adopt a transaction-based segmentation as activities may be multiplexed. Given a set of sensory events $E = \{e_1, e_2, \ldots e_E | e_i \in E\hat{S}\}$, we segment it into multiple transactions, denoted by $tr_i = \{e_i, e_{i+1}, \ldots, e_{i+j}\} \in Tr$. Suppose ProperCut is the transaction tr_i that matches exactly with activity a_i. OverCut includes the transactions that contain incomplete activities, and UnderCut covers those transactions that involve multiple activities. Then, our goal becomes to minimize the number of overcutting and undercutting transactions. To this end, we identify the minimal transactions of sensory events that contain complete activities for our downstream processing, the activity prediction, and use the *MinMax* algorithm to embed and cluster contextual information of sensors and IoT devices, where we use distances and temporal sequences for segmentation.

Activity Prediction. We infer a user's possible next moves for our downstream processing, such as giving commands to robotic assistants. Then, we employ two stages of the method proposed by Altulyan et al. [1] to suggest the next items to be used by the human:

- Complex activity recognition: At the current stage, the system learns to recognize simple activities, such as the posture and movement of human. The next step is to recognize complex activities based on predefined ontology and rules.
- Recommendation: At the current stage, the system prompts activities and items to be used by human or robot in the next step. We learn from past trajectories of activities with Q-learning.

Semantic Searching and Context-Aware Interactions

Semantic Searching for Interactive Internet of Things. The system uses semantic search to identify the suitable objects and generate the procedure for a robot to act toward the inferred human intent. We use Mask R-CNN [4], a widely used pixel-level object segmentation model that outputs 1 or 0 to indicate whether a pixel belongs to an object, for object detection. We also combine objective detection with depth information to get 3D positions of objects of interest. Such position information is then used to adapt the learning goals and training/running processes of robots.

Context-Aware Hypermedia Interactions. We introduce an RL-based approach named Policy Continuation with Hindsight Inverse Dynamics (PCHID) to generate hardware commands for instructing robotic arms' movements.

Policy Continuation with Hindsight Inverse Dynamics. PCHID [18] supports self-supervised learning for goal-conditional tasks and can extrapolate the learned policy to complex and nonlinear Hindsight Inverse Dynamics (HID) applications. Specifically, PCHID introduces the goal into inverse dynamics as Hindsight Inverse Dynamics and outputs the minimal k-step actions to achieve the goal under the optimal policy. This enables us to complete a complex task in multiple steps, each achieving a different subgoal.

Multistep Goals with Policy Continuation. While PCHID [18] makes the system aware of the hindsight goal, more sophisticated settings are introduced and it is considerable challenging. We extend the original Hindsight Experience Replay (HER) model with the ideal proposed by Sun et al. [18] to let HID embrace k-step solubility for better optimization. As in the Universal Value Function Approximators (UVFA) [15], we have possible goals $g \in G$ and a corresponding reward $r_g : S \times A \rightarrow R$, where S, A are the state space and action space, respectively. At timestamp t, we have $r_t = r_g(s_t, g_t)$ and policy $\pi : S \times G \rightarrow A$. The reward is extended from the (0, 1) binary problem set to the following:

$$r(s_t, a_t, g) = \lambda \left| g - s_t^{object} \right|^p - \left| g - s_{t+1}^{object} \right|^p . \tag{9.7}$$

This reward function encourages the system to move closer to the goal object at each step, where the hyperparameter $p \in \{1, 2\}$ determines the distance metric (Manhattan or Euclidean), and λ controls the reward scaling.

Based on the UVFA model of HID, we apply the k-step solvable extension, decomposing the state-goal space into multiple subspaces that correspond to different temporal horizons (see Sun et al. [18] for more technical details). Our objective is to find the optimal policy that consists of multiple sub-policies, where each sub-policy at a given timestamp leads to the next sub-goal. This optimization problem is effectively solved using stochastic gradient descent (SGD) models that minimize the prediction error between the learned function and the actual actions across multiple training episodes.

9.3.3 Experimental Evaluation and Results

We have implemented live demonstrations of some selected activities and evaluate the feasibility of our system in real-life applications based on simulation, with particular attention to tasks relevant to elderly assistance.

We test the task learning process of robotic assistants based on RLBench [7], an open source robotics-related manipulation benchmark that contains 100 daily activities. The selected tasks—picking and lifting objects, placing and removing cups, and pressing switches—represent common manipulation scenarios that can benefit various user groups, including elderly individuals with limited mobility or dexterity. While RLBench uses the PyRep simulator, we implement our system with the Deepbot framework [8] in the OpenAI Gym environment [2], which enables us to synchronize the simulation with Robot Operating System (ROS). Our setting involves a Lynx-motion AL5D robotic arm, a TurtleBot waffle Pi equipped with a 3D stereo camera, and various interactive items, such as kitchen utensils.

As aforementioned, the robotic assistant actuates based on the UVFA model of HID, an extension to DQN [12]. We compare PCHID with DQN and its successor HER to demonstrate the effectiveness of our framework in RLBench tasks. Specifically, we set the reward to 0 when the final state is within the tolerable range of the subgoal for each step and –1 otherwise.

Figure 9.3 shows the overall success rates and rewards with respect to episodes of training. The PCHID method is effective and learns significantly faster than HER and the original DQN methods. Figure 9.4 shows some intermediate learning outcomes: (a) and (b) failed to complete the task of "Pick and lift" while (c) succeeded at episode 20, 50, and 100. Figure 9.5 further demonstrates the effectiveness of PCHID in some selected tasks: (a) Pick and lift; (b) Place cups; (c) Remove cups; (d) Press switch. In our experiments, we set the steps k to 5—we observed a larger step tended to improve the results.

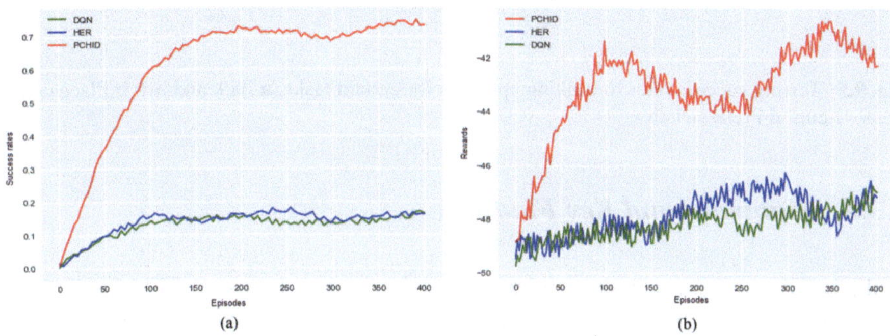

Fig. 9.3 **a** Overall testing success rate to training episodes. **b** Overall learning rewards obtained to training episodes

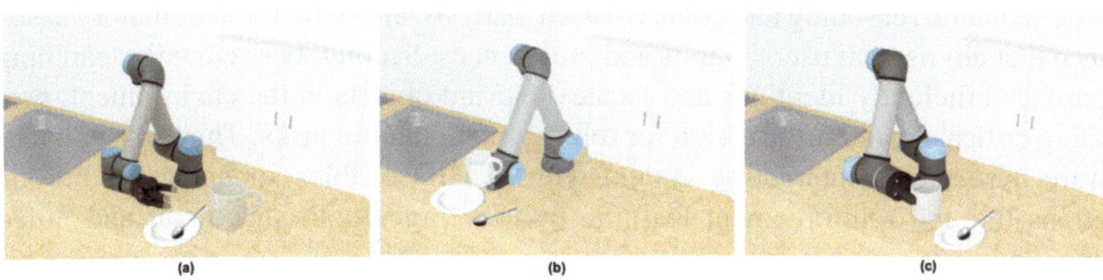

Fig. 9.4 Learning results for the task "Pick and lift" on some selected intermediate episodes, where **a** and **b** failed to complete the task while, **c** succeeded at episode 20, 50, and 100

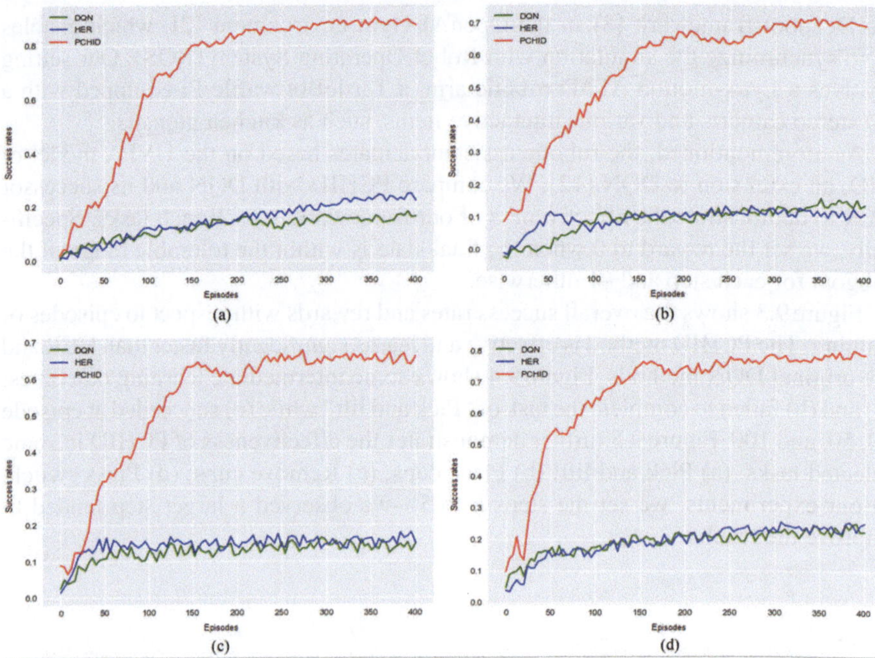

Fig. 9.5 Testing success rates to training episodes for certain tasks. **a** Pick and lift. **b** Place cup. **c** Remove cup. **d** Press switch

9.3.4 Summary and Key Findings

In this section, we presented the Intent-Aware Interactive Internet of Things (IAIoT) framework, which demonstrates several significant achievements in human-robot collaborative intelligence. Our framework successfully integrates multiple key components that work together to create a truly interactive ambient intelligence system. First, the intent-awareness methodology effectively predicts human activities using semantic reasoning and context-based analysis, allowing for anticipatory assistance that aligns with users' habits and preferences. Second, our semantic searching approach efficiently identifies and locates relevant objects in the environment, providing critical spatial information for robotic manipulation tasks. Third, the context-aware hypermedia interaction system with PCHID enables sophisticated robotic actions through reinforcement learning that leverages both successful and failed experiences.

Our experimental evaluation demonstrates that the PCHID method significantly outperforms traditional DQN and HER approaches in various manipulation tasks, with substantially faster learning rates and higher success rates. The framework's ability to complete everyday tasks like picking, placing, and manipulating objects shows promising potential for real-world smart home applications, particularly in elderly care scenarios where anticipatory assistance can enhance independence and safety. These results validate our approach to creating an end-to-end solution for interactive ambient intelligence that can bridge the gap between digital sensing and physical assistance.

9.4 Discussion and Future Directions

The Intent-Aware Interactive IoT framework presented in this chapter advances interactive and cooperative ambient intelligence through the integration of intent recognition, semantic reasoning, and robotic actuation. Our experimental evaluation demonstrates the technical feasibility of creating collaborative human-robot environments that can understand, predict, and respond to human intentions in real time.

Our framework makes several key technical contributions to interactive ambient intelligence. The integration of semantic reasoning with reinforcement learning enables robots to understand human activities and predict future intentions based on contextual information and historical patterns. The PCHID methodology demonstrates significant improvements in learning efficiency, with success rates exceeding 90% in complex manipulation tasks. The standardized Web-based abstraction for IoT device interactions provides a scalable foundation for deploying such systems across diverse environments.

The framework's design principles are well-suited for applications requiring anticipatory assistance and physical interaction support. This includes smart aging scenarios where users benefit from systems that reduce cognitive load, provide physical assistance, and enhance safety through predictive monitoring. However, the framework's utility extends beyond age-specific applications to any environment where human-robot collaboration can enhance productivity, safety, or quality of life.

Despite promising results, several challenges must be addressed for widespread deployment. Real-world environments present unstructured, highly variable conditions that differ substantially from controlled test settings. Current object recognition and manipulation capabilities struggle with the visual and physical complexity of actual home environments, including dynamic lighting conditions, cluttered spaces, and diverse household objects. Building user trust through reliable operation, transparent decision-making, and appropriate system autonomy remains critical. Intent prediction systems inevitably collect intimate behavioral data about users' daily activities, requiring careful consideration of privacy protection and data security practices.

Future research should focus on several key directions. Adaptive learning mechanisms that enable continuous evolution with changing user needs and environmental conditions are essential. Cross-domain knowledge transfer capabilities could significantly reduce setup time and improve performance across diverse scenarios. Explainable AI techniques must be incorporated to provide clear insights into system reasoning, particularly for applications involving healthcare or safety-critical domains. Multi-modal intent recognition integrating natural language processing, gesture recognition, and physiological monitoring could enhance accuracy and enable more sophisticated interactions. Edge computing architectures could improve responsiveness while addressing privacy concerns by keeping sensitive data local.

In summary, this chapter presents a comprehensive framework for intent-aware interactive IoT that demonstrates the feasibility of creating collaborative ambient intelligence systems. Our technical contributions provide a foundation for advancing interactive and cooperative ambient intelligence, with applications spanning from smart aging to general human-robot collaboration environments. Through continued research addressing the identified challenges, we envision ambient intelligence systems that seamlessly blend digital sensing, intelligent reasoning, and physical actuation to support human activities in natural, unobtrusive ways.

References

1. Altulayan, M.S., Huang, C., Yao, L., Wang, X., Kanhere, S.: Contextual bandit learning for activity-aware things-of-interest recommendation in an assisted living environment. In: Proceedings of the 32nd Australasian Database Conference (ADC), pp. 37–49. Springer (2021)
2. Brockman, G., Cheung, V., Petzke, L., Schulman, J., Yiyang, S., et al.: Openai gym (2016). arXiv:1606.01540
3. Cook, D.J., Crandall, A.S., Thomas, B.L., Krishnan, N.C.: CASAS: a smart home in a box. IEEE Comput. **46**(7), 62–69 (2013)
4. He, K., Gkioxari, G., Dollár, P., Girshick, R.: Mask R-CNN. In: Proceedings of the IEEE International Conference on Computer Vision (ICCV), pp. 2961–2969 (2017)
5. Huang, C., Yao, L.: Active object estimation for human-robot collaborative tasks. In: Proceedings of the International Conference on Neural Information Processing (ICONIP), pp. 750–761. Springer (2020)
6. Huang, C., Yao, L., Wang, X., Sheng, Q.Z., Dustdar, S., Wang, Z., Xu, X.: Intent-aware interactive internet of things for enhanced collaborative ambient intelligence. IEEE Internet Comput. **26**(5), 68–75 (2022)
7. James, S., Ma, Z., Arrojo, D.R., Davison, A.J.: RLBench: the robot learning benchmark & learning environment. IEEE Robot. Autom. Lett. **5**(2), 3019–3026 (2020)
8. Kirtas, M., Tsampazis, K., Passalis, N., Tefas, A.: Deepbots: a webots-based deep reinforcement learning framework for robotics. In: Proceedings of the IFIP International Conference on Artificial Intelligence Applications and Innovations, pp. 64–75. Springer (2020)
9. Lu, H., Cao, D., Tao, D., Dustdar, S., Ho, P.: Guest editorial for special issue on cognitive computing for collaborative robotics. IEEE/CAA J. Autom. Sinica **8**(7) (2021). Article no. 1221
10. Mahieu, C., Ongenae, F., Backere, F.D., Bonte, P., Turck, F.D., Simoens, P.: Semantics-based platform for context-aware and personalized robot interaction in the internet of robotic things. J. Syst. Softw. **149**, 138–157 (2019)
11. Mallick, M., Kodeswaran, P., Sen, S., Kokku, R., Ganguly, N.: TSFS: an integrated approach for event segmentation and ADL detection in IoT enabled smart-homes. IEEE Trans. Mob. Comput. **18**(11), 2686–2700 (2019)
12. Mnih, V., Kavukcuoglu, K., Silver, D., Rusu, A.A., Veness, J., et al.: Human-level control through deep reinforcement learning. Nature **518**, 529–533 (2015)
13. Ricci, A., Piunti, M., Viroli, M., Omicini, A.: Environment programming in CArtAgO. In: Multi-Agent Programming, pp. 259–288. Springer (2009)

14. Ruan, W., Sheng, Q.Z., Yao, L., Gu, T., Ruta, M., Shangguan, L.: Device-free indoor localization and tracking through human—Object interactions. In: Proceedings of the 17th IEEE International Symposium on a World of Wireless, Mobile and Multimedia Networks (WoWMoM), pp. 1–9. IEEE (2016)
15. Schaul, T., Horgan, D., Gregor, K., Silver, D.: Universal value function approximators. In: Proceedings of the 32nd International Conference on Machine Learning (ICML), pp. 1312–1320 (2015)
16. Shemshadi, A., Sheng, Q.Z., Qin, Y., Sun, A., Zhang, W.E., Yao, L.: Searching for the internet of things: where it is and what it looks like. Pers. Ubiquit. Comput. **21**(6), 1097–1112 (2017)
17. Sheng, M., Qin, Y., Yao, L., Benatallah, B. (eds.): Managing the Web of Things: Linking the Real World to the Web. Morgan Kaufmann (2017)
18. Sun, H., Li, Z., Liu, X., Zhou, B., Lin, D.: Policy continuation with hindsight inverse dynamics. In: Proceedings of the 33rd Conference on Neural Information Processing Systems (NeurIPS), pp. 10265–10275 (2019)
19. Tran, N.K., Sheng, Q.Z., Babar, M.A., Yao, L.: Searching the web of things: state of the art, challenges, and solutions. ACM Comput. Surv. **50**(4), 55:1–55:34 (2017)
20. Tran, N.K., Sheng, Q.Z., Babar, M.A., Yao, L., Zhang, W.E., Dustdar, S.: Internet of things search engine. Commun. ACM **62**(7), 66–73 (2019)
21. Triboan, D., Chen, L., Chen, F., Wang, Z.: A semantics-based approach to sensor data segmentation in real-time activity recognition. Futur. Gener. Comput. Syst. **93**, 224–236 (2019)
22. Yao, L., Sheng, Q.Z., Dustdar, S.: Web-based management of the internet of things. IEEE Internet Comput. **19**(4), 60–67 (2015)
23. Yao, L., Sheng, Q.Z., Falkner, N.J.G., Ngu, A.H.H.: ThingsNavi: Finding most-related things via multi-dimensional modeling of human-thing interactions. In: Proceedings of the 11th International Conference on Mobile and Ubiquitous Systems: computing, Networking and Services (MobiQuitous), pp. 20–29. ACM (2014)
24. Yao, L., Sheng, Q.Z., Falkner, N.J.G., Ngu, A.H.H., et al.: WITS: an IoT-endowed computational framework for activity recognition in personalized smart homes. Computing **100**(4), 369–385 (2018)

Chapter 10
Brain-Computer Interface for IoT Cognitive Interactivity

10.1 Introduction

10.1.1 Overview of BCI and IoT Integration

It is expected that billions of devices will be connected to the Internet. The proliferation of the Internet of Things (IoT) is expected to improve efficiency and impact various domains including home automation, manufacturing and industries, transportation, and healthcare [17]. Individuals will have the opportunity to interact and control a wide range of everyday objects through various means of interactions including applications running on their smartphone or wearable devices, voice, and gestures. Brain-computer interface (BCI) is emerging as a novel alternative for supporting interaction between IoT objects and individuals. BCI establishes a direct communication pathway between human brain and an external device thus eliminating the need for typical information delivery methods [16]. Recent trends in BCI research have witnessed the translation of human thinking capabilities into physical actions, such as mind-controlled wheelchairs and IoT-enabled appliances [3, 15]. These examples suggest that the BCI is going to be a major aiding technology in human-thing interaction [21].

A brain-computer interface (BCI) acquires brain signals, analyzes, and translates them into commands that are relayed to actuation devices for carrying out desired actions. With the widespread connectivity of everyday devices realized by the advent of the Internet of Things (IoT), BCI can empower individuals to directly control objects such as smart home appliances or assistive robots via their thoughts alone. This capability has broad applications across various domains, enabling enhanced independence without requiring complex physical interactions.

The integration of BCI with IoT systems creates new possibilities by enabling seamless interaction between individuals and their surroundings. This integration is especially valuable for people with diverse interaction needs who could control home automation systems, communicate more effectively, or operate assistive devices using

Q. Z. Sheng et al., *Harnessing Artificial Intelligence and Pervasive Internet of Things for an Empowered Aging*, https://doi.org/10.1007/978-3-032-16502-2_10

only their thoughts. This approach to human-thing cognitive interactivity offers several advantages, including enhanced independence, improved quality of life, and greater accessibility of technology for users with varying capabilities and preferences.

10.1.2 Challenges and Opportunities

The BCI-based human-thing cognitive interactivity faces several fundamental challenges. Brain signals can be measured using various technologies such as electroencephalogram (EEG) [16], functional near-infrared spectroscopy (fNIR) [13], and magnetoencephalography (MEG) [7], but all these methods are susceptible to low fidelity and are easily influenced by environmental factors and sentiment status (e.g., noise and concentration) [12]. In other words, brain signals generally have very low signal-to-noise ratios, and inherently lack sufficient spatial or temporal resolution and insight on activities of deep brain structures [21]. As a result, while current cognitive recognition systems can achieve about 70–80% accuracy, this is not sufficient for designing reliable practical systems, which is particularly important in applications like smart aging where dependability is essential.

Another significant challenge is that data preprocessing, parameter selection (e.g., filter type, filtering band, segment window, and overlapping), and feature engineering (e.g., feature selection and extraction both in the time domain and frequency domain) are all time-consuming and highly dependent on human expertise in the domain [5]. This complexity presents barriers to widespread implementation, especially in contexts where technical support may be limited.

Despite these challenges, BCI-based cognitive interactivity offers several unique opportunities. One is the inherent privacy arising from the fact that brain activity is invisible and thus impossible to observe and replicate [11]. Another is the convenience and real-time nature of the interaction, since users only need to think about the interaction rather than undertake the corresponding physical motions (e.g., speak, type, and gesture) [10]. These advantages are particularly valuable for users with limited mobility, dexterity, or speech capabilities, making BCI a promising technology for enhancing human-thing interaction across diverse application domains.

10.1.3 Contributions

In this chapter, we present several significant contributions to the field of brain-computer interfaces. We propose a unified deep learning framework that bridges BCI and IoT to enable end-to-end cognitive brain-to-thing interaction. To our best knowledge, this is the first work that systematically investigates this integration for human-thing cognitive interactivity, with applications in various domains including assistive technologies.

We introduce three complementary technical innovations that work together to overcome key challenges in brain signal processing. First, we develop a Replicate and Shuffle (RS) process that enhances feature representation by creating diverse combinations of signal dimensions. Second, we present a Selective Attention Mechanism (SAM) with focal zone optimization that identifies the most informative segments of brain signals using deep reinforcement learning. Third, we propose a Weighted Average Spatial LSTM (WAS-LSTM) that captures complex interdimensional relationships while providing enhanced classification stability through weighted averaging approaches.

We demonstrate the practical utility of our framework through two operational prototypes: a brain typing system and a cognitive robot control system. These implementations validate the framework's ability to enable intuitive human-thing interaction through direct brain-to-device communication, which can enhance independence and quality of life for users with diverse needs and capabilities. Our experimental evaluation shows that the framework achieves 93.6% recognition accuracy across six mental tasks while maintaining response times under one second, making it suitable for real-world deployment in various application domains.

10.1.4 Chapter Organization

Section 10.2 presents the background and related work on brain-computer interface technologies, IoT systems for human-thing interaction, and deep learning approaches for brain signal processing. This section establishes the theoretical foundations and reviews current approaches in BCI-IoT integration, identifying key research gaps and opportunities that motivate our work. Section 10.3 introduces our deep learning framework for brain-to-IoT cognitive interactivity. This section details our technical approach including the Replicate and Shuffle process, Selective Attention Mechanism, and Weighted Average Spatial LSTM, followed by comprehensive experimental evaluation and practical applications that demonstrate the framework's effectiveness. Section 10.4 discusses the broader implications of our work, including technical limitations of the current approach, application potential across various domains, and future research directions for advancing BCI-IoT integration technologies.

10.2 Background and Related Work

This section provides an overview of brain-computer interface technologies and their applications in IoT environments. We discuss the challenges in processing and interpreting brain signals, highlight existing approaches for BCI-based cognitive interactivity, and examine their potential relevance to various application domains, including smart aging contexts.

10.2.1 BCI Technologies and Methods

Brain-computer interface (BCI) systems establish direct communication pathways between the human brain and external devices [16]. The BCI mentioned in this chapter refers primarily to non-invasive BCI, which captures brain activity without requiring surgical implantation of electrodes. These non-invasive technologies include electroencephalogram (EEG) [16], functional near-infrared spectroscopy (fNIR) [13], and magnetoencephalography (MEG) [7].

Among these technologies, EEG has become particularly popular for practical BCI applications due to its relative affordability, portability, and ease of use. EEG captures electrical activity from the scalp using electrodes, providing temporal information about brain function. While fNIR and MEG offer alternative approaches with certain advantages in terms of signal quality or spatial resolution, they typically require more expensive equipment and controlled environments, limiting their applicability in everyday contexts including home environments, assistive technologies, and other scenarios where ease of deployment is essential.

10.2.2 IoT and Human-Thing Interaction

The Internet of Things (IoT) refers to the network of interconnected physical objects embedded with sensors, software, and other technologies that enable these objects to connect and exchange data [17]. IoT technologies have been deployed across numerous domains to enhance safety, support independence, monitor health, and improve quality of life for various user groups.

IoT applications include smart home automation systems that can adjust lighting, temperature, and security based on residents' needs; wearable devices that monitor vital signs and detect anomalies; personalized management systems that provide reminders and track adherence to schedules; and interactive robots that offer assistance with daily tasks. These technologies have particular relevance for smart aging contexts among other applications, as they can help extend independence and enhance quality of life. Currently, most IoT systems rely on conventional interaction methods such as touch interfaces, voice commands, or automated sensing to function [1, 18], creating opportunities for new interaction paradigms like BCI.

10.2.3 Deep Learning for BCI

Deep learning techniques have shown promising results in addressing the challenges of processing and interpreting brain signals. Convolutional neural networks (CNNs), recurrent neural networks (RNNs), and their variants have been applied to EEG signal classification tasks with increasing success [8]. These approaches can automatically learn hierarchical features from raw or minimally preprocessed brain signals, potentially reducing the need for extensive manual feature engineering.

However, many existing deep learning approaches for BCI still face challenges related to the high dimensionality of brain signal data, inter-subject variability, and limited training data availability. Additionally, most current approaches focus on specific classification tasks rather than providing comprehensive frameworks for enabling real-time cognitive interactivity in IoT environments.

10.2.4 Research Gaps and Opportunities in Smart Aging Applications

Despite advances in both BCI technologies and IoT applications, several research gaps remain in integrating these domains effectively:

- Most existing BCI systems have not been designed with diverse user needs and limitations in mind, potentially limiting their usability and acceptance across different application contexts, including but not limited to smart aging.
- There is limited research on end-to-end frameworks that bridge BCI and IoT to enable seamless cognitive interactivity for real-world applications, which could benefit various user groups with different interaction requirements.
- The challenges of low signal fidelity, high variability, and complex feature engineering in brain signal processing have not been adequately addressed for practical deployment in everyday environments where background noise and distractions are common.
- Few studies have demonstrated practical applications of BCI-IoT integration that effectively enhance human-thing interaction for users with diverse needs and capabilities.

These research gaps present opportunities to develop more effective, user-friendly, and practical BCI-IoT systems. Such systems could potentially transform how people interact with their environments, including applications in smart aging contexts where they could provide new avenues for maintaining independence and enhancing quality of life for individuals with varying physical capabilities.

10.3 Deep Learning Framework for Brain-to-IoT Cognitive Interactivity

10.3.1 Motivation and Overview of Deep Learning Framework

In this section, we present our unified deep learning framework for enabling human-thing cognitive interactivity [22]. The development of this framework is motivated by the need to overcome key challenges in brain signal interpretation, particularly the low signal-to-noise ratio and the complexity of feature engineering. These challenges are especially relevant for practical applications where reliability and ease of use are essential requirements.

As shown in Fig. 10.1, our framework measures the user's brain activities (such as EEG, fNIRS, and MEG) through specific brain signal collection equipment. The raw brain signals are forwarded to the cloud server via Internet access. The cloud server uses a person-dependent pretrained deep learning model for analyzing the raw signals. The analyzed and interpreted signals can then be used for actuating functions in a wide range of IoT applications, such as smart cities [2] (e.g., transportation control and agenda schedule), smart hospitals [4, 19] (e.g., emergency call and anomaly monitoring), and smart homes [1, 18] (e.g., appliances control and assistive robot

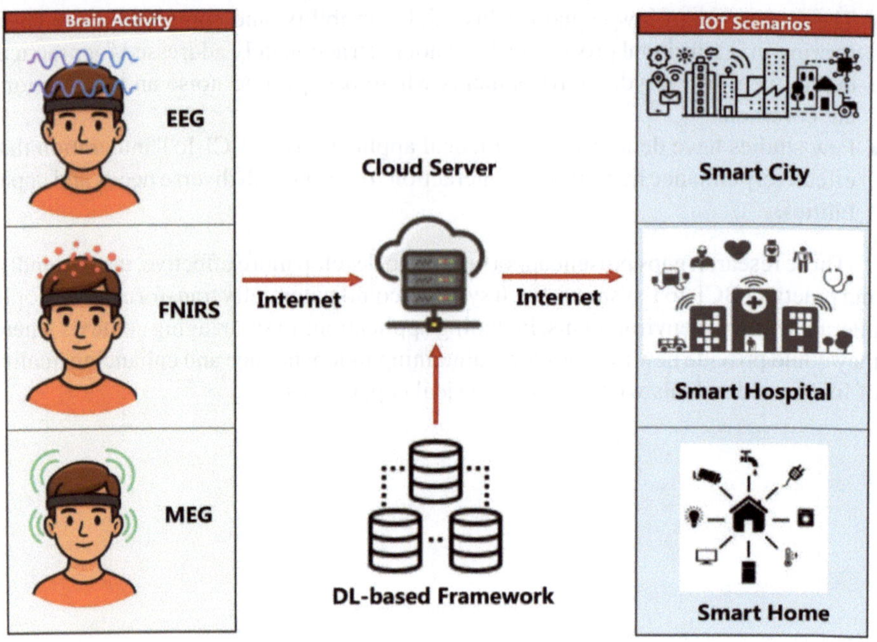

Fig. 10.1 Schematic of the cognitive IoT framework

control). These applications have particular relevance for enhancing independence and assistance in smart aging contexts.

Our unified deep learning framework aims to interpret the subjects' intent and decode it into corresponding commands that are discernible for IoT devices. Based on our previous study [20, 21], for each single brain signal sample, the self-similarity is always higher than the cross-similarity, which means that the intraintent cohesion of the samples is stronger than the interintent cohesion. To leverage this characteristic, we propose a weighted average spatial long short-term memory (WAS-LSTM) approach to exploit the latent correlation between signal dimensions. The proposed end-to-end framework is capable of modeling high-level, robust, and salient feature representations hidden in the raw human brain signal streams and capturing complex relationships within data.

The key innovation of our approach is addressing the dual challenges of low signal fidelity and complex feature engineering through an integrated deep learning solution. Our framework eliminates the need for extensive manual preprocessing and feature engineering, making BCI technology more accessible and practical for everyday use by diverse user groups. This accessibility is particularly valuable in applications requiring intuitive and reliable interaction, such as assistive technologies, including those designed for smart aging contexts.

10.3.2 Deep Learning Methodology for BCI-IoT Integration

Our cognition detection framework exploits EEG signals due to their unique features that make them suitable for practical applications, such as low-cost, low-energy consumption, privacy, and portability. The proposed framework is depicted in Fig. 10.2. The main focus of our approach is to exploit the latent dependency among different signal dimensions, which is critical for accurate brain signal interpretation.

Our framework contains three key components: (1) the replicate and shuffle (RS) processing to enhance feature representation; (2) the selective attention learning to focus on the most relevant signal components; and (3) the sequential LSTM-based classification to capture complex interdimensional dependencies.

Framework Design Considerations. The effective interpretation of brain signals for cognitive interactivity presents unique challenges. Our key insight is that signals belonging to different cognitions have distinct interdimensional dependency relationships containing rich and discriminative information. EEG signals are typically arranged as 1-D vectors, but this representation is limited by fixed element arrangements that may not capture the complex relationships between signal dimensions.

To address these challenges, we propose three complementary techniques designed to enhance BCI performance, making our framework suitable for a wide range of applications where signal quality and interpretation challenges can impact system performance.

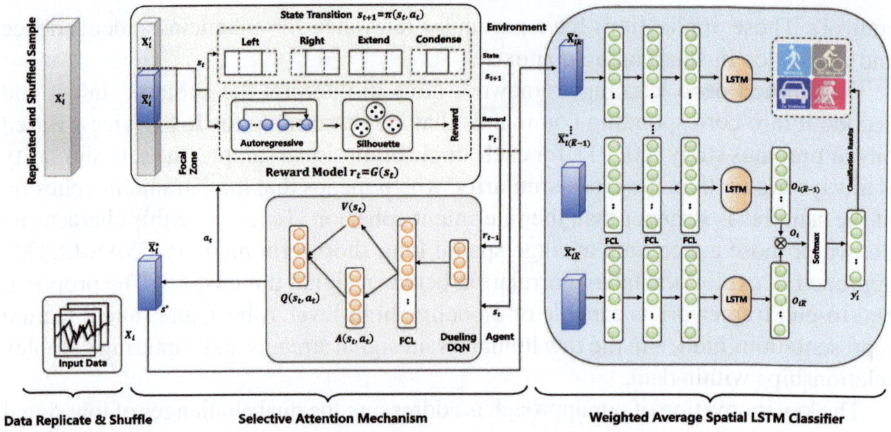

Fig. 10.2 Flowchart of the proposed framework. The focal zone $\tilde{x}_t$ is a selected fragment from x'_t to feed in the state transition and the reward model. In each step t, one action is selected by the state transition to update s_t based on the agent's feedback. The reward model evaluates the quality of the focal zone to the reward r_t. The dueling DQN is employed to find the optimal focal zone $\tilde{x}_t^+$ which will be feed into the LSTM-based classifier to explore the interdimension dependency and predict the sample's label y'_t. FCL denotes fully connected layer. The state transition contains four actions: left shifting, right shifting, extend, and condense. The dashed line indicates the focal zone before the action while the solid line indicates the position of the focal zone after the action

Data Replication and Shuffling. We introduce a data Replicate and Shuffle (RS) technique that creates more diverse feature combinations. This approach is particularly valuable in applications where maximizing the information extracted from limited or noisy signals is essential.

The input EEG data is represented as $\mathbf{X} = \{(\mathbf{x}_i, y_i),\ i = 1, 2, \ldots, I\}$ where each pair represents a 1-D EEG signal sample with its corresponding category label. Our RS method transforms the original signal $\mathbf{x}_i \in \mathbb{R}^K$ into an enhanced representation $\mathbf{x}'_i \in \mathbb{R}^{K'}$ with more complete element combinations, where $K' > K$.

Selective Attention Mechanism. After enhancing the signal representation through the RS process, we introduce a Selective Attention Mechanism (SAM) that focuses on the most informative portions of the signal. We define a "focal zone" that represents a particularly informative fragment of the enhanced signal. To optimally position this focal zone, we employ deep reinforcement learning, which can automatically adapt to individual differences in brain signal patterns.

Our focal zone optimization framework includes the environment (including state transition and reward model) and the agent. The agent can perform four types of actions to adjust the focal zone: left shifting, right shifting, extending, or condensing the zone. We employ a dueling deep Q-network (DQN) that efficiently learns the state-value function, providing faster convergence beneficial for real-time applications.

Weighted Average Spatial LSTM. We introduce a Weighted Average Spatial LSTM (WAS-LSTM) approach designed to capture complex interdimensional relationships in brain signals while providing enhanced stability. Our innovation lies in repurposing LSTM models to analyze spatial relationships within brain signals rather than temporal sequences.

The WAS-LSTM achieves enhanced stability by calculating outputs using a weighted average of the past two outputs rather than only the final one. This weighted averaging approach helps mitigate fluctuations in neural network convergence, resulting in more consistent and reliable classification performance.

Through this approach, our framework can reliably interpret diverse brain signals and translate them into appropriate commands for IoT devices, enabling intuitive cognitive interactivity that can significantly enhance independence and quality of life in various application contexts.

10.3.3 Experimental Validation and Performance Analysis

Experimental Setting: We conducted EEG data collection using a portable Emotiv Epoc+ headset with 14 channels at a sampling rate 128 Hz. The experiment involved seven subjects (four males and three females) aged from 23 to 26. During the experiments, subjects wore the EEG headset and focused on corresponding hints displayed on the screen while imaging certain actions without physical movement. Six categories of mental tasks were recorded: upward arrow, downward arrow, leftward arrow, rightward arrow, middle cycle, and eye-closed relaxation state. The imagery actions, labels, and corresponding commands used in our case studies are listed in Table 10.1. The dataset contains 241,920 samples with 34,560 samples per subject. For each participant, the dataset was divided into a training set (31,104 samples) and a testing set (3,456 samples).

Performance Analysis: To validate our framework's effectiveness, we compared our approach with several competitive baselines including non-deep learning methods (SVM, Random Forest, KNN, AdaBoost, LDA), deep learning methods (LSTM,

Table 10.1 Imagery action, label, and corresponding commands in case studies

Imagery action	Label	Typing commands	Robot commands
Upward	0	Up	Forward
Downward	1	Cancel	Turn left
Leftward	2	Left	Grasp
Rightward	3	Right	Loose
Middle cycle	4	Nothing	Nothing
Eye-closed	5	Confirm	Stop/start

Table 10.2 Overall comparison with the state-of-the-art baselines. DL denotes deep learning

Baselines	Methods	Acc	Pre	Rec	F1-score
Non-DL	SVM	0.2569	0.2737	0.2569	0.2577
	RF	0.8041	0.8071	0.8041	0.8048
	KNN	0.8539	0.8563	0.8539	0.8544
	AB	0.2506	0.2039	0.2506	0.1557
	LDA	0.2595	0.2761	0.2595	0.2618
DL	LSTM	0.2609	0.2447	0.2348	0.2354
	GRU	0.2521	0.271	0.2696	0.2701
	CNN	0.725	0.724	0.7237	0.7238
The state-of-the-art	[6]	0.8965	0.9011	0.8926	0.8968
	[14]	0.7894	0.7938	0.8013	0.7975
	[9]	0.8891	0.8932	0.8765	0.8848
	WAS-LSTM	0.9026	0.9125	0.9003	0.9064
	SAM+WAS-GRU	0.9135	0.9188	0.9395	0.9378
Ours	SAM+WAS-LSTM	0.9363	0.9394	0.9398	0.9396

GRU, CNN), and state-of-the-art approaches [6, 9, 14]. The classification results were evaluated using multiple metrics including accuracy, precision, recall, and F1-score.

Table 10.2 presents the overall comparison results. Our evaluation demonstrates several key advantages of the proposed SAM+WAS-LSTM framework:

- *Superior Accuracy*: Our framework achieved 93.63% accuracy in the six-class classification task, significantly outperforming both traditional machine learning approaches and other deep learning models.
- *Consistent Performance*: Our approach performs consistently well across all cognitive tasks, demonstrating robust recognition capabilities with balanced precision (93.94%), recall (93.98%), and F1-score (93.96%).
- *Low Latency*: The framework achieves a response time of less than one second, essential for providing a natural interaction experience.
- *Computational Efficiency*: Our efficient reward model significantly reduces the computational burden, with training time reduced by approximately 98.3% compared to direct classification-based approaches.

As shown in Table 10.2, our approach outperforms all baselines by achieving the highest accuracy of 0.9363 on the six-class classification. Our model (SAM+WAS-LSTM) performs better than the solo WAS-LSTM, which demonstrates that the SAM has a positive contribution to the classification. The confusion matrix, ROC curves, and AUC scores of the proposed framework are reported in Fig. 10.3. We

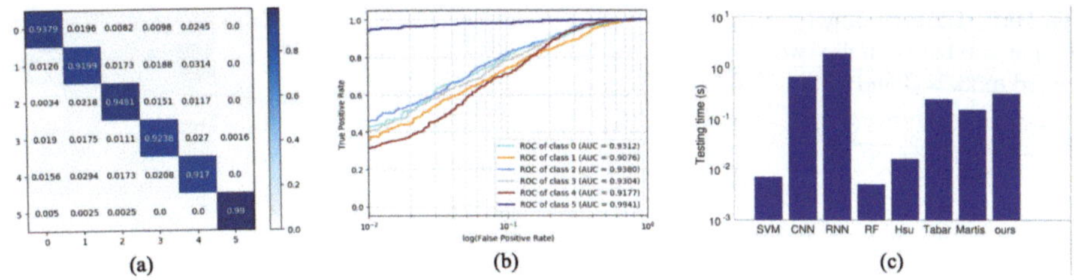

Fig. 10.3 Recognition results. **a** Confusion matrix. **b** ROC curves with AUC scores. **c** Latency

observe that the eye-closed state obtains the best performance compared to other classes, which is reasonable as all other classes are in eye-open state and are more susceptible to environmental factors. Through the results comparison of SAM+WAS-GRU and SAM+WAS-LSTM (Table 10.2), we observe that the latter achieves higher performance (0.9363 > 0.9135), indicating that LSTM slightly outperforms GRU in our scenarios due to its ability to remember longer sequences.

Impact of Key Factors: To design effective real-world cognitive interactive applications, both accuracy and latency are equally important. We compared the latency of our framework with several state-of-the-art algorithms, with results presented in Fig. 10.3c. Our approach has competitive latency compared with other methods, with overall latency less than 1 s, demonstrating that the deep learning-based techniques do not explicitly lead to extra latency.

Furthermore, we conducted extensive experiments to demonstrate the efficiency of the proposed reward model. We measured data pairs of the reward (from model $\mathcal{G}$) and the WAS-LSTM classifier accuracy (from model $\mathcal{F}$). The relationship between the reward and accuracy is shown in Fig. 10.4. The figure illustrates that the accuracy has an approximately linear relationship with the reward, with a correlation coefficient of 0.8258 (p-value = 0.0115), showing that accuracy and reward are highly positively related. As a result, we can estimate $\arg\max_{\bar{x}^*} \mathcal{F}$ by $\arg\max_{\bar{x}^*} \mathcal{G}$. Moreover, we measured the single-step training time of the two reward models $\mathcal{G}$ and $\mathcal{F}$.

Fig. 10.4 The relationship between the reward and the WAS-LSTM classifier accuracy

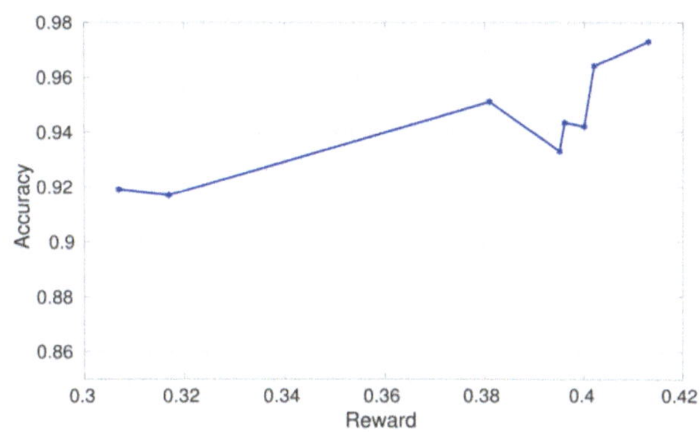

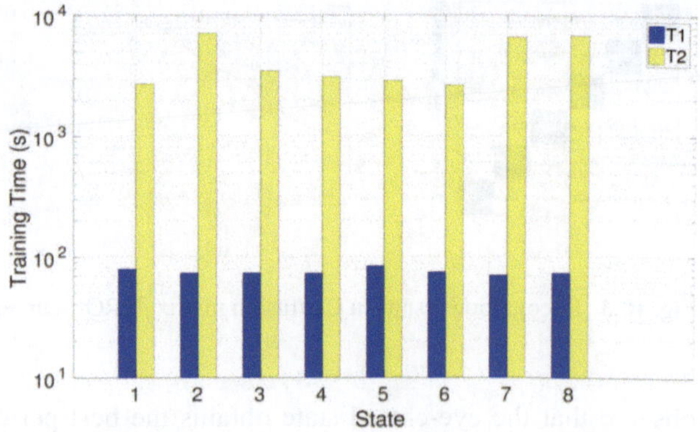

Fig. 10.5 Training time comparison between the two reward models $\mathcal{G}$ and $\mathcal{F}$

Figure 10.5 qualitatively shows that the training time of $\mathcal{F}$ (T2) is much higher than that of $\mathcal{G}$ (T1). Quantitatively, the sum of T1 over eight states is 601.58 s while the sum of T2 is 35,237.41 s. These results demonstrate that the proposed approach of designing $\mathcal{G}$ to approximate $\mathcal{F}$ saves 98.3% training time in focal zone optimization.

These results validate the effectiveness of our approach for enabling reliable human-thing cognitive interactivity in real-world applications.

Practical Applications: To demonstrate the practical utility of our framework, we implemented two prototypes that showcase BCI-IoT integration: a brain typing system and a mind-controlled assistive robot. These applications illustrate the potential for enhancing independence and communication through direct brain-to-device interaction.

The brain typing system, shown in Fig. 10.6a, enables users to compose text using only their thoughts. It features a hierarchical interface that provides access to all 26 English letters plus a space character using just six mental commands, prioritizing reliability over speed. The system employs several reliability-enhancing strategies, including data windowing and confirmation requirements to prevent false activations, resulting in robust performance suitable for users with limited physical abilities.

Our second prototype demonstrates cognitive robot control in a smart home setting. Using six mental commands (upward, downward, leftward, rightward, middle cycle, and eye-closed), users can direct a PR2 robot to perform tasks such as retrieving objects. In our demonstration scenario, a user mentally guides the robot to fetch a beverage, with the system translating brain signals into navigation and manipulation commands. Despite being implemented in a simulated environment using the Gazebo platform and Robot Operating System, the system achieved 100% task completion accuracy when following mentally-planned paths.

These applications demonstrate how BCI-IoT integration can create new possibilities for human-thing interaction, particularly for individuals who might benefit from alternative control methods. By enabling direct brain-to-device communication, our approach bridges the gap between user intentions and environmental control, potentially enhancing independence and quality of life.

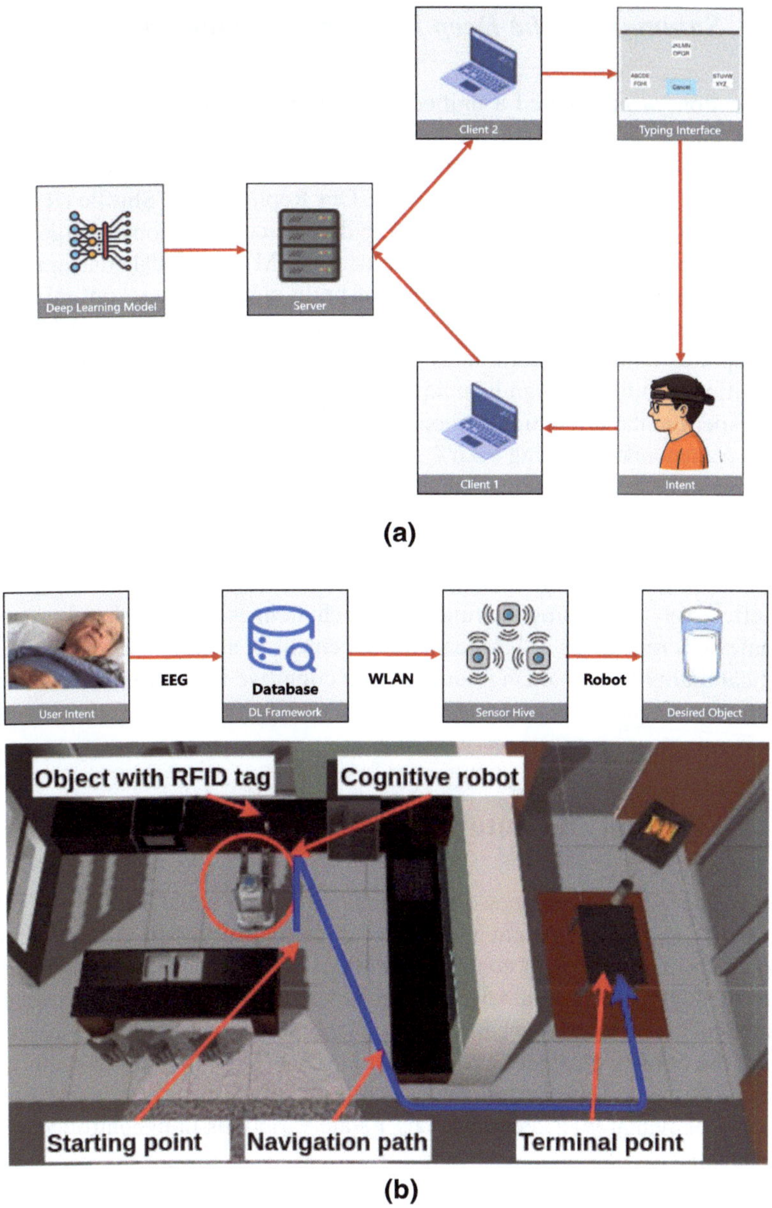

Fig. 10.6 Human-thing cognitive applications. **a** Brain typing system. **b** Cognitive robot in IoT scenario

10.3.4 Summary of the Deep Learning Framework

In this section, we presented a unified deep learning framework for human-thing cognitive interactivity through the integration of BCI and IoT technologies. The framework addresses several key challenges in brain signal interpretation through three complementary technical innovations. Our Replicate and Shuffle (RS) process enhances feature representation by creating diverse combinations of signal dimensions, while the Selective Attention Mechanism (SAM) with focal zone optimization identifies the most informative segments of brain signals. These optimized signal features are then processed by our Weighted Average Spatial LSTM (WAS-LSTM), which captures complex interdimensional relationships while providing enhanced classification stability through its unique weighted averaging approach.

Our experimental evaluation demonstrated the effectiveness of these innovations, with the framework achieving 93.6% recognition accuracy across six mental tasks and maintaining response times under one second. The practical applications we implemented—a brain typing system and a cognitive robot control system—further validated the framework's ability to enable intuitive human-thing interaction through direct brain-to-device communication.

By effectively addressing the fundamental challenges of brain signal processing, our framework represents a significant advancement in making BCI-IoT integration a practical reality for enhancing human-thing cognitive interactivity across various application domains.

10.4 Discussion and Future Directions

Our unified deep learning framework demonstrates the potential for BCI-IoT integration to enable cognitive ambient intelligence through direct brain-to-device communication. While promising in controlled settings, several considerations emerge for broader deployment. The framework faces key technical limitations: experimental validation involved only seven participants in laboratory conditions, limiting generalizability; the Selective Attention Mechanism increases computational requirements that may affect real-time performance; and brain signal quality remains susceptible to environmental interference and user state variations in uncontrolled ambient environments.

The demonstrated capabilities suggest promising directions for interactive ambient intelligence. The brain typing and robot control applications illustrate potential for intuitive environmental interaction without traditional interfaces, enhancing accessibility while maintaining privacy. The person-dependent modeling approach enables adaptive systems that could support customized ambient intelligence experiences. For smart aging contexts, the framework's emphasis on reduced physical interaction requirements suggests relevance for communication assistance and daily task support, though age-related factors would require careful evaluation in future research.

Key research directions include: (1) extended validation in real-world environments to assess long-term usability and stability; (2) multimodal integration with existing IoT ecosystems to enhance robustness; (3) development of privacy-preserving approaches for sensitive neural data; and (4) examination of framework performance across diverse user populations to maximize inclusivity.

Our framework represents a step toward practical BCI-IoT integration for cognitive ambient intelligence, with potential to contribute to more accessible and intuitive ambient systems that enhance quality of life across diverse application contexts.

References

1. Al-Ali, A.R., Zualkernan, I.A., Rashid, M., Gupta, R., Alikarar, M.: A smart home energy management system using IoT and big data analytics approach. IEEE Trans. Consum. Electron. **63**(4), 426–434 (2017)
2. Angelidou, M.: Smart city planning and development shortcomings. TEMA J. Land Use Mob. Environ. **10**(1), 77–94 (2017)
3. Bandaru, J., Kiran, M.S., Rajalakshmi, P.: A novel system architecture for brain controlled iot enabled environments. In: 19th IEEE International Conference on e-Health Networking, Applications and Services (HealthCom), pp. 1–5. IEEE (2017)
4. Dhariwal, K., Mehta, A.: Architecture and plan of smart hospital based on internet of things (IoT). Int. Res. J. Eng. Technol. **4**(4), 1976–1980 (2017)
5. Haselsteiner, E., Pfurtscheller, G.: Using time-dependent neural networks for EEG classification. IEEE Trans. Rehabil. Eng. **8**(4), 457–463 (2000)
6. Hsu, W.Y.: Assembling a multi-feature EEG classifier for left–right motor imagery data using wavelet-based fuzzy approximate entropy for improved accuracy. Int. J. Neural Syst. **25**(8) (2015)
7. Iijima, M., Nishitani, N.: Cortical dynamics during simple calculation processes: a magnetoencephalography study. Clin. Neurophys. Pract. **2**, 54–61 (2016)
8. LeCun, Y., Bengio, Y., Hinton, G.: Deep learning. Nature **521**(7553), 436–444 (2015)
9. Martis, R.J., Tan, J.H., Chua, C.K., Loon, T.C., Yeo, S.W.J., Tong, L.: Epileptic EEG classification using nonlinear parameters on different frequency bands. J. Mech. Med. Biol. **15**(3) (2015)
10. Nakamura, T., Goverdovsky, V., Mandic, D.: In-ear EEG biometrics for feasible and readily collectable real-world person authentication. IEEE Trans. Inf. Forensics Secur. **13**(3), 648–661 (2018)
11. Nguyen, B., Nguyen, D., Ma, W., Tran, D.: Investigating the possibility of applying EEG lossy compression to EEG-based user authentication. In: International Joint Conference on Neural Networks (IJCNN), pp. 79–85. IEEE (2017)
12. Rahman, M.A., Ahmad, M.: A straight forward signal processing scheme to improve effect size of FNIR signals. In: International Conference on Informatics, Electronics & Vision (ICIEV), pp. 439–444 (2016)
13. Rahman, M.A., Ahmad, M.: Evaluating the connectivity of motor area with prefrontal cortex by FNIR spectroscopy. In: IEEE Energy Conversion Congress and Exposition (ECCE), pp. 296–300 (2017)
14. Tabar, Y.R., Halici, U.: A novel deep learning approach for classification of EEG motor imagery signals. J. Neural Eng. **14**(1) (2016)
15. Teles, A., Antunes, M., Luz, P., Ao Paulo, J.: Using brain–Computer interface and internet of things to improve healthcare for wheelchair users. In: Proceedings of the 11th International Conference on Mobile Ubiquitous Computing, Systems, Services and Technologies (UBICOMM), pp. 92–94 (2017)

16. Vallabhaneni, A., Wang, T., He, B.: Brain–computer interface. In: Neural Engineering, pp. 85–121. Springer, Boston, MA, USA (2005)
17. Yao, L., Sheng, Q.Z., Dustdar, S.: Web-based management of the internet of things. IEEE Internet Comput. **19**(4), 60–67 (2015)
18. Yao, L., Sheng, Q.Z., Li, C., Ruan, W., Kanhere, S.S., Wang, X.: Wits: an IoT-endowed computational framework for activity recognition in personalized smart homes. Computing **100**(4), 369–385 (2018)
19. Zhang, X., Yao, L., Huang, C., Sheng, Q.Z., Gu, T.: Multi-modality sensor data classification with selective attention. In: Proceedings of the 27th International Joint Conference on Artificial Intelligence (IJCAI), pp. 3111–3117. IJCAI (2018)
20. Zhang, X., Yao, L., Huang, C., Sheng, Q.Z., Wang, X.: Intent recognition in smart living through deep recurrent neural networks. In: International Conference on Neural Information Processing (ICONIP), pp. 748–758. Springer (2017)
21. Zhang, X., Yao, L., Sheng, Q.Z., Kanhere, S., Gu, T., Zhang, D.: Converting your thoughts to texts: Enabling brain typing via deep feature learning of EEG signals. In: IEEE International Conference on Pervasive Computing and Communications (PerCom), pp. 1–10. IEEE Computer Society (2018)
22. Zhang, X., Yao, L., Zhang, S., Kanhere, S.S., Sheng, M., Liu, Y.: Internet of things meets brain-computer interface: a unified deep learning framework for enabling human-thing cognitive interactivity. IEEE Internet Things J. **6**(2), 2084–2092 (2019)

Part IV
AI-empowered IoT Solutions

This part represents the culmination of the book's technological progression, demonstrating how artificial intelligence (AI) can be integrated with IoT systems to create comprehensive solutions for smart aging applications. Building upon the sensing foundations (Parts I–II) and interactive technologies (Part III), this part showcases advanced AI methodologies that transformraw data into actionable insights and intelligent decision-making capabilities.

Chapter 11 addresses personal health management through sophisticated data mining approaches applied to geriatric medical examination records. The chapter presents MyPHI and SHG-Health systems that tackle fundamental challenges in healthcare data analysis, including label uncertainty, class imbalance, and heterogeneous health parameters. These approaches achieve remarkable performance with 89.95% AUC under severely imbalanced conditions and over 96% precision for high-risk identification, demonstrating how AI can extract meaningful health insights from large-scale longitudinal data.

Chapter 12 explores advanced identity management through multimodal biometric authentication, presenting the DeepKey system that combines EEG and gait biometrics for enhanced security. The system achieves zero false acceptance rate and minimal false rejection rate through attention-based deep learning architectures, addressing critical security needs in smart aging environments while accommodating the physical and cognitive considerations of elderly users.

Chapter 13 examines the transformative potential of large language models (LLMs) in creating conversational AI interfaces for smart aging systems. The chapter explores how these technologies can provide natural language interactions, personalized assistance, and intelligent interpretation of complex IoT data streams, making smart environments more accessible and intuitive for elderly users.

Chapter 14 investigates intelligent agent-based emergency response systems that integrate multimodal sensing, large language models, and distributed coordination mechanisms. These systems demonstrate how AI agents can provide comprehensive situational awareness, adaptive response management, and sophisticated communication capabilities to enhance safety and emergency preparedness for aging populations.

Together, these chapters establish AI as the critical enabling technology that transforms basic IoT infrastructure into intelligent, adaptive, and responsive systems that are capable of supporting independent living, health management, security, and emergency response in smart aging environments.

Chapter 11
Personal Health Management

11.1 Introduction

11.1.1 Overview of Personal Health Management

Modern societies have experienced dramatic growth in elderly population over recent decades, implying increasing healthcare needs and government expenditure. Healthcare spending for elderly populations has shown substantial increases, with annual geriatric medical examination (GME) becoming an integral part of elderly healthcare for many developed countries.

Huge amounts of Electronic Health Records (EHRs) collected over the years have provided a rich base for risk analysis and prediction [3, 9]. An EHR contains digitally stored healthcare information about an individual, such as observations, laboratory tests, diagnostic reports, medications, procedures, patient identifying information, and allergies [6]. A special type of EHR is the Health Examination Records (HER) from annual general health check-ups.

With the availability of large volumes of data collected from multiple sources over years through the *big data* era, effectively evaluating personal health status from-cradle-to-grave is becoming possible. Predicting personal health status based on medical examinations reveals a promising and important trend in healthcare research, particularly relevant for smart aging environments.

11.1.2 Challenges and Opportunities

However, it is always a difficult task for healthcare professionals to provide an overall report on personal health after a comprehensive medical check-up is performed with hundreds of parameters. Moreover, the richness of GME records, such as correlations amongst test results, their longitudinal progression, and their relationships to other

Q. Z. Sheng et al., *Harnessing Artificial Intelligence and Pervasive Internet of Things for an Empowered Aging*, https://doi.org/10.1007/978-3-032-16502-2_11

participants that have similar patterns of health development, is often left unexplored. In fact, such exploration is manually impossible, because the complexity of the combined effects grows exponentially with the growth of the number of different test results, the available number of longitudinal records, and the total number of participants.

General health examination is an integral part of healthcare in many countries. Identifying the participants at risk is important for early warning and preventive intervention. The fundamental challenge of learning a classification model for risk prediction lies in the unlabeled data that constitutes the majority of the collected dataset. Particularly, the unlabeled data describes the participants in health examinations whose health conditions can vary greatly from healthy to very-ill. There is no ground truth for differentiating their states of health.

The key challenges in health examination records include heterogeneity and sparsity. Health examination records contain test items that are naturally in categories, each conveying different semantics and possibly contributing differently in risk identification. A participant may have a sequence of irregularly time-stamped longitudinal records, each of which is likely to be sparse in terms of abnormal results. Therefore this heterogeneity should be respected in the modeling.

11.1.3 Contributions

This chapter presents two complementary approaches to personal health management in smart aging environments. Our first major contribution is MyPHI, a novel data mining method that predicts personal health index (PHI) from geriatric medical examination records. This work is the first of its kind in predicting personal health scores by mining large medical examination data, effectively handling the infrequent, incomplete, and sparse nature of geriatric medical records through novel feature extraction and temporal weighting approaches.

Our second contribution is SHG-Health (Semi-supervised Heterogeneous Graph on Health), an innovative graph-based algorithm for risk prediction from longitudinal health examination records. This approach pioneers risk prediction with large volumes of unlabeled data, demonstrating effectiveness in identifying high-risk participants and classifying them into specific disease categories.

Both methods introduce novel methodological innovations including soft-label learning for handling label uncertainty in medical data and heterogeneous graph construction that respects the natural heterogeneity in health examination items. Comprehensive validation on large-scale real-world datasets containing 262,424 records from 102,258 participants demonstrates significant performance improvements over conventional approaches in both risk identification and disease categorization tasks.

11.1.4 Organization

The remainder of this chapter is organized as follows. Section 11.2 reviews the background and related work in health indexing systems, data mining on health examination records, and classification with unlabeled healthcare data. Section 11.3 presents the MyPHI method for personal health indexing via data mining. Section 11.4 introduces the SHG-Health algorithm for graph-based health risk prediction. Section 11.5 provides discussion and future directions for personal health management in smart aging.

11.2 Background and Related Work

11.2.1 Health Indexing and Scoring Systems

Health indices provide numerical expressions of health status [13]. Many scoring systems were introduced to assist clinical decision-making, for example, the APACHE, SAPS, and MPM for Intensive Care Unit patients [8] and the survival prediction tools for palliative care [10]. A systematic review conducted in 2012 [1] showed that clinical decision support systems (CDSSs) improved healthcare process for preventive and other types of services.

Indices or scores calculated based on patient conditions are commonly used in clinical practice, for example the severity of illness scoring systems for Intensive Care Unit (ICU) [8] and survival prediction tools for palliative care [10]. These tools often serve as a starting point for clinical diagnosis or prognosis [8]. However, existing studies are generally based on statistical analysis on a small set of factors manually selected by medical experts, but in an era of information explosion, it is no longer possible to process all the information available and select factors manually.

Generally, these methods are defined based on factors selected with expert knowledge and validated via population-based studies [25]. However, as discussed earlier, it becomes problematic when the dimensionality increases and the longitudinal aspect is involved. Yi et al. [27] developed a bio-mark based system to grade personal health status. Again the model relies on the experts to define factors and the associated weights.

11.2.2 Data Mining for Health Examination Records

Although Electronic Health Records have attracted increasing research attention in the data mining and machine learning communities in recent years [3, 14–16, 18, 22, 29], mining general health examination data is an area that has not yet been well-explored, except a few studies on risk prediction such as the chronic disease early warning system proposed in [11] and our previous work on health score classification framework [3, 4]. However, none of them considered unlabeled data. In addition, the approach presented in [3] is limited to a binary classification problem (using alive/deceased labels) and consequently it is not informative about the specific disease area in which a person is at risk.

In the last decade, increasing number of data mining applications has been developed to support healthcare decision making [7]. Of particular focus in recent years is the clinical risk classification [23]. These studies generally treat class labels with 100% certainty. However, label uncertainty is commonly found in clinical judgments due to expert subjectivity and inadequate information [20].

11.2.3 Semi-Supervised Learning and Graph-Based Methods in Healthcare

The existing studies on healthcare data that handled unlabeled data focus on semi-supervised learning techniques. Situations arise when unlabeled data may belong to unknown or known classes. Nie et al. introduced a scholastic graph-based semi-supervised learning method for novel class discovery or outlier detection. By introducing an instance-level parameter that assigns different weights to labeled versus unlabeled data, this approach allows the label scores of unlabeled vertices to be updated according to their connectivities to labeled vertices.

Wang et al. [24] further modified the model to discover more than one unseen class for patient risk stratification based on a patient graph constructed using ICD codes. Recently Zhao et al. [28] extended GGSSL for classification on Alzheimer's Disease, by introducing a compact graph construction strategy via minimizing local reconstruction error. However, all of the above algorithms are limited to homogeneous graphs, where vertices belong to one object type, and thus are by themselves not capable of handling the heterogeneity embedded in health examination records.

Recently in the field of Computer Vision, Yi et al. introduced a soft-label learning model for complex event detection on Web videos [26]. For a given small number of target event instances, the model leverages related instances whose "relativeness" is uncertain and to be learned. Inspired by this work, the PHI prediction problem can be formulated as a soft-label optimization problem.

11.2.4 Research Gaps and Opportunities in Smart Aging Applications

In the context of smart aging, several research gaps and opportunities exist in the field of personal health management and health data mining:

- *Label Uncertainty*: Most existing methods treat medical labels with absolute certainty, failing to account for the inherent uncertainty in clinical judgments and comorbidity conditions. This is particularly problematic for elderly patients who often present with multiple concurrent conditions, making precise categorization difficult and potentially misleading.
- *Heterogeneity Handling*: Current approaches inadequately address the natural heterogeneity in health examination data, where different types of tests convey different semantic meanings. The complex interrelationships between various health parameters in older adults require more sophisticated modeling approaches that can respect the inherent heterogeneous structure of medical examination data.
- *Longitudinal Sparsity*: Existing methods struggle with the sparse, infrequent, and incomplete nature of geriatric medical examination records. As older adults undergo different tests at irregular intervals, capturing meaningful temporal patterns becomes challenging yet crucial for accurate health monitoring and risk prediction.
- *Unlabeled Data Utilization*: Limited work has been done on effectively leveraging the large volumes of unlabeled health examination data for risk prediction. Semi-supervised approaches that can maximize the value of unlabeled data have significant potential to improve predictive models, especially in resource-constrained healthcare settings serving aging populations.
- *Comprehensive Health Indexing*: There is a lack of systematic approaches to generate comprehensive personal health indices that can benefit multiple stakeholders in the healthcare ecosystem. Holistic health indices that integrate various dimensions of elderly health could provide valuable decision support for clinicians, caregivers, and older adults themselves.

These gaps highlight the importance of developing more sophisticated, flexible, and integrated approaches to health data mining for smart aging applications. The methods presented in this chapter–MyPHI for personal health indexing and SHG-Health for graph-based mining—directly address these challenges and demonstrate the potential to transform health monitoring and assessment for aging populations.

11.3 Personal Health Indexing via Data Mining

11.3.1 Motivation and Overview of MyPHI System

Computing comprehensive health scores for elderly citizens presents significant challenges due to the infrequent, incomplete, and sparse nature of geriatric medical examination records. To address these challenges, we propose MyPHI [4], a novel data mining approach that predicts personal health indices to identify at-risk individuals for early intervention. MyPHI defines PHI as a vector of scores, each reflecting the health risk in a particular disease category. The PHI prediction is formulated as an optimization problem that finds the optimal soft labels as health scores based on medical records that are infrequent, incomplete, and sparse.

To the best of our knowledge, this work is the first of this kind in predicting personal health scores by mining large medical examination data. PHI provides an important benchmark for understanding health status of the elderly people. Particularly, governments, organizations such as hospitals, insurance companies, nursing homes, and individuals can benefit from PHI for population health policies, clinical decision support, risk assessment, and personal health tracking respectively.

The PHI prediction problem is formulated as a soft-label optimization problem that distinguishes three types of instances: participants with a target COD label, participants with a non-target COD label, and participants without a COD label. Our proposed method can capture the differences amongst these three types of instances and handle label uncertainty commonly found in clinical judgments due to expert subjectivity and comorbidity conditions. This work substantially extends our previous binary classification approach to a vector of scores across multiple disease categories using soft-label learning techniques.

11.3.2 MyPHI: A Soft-Label Optimization Approach

The proposed MyPHI prediction method computes personal health index (PHI) for elderly healthcare through a comprehensive data mining approach. As shown in Fig. 11.1, the method contains three key components: data preprocessing, feature extraction using chi-squared kernels for temporal weighting, and model learning with soft-label optimization for handling label uncertainty. The inputs are geriatric medical examination (GME) records linked to cause of death (COD) database, and the output is a vector of predicted scores in the range [0, 1], reflecting personal health risks across multiple disease categories.

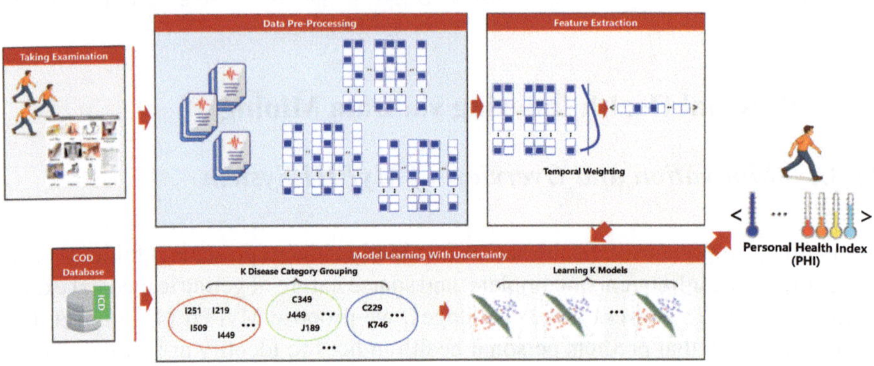

Fig. 11.1 The process of personal health index (PHI) prediction

Data and Preprocessing. We employ two linked datasets: a geriatric medical examination (GME) dataset containing 262,424 check-ups from 102,258 participants aged 65 or above, collected over six years by the Taipei City Government, and a cause of death (COD) dataset with 7,569 participants having COD labels using WHO ICD standards.

Our GME data exhibits three key characteristics: infrequency (yearly examinations), incompleteness (sparse temporal coverage with an average of 2.56 records per participant), and sparsity (most examination results are normal). We applied comprehensive preprocessing including standardization, noise correction, and feature extraction, resulting in a refined dataset of 221,074 records from 60,881 participants.

We adopted an event-based view treating observed abnormal results as events, following evidence-based medicine principles. Variables are binarized with abnormality encoded as 1, and 0 otherwise. Participant longitudinal records are represented as sequences of time-stamped records with normalized temporal mapping.

Feature Extraction. A central challenge is effectively representing participants' records with varying lengths and temporal patterns. We employ a feature-based approach to transform irregular record sequences into standardized feature vectors using a chi-squared kernel for temporal weighting that accounts for diminishing relevance of older records while capturing meaningful longitudinal health patterns.

The temporal weighting kernel assigns higher weights to more recent examination records while maintaining appropriate representation of historical health patterns, systematically transforming each participant's record sequence into a feature vector that effectively represents their health trajectory.

Model Learning. To build an effective PHI prediction model, we train multiple models for different target disease categories. The approach handles label uncertainty by distinguishing three types of instances: participants with target disease labels, participants with non-target disease labels, and participants without disease labels.

The problem is formulated as a soft-label optimization problem that finds optimal soft labels for every instance. This regularized optimization approach efficiently handles label uncertainty through principled mathematical optimization while maintaining computational efficiency. The optimization alternately updates weight matrices and soft labels until convergence, with theoretical guarantees for reaching optimal solutions.

The final prediction function generates a vector of risk scores across all disease categories, providing comprehensive health risk assessment after calibration through z-normalization and transformation using generalized extreme value distribution.

11.3.3 Experimental Validation and Performance Analysis

Disease Category Grouping. We selected top 10 disease categories that have the highest frequency counts in the GME dataset based on the linked Cause of Death (COD) labels encoded in ICD-9 and ICD-10, as shown in Table 11.1. The "Other"

Table 11.1 Numbers of positive cases in disease categories

Top k	Disease category	Count
1	Lung	649
2	Heart	296
3	Cerebrovascular	153
4	Diabetes	112
5	Stomach	105
6	Colon	101
7	Liver	83
8	Pancreas	61
9	Septicemia	60
10	Hypertension	42
11	Other	1,314

category is defined to contain all the rest health-related ICD codes not in the top 10 disease categories.

Experiment Setup. We compare MyPHI with established classification methods including linear support vector machines (LinSVM) and logistic regression (LR), both in standard and class-weighted versions (LinSVM-W and LR-W). We trained a model for each of the 11 disease categories, following a 35:35:30 stratified train/validate/test split ratio. The negative (alive) cases were sub-sampled according to positive versus negative ratios of 1:1, 1:10 and 1:100. The experiments examine both "clean" scenarios (with only positive and negative instances) and realistic "noisy" scenarios (including non-target disease instances).

Results. Table 11.2 presents the averaged AUC (%) across 11 disease categories under various positive versus negative ratios. The results demonstrate that MyPHI consistently outperforms baseline methods across different scenarios.

In the clean case (left of Table 11.2), where there are only positive instances (those whose main cause of death is the target disease) and negative instances (those who are alive), MyPHI outperforms all other methods in most cases. The approach

Table 11.2 The averaged AUC (%) of 11 disease categories of various positive versus negative ratios. The proposed MyPHI significantly outperforms all the other algorithms in most cases. The bold values indicate the best performance for a given case-ratio scenario

Ratio	Clean case					Noisy case				
	MyPHI	LinSVM	LinSVM-W	LR	LR-W	MyPHI	LinSVM	LinSVM-W	LR	LR-W
1:1	**83.48**	82.11	82.11	82.79	82.79	**74.07**	71.23	71.23	70.47	70.47
1:10	**85.65**	77.99	**85.66**	78.72	85.19	**85.14**	75.03	81.56	75.65	80.32
1:100	**89.95**	68.57	85.91	70.42	85.99	**89.37**	69.10	83.83	70.45	84.04

achieves the highest performance at 89.95% averaged AUC under severely imbalanced conditions (1:100 ratio), substantially better than standard classifiers. Baseline methods without considering class weighting perform poorly at ratio 1:100, while class-weighted versions (LinSVM-W and LR-W) can better handle class imbalance, though not as effectively as MyPHI.

More importantly, in noisy cases (right of Table 11.2) that better reflect real-world clinical scenarios, where non-target disease instances are introduced, MyPHI maintains its superior performance with 89.37% AUC at 1:100 ratio, while other methods show significant performance drops. The performance is greatly compromised in the case of 1:1 ratio for all algorithms, showing that non-target cases confuse algorithms given limited learning instances. However, when the portion of negative instances increases, the performance recovers. The gap between MyPHI and other methods is enlarged in the noisy case, demonstrating the robustness of our approach when dealing with uncertain labels and class imbalance—common challenges in medical data analysis.

When examining individual disease categories, our analysis shows that MyPHI performs particularly well for heart-related, cerebrovascular, and digestive system diseases. The best performance for a single disease category was achieved for lung-related conditions at 96.95% AUC (Fig. 11.2). The ROC curves (Fig. 11.3) further confirm the superior performance at a fine-grained level. These strong results across different disease types demonstrate the versatility and effectiveness of our approach.

Further experiments confirm that our technique of introducing trace norm constraints for handling label uncertainty significantly improves performance, particularly at extreme class imbalance ratios (Fig. 11.4). The figure shows that applying

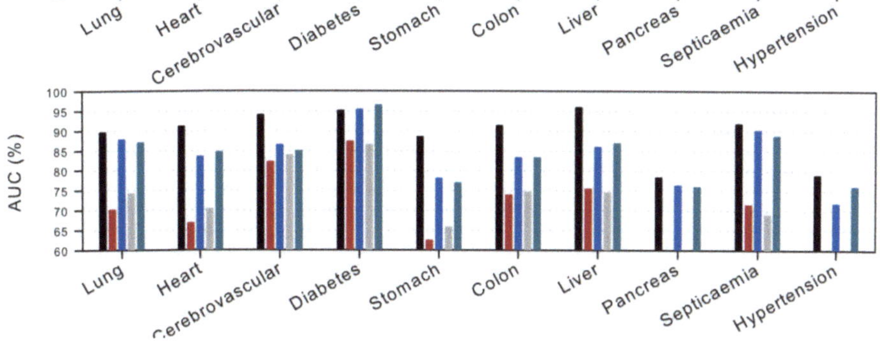

Fig. 11.2 AUC scores for individual disease categories at 1:100 ratio in the noisy case, showing MyPHI's superior performance across different disease types

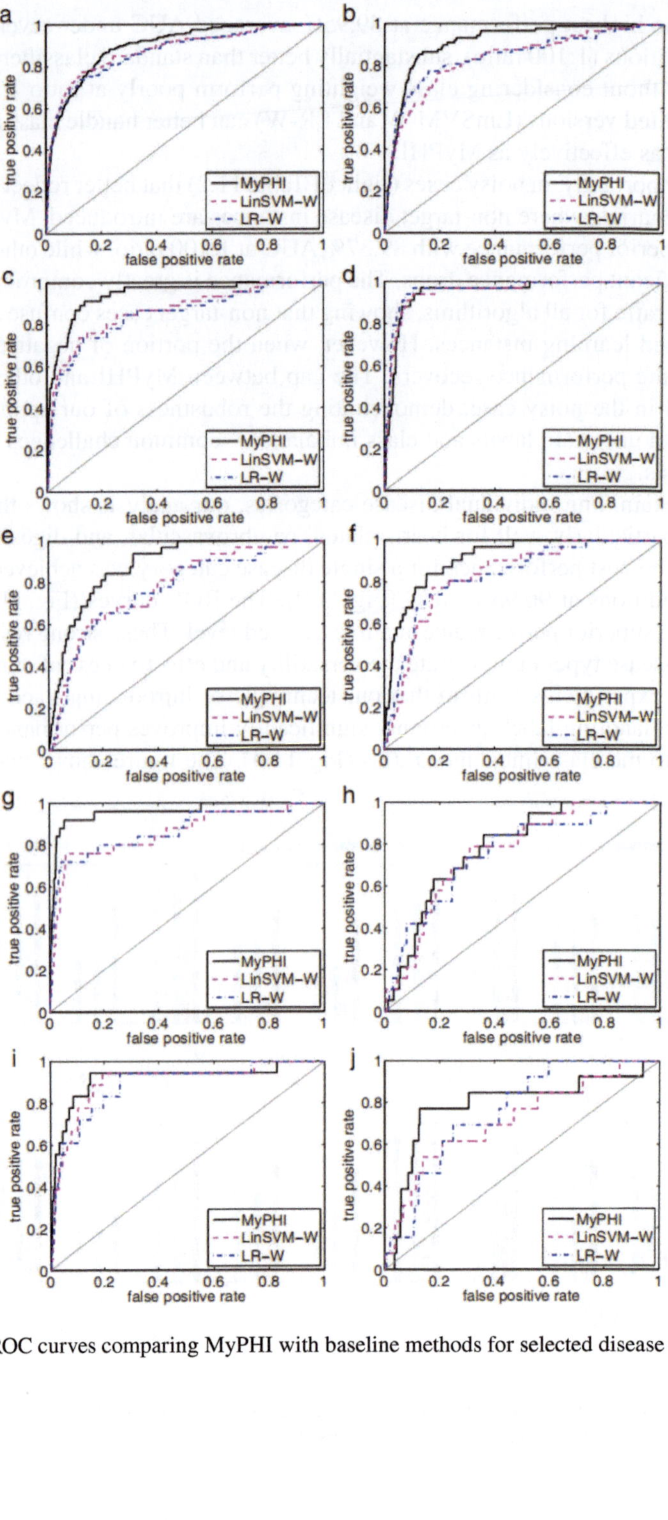

Fig. 11.3 ROC curves comparing MyPHI with baseline methods for selected disease categories

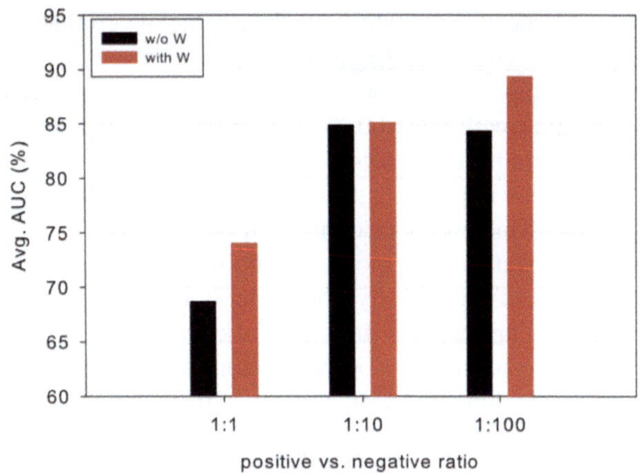

Fig. 11.4 Impact of trace norm regularization on model performance across different class imbalance ratios

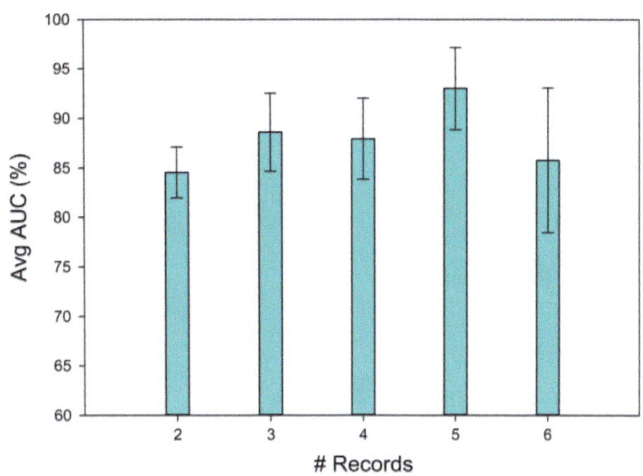

Fig. 11.5 Effect of record sequence length on prediction accuracy, showing optimal performance at 5 records

trace norm regularization consistently improves AUC scores across different positive-to-negative ratios, with the most significant gains observed at higher imbalance ratios.

Additionally, our investigation into the effects of record sequence length revealed that predictions based on 5 records achieve the highest accuracy (Fig. 11.5), confirming that longitudinal data improves prediction performance, though even with just 2-3 records, the model maintains reasonable accuracy. This finding has practical implications for deployment, as it suggests that meaningful risk predictions can be made even when participants have limited examination history.

Discussion of Results. Our extensive experiments on a large GME dataset with 262,424 check-ups of 102,258 participants have demonstrated the robustness and effectiveness of our approach. The superior performance of MyPHI over standard classifiers confirms that our soft-label learning model effectively handles label-uncertain data common in medical applications. The parameter for soft-labeling enables the algorithm to learn the degree of certainty for each data instance based on the underlying data structure.

The improved performance from applying regularization techniques suggests that in dealing with uncertainty, expert knowledge about which types of labels may be more certain than others plays an important role in building effective models. This finding has implications for developing practical clinical decision support systems that can handle imperfect medical data.

While our current model was built and validated on the GME dataset from elderly residents of Taipei City, the methodology is applicable to other medical datasets with similar characteristics. We acknowledge the potential for misinterpretation of predictive results by non-professionals and recommend that interpretation of PHI scores be conducted with assistance from healthcare providers.

PHI Visualization. We also provide a visualization interface that allows health state analysis at the personal level, as well as the population level.

Health analysis at a personal level provides insights into individual's health conditions and lays the foundation of effective health monitoring [19]. With MyPHI, a person's PHI scores in disease categories can be computed, and the results can be displayed as a fingerprint chart on the left of Fig. 11.6, where an annulus represents

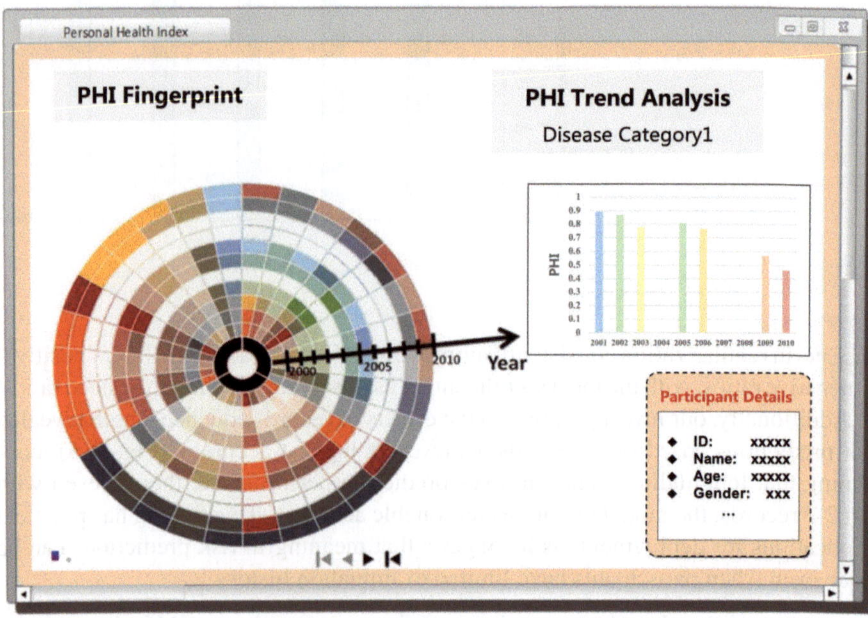

Fig. 11.6 A dashboard of personal health analysis. The fingerprint on the left gives the breakdown PHI scores in disease categories, where an annulus of the concentric circle represents the PHI scores of a year and a sector in an annulus denotes the score of a particular disease category of that year. Color indicates severity and the white annuluses denote no attendance. In addition, yearly PHI scores of a disease category are summarized in the bar chart on the right

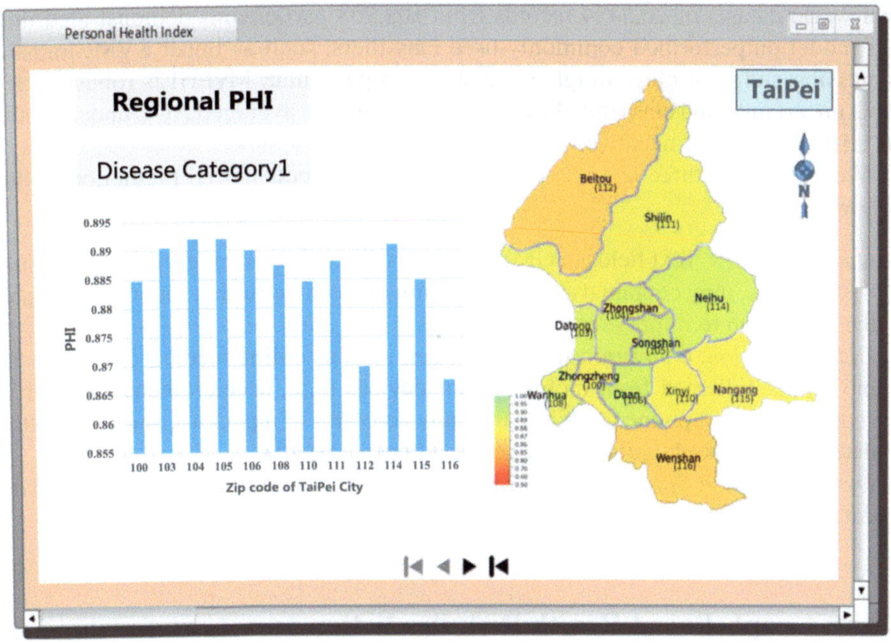

Fig. 11.7 A dashboard of Taipei City's regional health based on the averaged PHI scores of a disease category for the 12 districts indexed by their zip codes. The colors on the district map reflect the degree of healthiness based on the PHI scores

the PHI scores of a year and a colored cell reflects the degree of severity for a disease category in that year. The white annuluses denote the years with no examinations taken. Yearly PHI scores of a particular disease category can be compared in the top-right chart for trend analysis. This visualization of PHI can make it easier for clinical professionals to grasp a person's health status.

Health analysis at a population level can reveal regional health conditions and assist local government's health policy making [5]. Figure 11.7 shows a dashboard of regional health based on the averaged PHI scores of a disease category for the 12 districts of Taipei City, indexed by their zip codes. The colors on the district map reflect the degree of regional health using a color spectrum from red to green denoting PHI in the [0.5, 1.0] range. Note that since the current model is trained based on the senior population of Taipei City, the use of the computed PHIs should be limited to this context.

11.3.4 Summary of MyPHI

In this section, we described MyPHI, a data mining-based method that predicts personal health index (PHI) based on GME records. The extensive experiments on a real-world dataset of 262,424 records from 102,258 participants demonstrated that our model outperformed commonly-used classifiers, such as linear SVM, logistic regression and their class-weighted versions. In particular, MyPHI is robust under label uncertainty and class imbalance, achieving 89.95% averaged AUC under a ratio of 1:100 positive vs. negative.

We foresee the three key areas for future improvements in PHI prediction as the following:

- *Data semantics*. Text fields in GME records, such as doctor suggestions and result descriptions, may contain useful information that can be further incorporated into the evaluation to improve the effectiveness.
- *Data expansion*. Other information sources, such as online medical information, bio-marks collected from mobile sensor devices (e.g., accelerometer and gyroscope on a smart phone recording the daily activities of a person), and in-hospital data, can be linked to obtain more comprehensive results.
- *Dynamic system*. In current work, PHI is computed based on the archived GME database, which can be extended to an online dynamical version.

11.4 Graph-Based Health Risk Prediction

11.4.1 Motivation and Overview of the SHG-Health System

Identifying participants at risk is critical for early warning and preventive intervention in healthcare systems serving elderly populations. However, the fundamental challenge in developing effective risk prediction models lies in the unlabeled data that constitutes the majority of collected datasets. Particularly, unlabeled health examination records represent participants whose health conditions vary greatly from healthy to very-ill, with no ground truth for differentiating their states of health.

In this section, we propose SHG-Health (Semi-supervised Heterogeneous Graph on Health) [2], an innovative graph-based, semi-supervised learning algorithm specifically designed for risk prediction using longitudinal health examination records. SHG-Health addresses two critical challenges in mining health examination data: heterogeneity and large volumes of unlabeled data.

The key innovation of SHG-Health lies in its heterogeneous graph structure that models different types of examination items as distinct node types, respecting the inherent heterogeneity in health records. This approach captures complex relationships between various health parameters and their contributions to different disease risks. Additionally, our semi-supervised learning framework effectively leverages both labeled and unlabeled data, making it possible to identify not only known high-risk categories but also to classify cases into an "unknown" category when appropriate.

11.4.2 SHG-Health: Framework Design and Components

To solve the problem of health risk prediction based on health examination records with heterogeneity and large unlabeled data issues, we present SHG-Health, a semi-supervised heterogeneous graph-based algorithm. The method addresses the challenge of predicting health risks when most data is unlabeled and examination records contain heterogeneous types of medical tests. The approach can classify participants into known high-risk disease categories or identify them as belonging to an "unknown" class when their patterns do not match established risk profiles.

An overview of our proposed solution to the problem is included in Fig. 11.8, above. Our SHG-Health algorithm takes health examination data and the linked cause of death labels described previously as inputs. Its key components are a process of Heterogeneous Health Examination Record graph construction and a semi-supervised learning mechanism with label propagation for model training. Given the records of a participant as a query, SHG-Health predicts whether the participant falls into any of the high-risk disease categories or "unknown" class whose instances do not share the key traits of the known instances belonging to a high-risk disease class.

HeteroHER Graph

A graph representation allows us to model data that is sparse. To capture the heterogeneity naturally found in health examination items, we constructed a graph called HeteroHER consisting of multi-type nodes based on health examination records.

Graph Construction. The process of HeteroHER graph construction includes the following steps:

1. Binarization. As a preparatory step, all the record values are first discretized and converted into a 0/1 binary representation, which serves as a vector of indicators for the absence/presence of a discretized value. Specifically, real values, such as age, are first binned into fixed intervals (e.g., 5 years). Then, all the ordinal and categorical values are converted into binary representations.

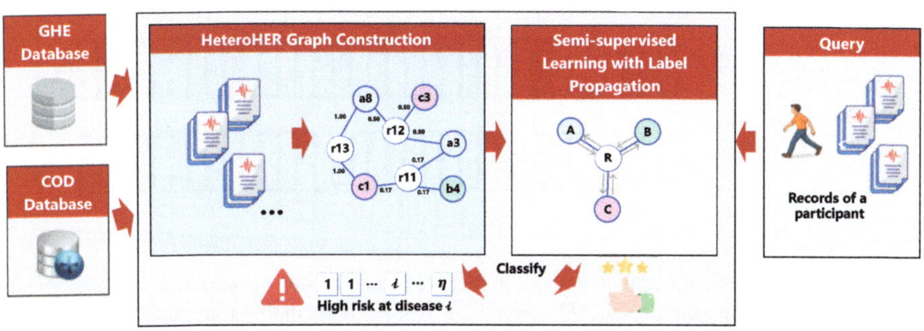

Fig. 11.8 An overview of the proposed SHG-Health algorithm for risk prediction

2. Node Insertion. Every element in the binary representation obtained in Step 1 with a value "1" is modeled as a node in our HeteroHER graph, except that only the abnormal results are modeled for examination items (both physical and mental). This setting is primarily based on the observation that physicians make clinical judgements generally based on the reported symptoms and observed signs, and secondarily for the reduction of graph density.
3. Node Typing. Every node is typed according to the examination category that its original value belongs to, for example, the Physical tests (A), Mental tests (B), and Profile (C) in Fig. 11.9. In addition, a new type of nodes is introduced to represent individual records such as r_{11}, r_{12}, and r_{13} in the same figure. All the other non-Record type nodes that are linked to the Record type nodes can be seen as the attribute nodes of these Record type nodes. In other words, categories A, B, and C in Fig. 11.9 can be regarded as the attributes of the Record type at a schema level. This leads to a graph schema with a star shape as shown on the right of Fig. 11.10 below, which is known as a star schema [21]. Note that types can often be hierarchically structured and thus choosing the granularity of node type may require domain knowledge or be done experimentally.
4. Link Insertion. Every attribute (non-Record) type node is linked to a Record type node representing the record that the observation was originally from. The weight of the links is calculated based on temporal importance, where newer records receive higher weights in terms of risk prediction. A simple temporal weighting function assigns weights proportional to the recency of each record within the specified time window.

For example, in the simplified case shown in Fig. 11.10, different types of examination items are treated as different types of nodes on the graph. An abnormal result creates a weighted link between the corresponding record node and examination

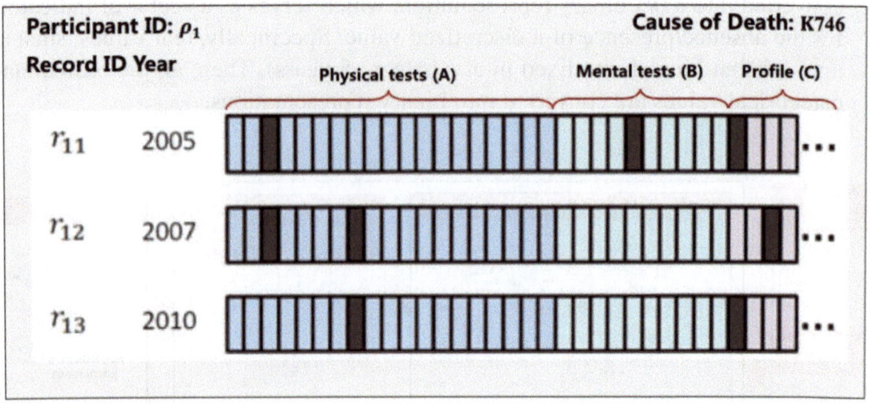

Fig. 11.9 An example of health examination records of participant p_1 who took examinations in three non-consecutive years, 2005, 2007, and 2010. Test items are in different categories (A, B, ...) and the abnormal results are marked black. The main cause of death of p_1 was cirrhosis of liver encoded as $K746$

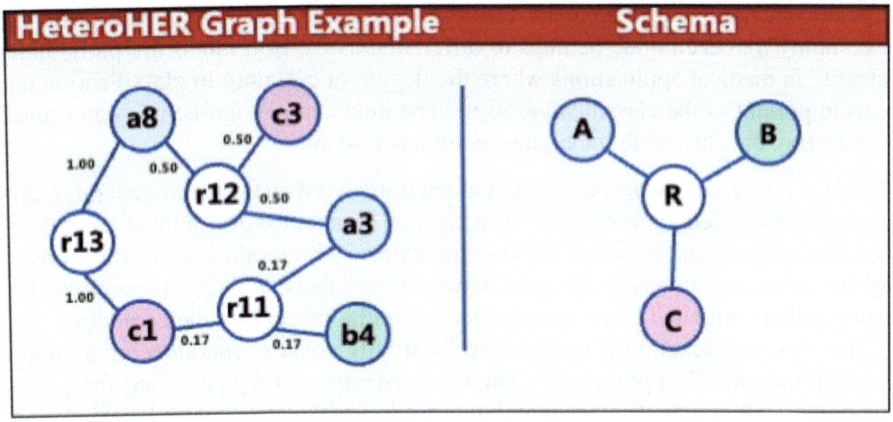

Fig. 11.10 The graph on the left shows a HeteroHER graph extracted from the example in Fig. 11.9. For instance, there is a link between r_{11} (the first record of p_1) and a_3 (the third item of category A) if the result of a_3 is abnormal in r_{11}. The star-shaped schema on the right is a type-level schema of such a graph

item node, with weights reflecting temporal importance. The output of the graph construction process is a heterogeneous graph represented as a set of sparse matrices for any two node types that are linked to each other in the schema.

Normalized Weights. To balance the influence of nodes in different density regions, the link weights are further normalized using standard graph normalization techniques. This normalization strengthens weights in low density regions while weakening weights in high density regions, improving the overall graph-based learning performance.

Semi-Supervised Learning on HeteroHER Graph

The second component of our method is a semi-supervised learning algorithm for the constructed HeteroHER graph. The algorithm combines the advantages of [17] for class discovery and [12] for handling heterogeneity to solve a specific problem induced by evidence-based risk prediction from health examination records.

In this section, we first define an objective function for the learning problem and show its convexity, followed by an optimization procedure to solve the problem. Then we derive an efficient iterative algorithm and show its convergence. Finally, time complexity is discussed.

Notations. In our framework, we consider multiple disease classes plus one "unknown" class. Label information is represented in a structured format where each node is assigned to the appropriate class based on available ground truth data. For unlabeled nodes, we initially assign them to the "unknown" class.

A key innovation in our approach is the use of soft labels, which indicate the degree of certainty that each node belongs to different classes. Soft labels are particularly valuable in medical applications where the degree of certainty in classification can be as important as the classification itself. The final class assignment is determined by selecting the class with the highest confidence score.

Objective Function. We develop a regularized framework on the heterogeneous graph for semi-supervised learning. The classification problem is formulated as an optimization problem that balances two key constraints: (1) smoothness constraint ensuring that connected nodes in the graph have similar labels, and (2) fitness constraint ensuring that computed labels remain close to initial labels for labeled nodes.

The objective function is designed to be strictly convex, guaranteeing a unique global minimum. The optimization can be solved either through a closed-form solution or more efficiently through an iterative algorithm that propagates label information between connected nodes until convergence.

Iterative Solution

An iterative algorithm provides a more efficient solution than matrix inversion. The algorithm follows a label propagation interpretation where each node iteratively spreads label information to its neighbors until a global stable state is achieved.

The iterative update rule for soft labels incorporates two key factors: (1) computed label scores from neighboring nodes propagated via graph links, and (2) initial labels for labeled nodes. A tunable parameter controls the trade-off between these influences, providing a mechanism to learn an additional "unknown" class for nodes that are less connected to labeled high-risk disease nodes. The iterative algorithm is proven to converge to the optimal solution, ensuring reliable performance. The computational complexity is manageable for large-scale health datasets, making the approach efficient and scalable for practical applications.

The complete SHG-Health algorithm first constructs the HeteroHER graph from health examination records, then normalizes the link weights, and initializes soft labels uniformly for all node types. The core iterative process updates soft labels by combining information from connected nodes until convergence, ultimately producing optimal soft label assignments for risk prediction.

11.4.3 Experimental Results and Performance Analysis

We evaluate the SHG-Health algorithm using both real-world geriatric health examination data and synthetic datasets. The real dataset contains health records from over 100,000 elderly participants collected over six years, linked to health outcome data for validation. The evaluation focuses on two key tasks: identifying high-risk cases and classifying them into specific disease categories. We compare SHG-Health against

Table 11.3 Sizes of 10 disease categories and unlabeled cases in terms of participant (p) and record (R)

Class	ICD10	Name	ICD9	Size (P)	Size (R)
1	J18	Pneumonia, organism unspecified	481,485,486,514	434	851
2	J40-J44	Chronic lower respiratory diseases	490-493,496	277	531
3	C34	Malignant neoplasm of bronchus and lung	162	253	586
4	C22	Malignant neoplasm of liver and intrahepatic bile ducts	155	219	375
5	C16	Malignant neoplasm of Stomach	151	193	355
6	C18	Malignant neoplasm of colon	153	186	371
7	I25	Chronic ischaemic heart disease	412,414,429	185	330
8	C25	Malignant neoplasm of pancreas	157	123	242
9	C23	Malignant neoplasm of gallbladder	156	74	126
10	G20	Parkinson's disease	332	37	73
Unlabeled (alive) cases				26,771	69,802

established algorithms including Support Vector Machines (SVM), K-Nearest Neighbors (KNN), and other graph-based semi-supervised learning methods.

Disease Categories and Data Distribution

We selected 10 ICD disease categories as high-risk disease classes, shown in Table 11.3. The disease categories were determined to maximize coverage while ensuring sufficient instances per class for reliable classification. Based on clinical expert suggestions, we excluded diabetes mellitus (known complications) and acute myocardial infarction (acute disease nature). The final selection includes major causes of elderly mortality such as pneumonia, chronic respiratory diseases, and various malignancies, along with two minority classes (gallbladder cancer and Parkinson's disease) to represent real-world imbalanced scenarios.

The unlabeled cases were randomly selected from alive participants with a ratio matching the overall deceased/alive distribution (7.4%/92.6%), resulting in 69,802 records from 26,771 unlabeled participants. This large proportion of unlabeled data (approximately 13 times the labeled cases) presents a challenging but realistic scenario for semi-supervised learning in healthcare applications.

Binary Classification: High-Risk Case Identification

The first evaluation task assesses the algorithm's ability to identify high-risk cases regardless of specific disease categories. This binary classification treats all disease cases as a single high-risk class versus the unknown class. Table 11.4 presents the

Table 11.4 Evaluation on binary prediction (avg ± std%)

	Precision	Recall/Sensitivity	F-Score
Ours	96.24 ± 1.60	43.93 ± 1.11	60.32 ± 1.23
Ours-Chi2	99.33 ± 0.36	43.02 ± 1.40	60.02 ± 1.41
Ours-Gaus	96.99 ± 1.32	43.69 ± 1.14	60.23 ± 0.86
SVM	89.00 ± 10.19	0.49 ± 0.36	0.98 ± 0.71
KNN	37.52 ± 1.48	25.62 ± 1.30	30.45 ± 1.36
GNetMine	0.00 ± 0.00	0.00 ± 0.00	0.00 ± 0.00
GGSSL	5.21 ± 0.02	100.00 ± 0.00	9.91 ± 0.03

results, where our SHG-Health methods achieved superior performance with Ours-Chi2 reaching 99.33% precision, though recall remains moderate at around 43%.

The high precision but moderate recall indicates that SHG-Health operates as a conservative model, which is desirable for preventive care systems where false alarms carry significant costs. The method correctly identifies nearly all predicted high-risk cases, though it misses some true positive cases to maintain high confidence. In contrast, GGSSL achieved 100% recall but only 5.21% precision, indicating it predicted most cases as high-risk without discrimination. GNetMine showed complete bias toward the unknown class with zero scores across all metrics.

Multi-class Disease Category Prediction

The second evaluation task examines the algorithm's ability to correctly classify high-risk cases into specific disease categories. This conditional evaluation considers only cases predicted as one of the disease classes, using macro-averaging to ensure equal importance across all classes including minority diseases. Table 11.5 demonstrates that SHG-Health, particularly Ours-Chi2, significantly outperforms all comparison methods with 90.58% macro-precision and 90.73% macro-recall.

These results indicate that when SHG-Health identifies a case as high-risk, it can accurately determine the specific disease category with over 90% accuracy. The balanced macro-precision and macro-recall scores show that the method performs con-

Table 11.5 Evaluation on disease class prediction (avg ± std%)

	Macro-Precision	Macro-Recall
Ours	89.14 ± 0.38	89.62 ± 0.28
Ours-Chi2	90.58 ± 0.19	90.73 ± 0.15
Ours-Gaus	89.55 ± 0.56	90.30 ± 0.41
KNN	21.12 ± 1.49	59.92 ± 2.50
SVM	52.50 ± 39.41	62.33 ± 30.55
GNetMine	–	–
GGSSL	0.11 ± 0	9.09 ± 0

sistently across all disease categories, including minority classes with fewer training samples. KNN achieved only 21.12% macro-precision despite 59.92% macro-recall, indicating poor specificity in disease classification. SVM showed high variance with 52.50% ± 39.41% macro-precision, suggesting unstable performance across different folds.

Figure 11.11 presents detailed performance comparisons on balanced synthetic datasets with varying class sizes. The results show that SHG-Health maintains stable performance across different dataset sizes, consistently achieving the highest macro-precision and macro-recall scores for disease classification. Figure 11.12 demonstrates the algorithm's robustness under increasing amounts of unlabeled data, where our method shows the most graceful degradation compared to other approaches. Interestingly, the performance slightly improves when unlabeled cases increase from 10,000 to 20,000, suggesting that more unlabeled data helps better differentiate between disease classes through graph structure learning.

Figure 11.13 compares the training time efficiency across all algorithms. SHG-Health demonstrates superior computational efficiency, requiring only 1.41 s for training on datasets with 10,000 disease cases plus 20,000 unlabeled cases. This efficiency, combined with the method's superior effectiveness, makes SHG-Health

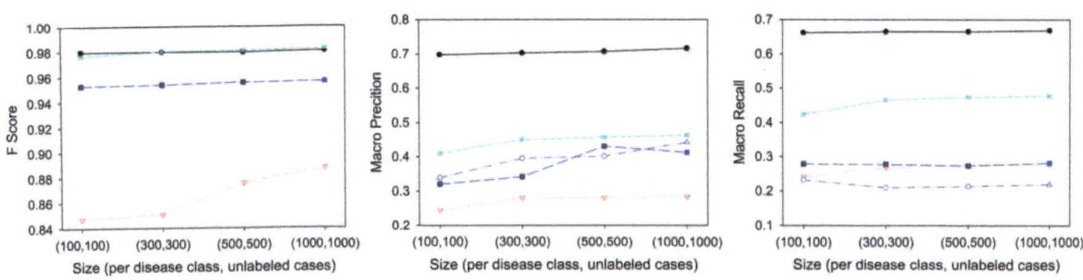

Fig. 11.11 Performance comparison on balanced synthetic datasets with varying class sizes, showing F-scores for high-risk identification (Task 1) and macro-precision/macro-recall for disease classification (Task 2). Marker shapes and colors represent different methods: black (Ours), red (1NN), cyan (SVM), purple (GNetMine), and blue (GGSSL)

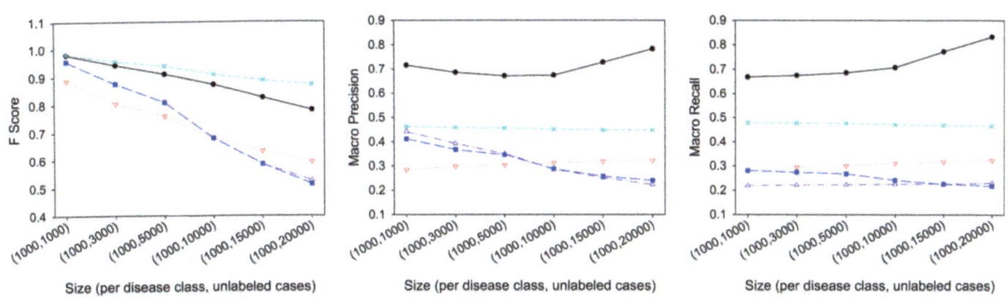

Fig. 11.12 Stability analysis with increasing unlabeled data scales, demonstrating SHG-Health's robustness under large proportions of unlabeled cases. Marker shapes and colors represent different methods: black (Ours), red (1NN), cyan (SVM), purple (GNetMine), and blue (GGSSL)

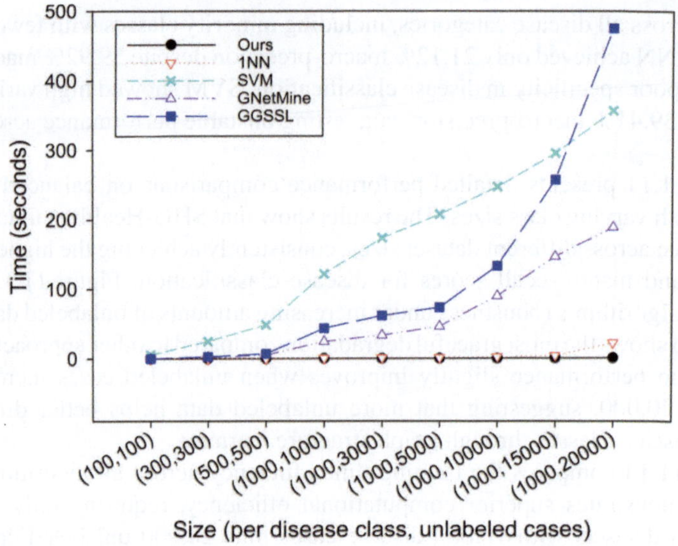

Fig. 11.13 Training time comparison with increasing data sizes, showing SHG-Health's superior computational efficiency

highly suitable for large-scale healthcare applications where both accuracy and scalability are critical requirements.

The comprehensive experimental results demonstrate that SHG-Health effectively addresses the challenges of health risk prediction with heterogeneous examination records and large unlabeled datasets, achieving both high accuracy and computational efficiency.

11.4.4 Summary of SHG-Health

Mining health examination data presents significant challenges due to its heterogeneity, intrinsic noise, and the large volume of unlabeled data. To address these challenges, we introduced SHG-Health, an effective and efficient graph-based semi-supervised algorithm with several key advantages.

Our approach represents health examination records as a graph that connects all relevant cases, particularly useful for modeling sparse abnormal results. The heterogeneous graph structure allows us to capture multi-typed relationships between data items, with different examination components represented as distinct node types. This enables our method to exploit the underlying heterogeneous subgraph structures of individual disease classes. Additionally, features are weighted within their own type through a label propagation process, contributing to effective classification through an iterative convergence process.

Our work demonstrates a novel approach to predicting health risks based on annual examinations. In future work, we plan to integrate health examination records with other data sources, such as hospital-based electronic health records and information about participants' living conditions (diet, exercise patterns, etc.). By combining data from multiple sources, we believe even more effective risk prediction can be achieved, furthering the potential of AI-empowered personal health management systems.

11.5 Discussion and Future Directions

This chapter has presented two data mining approaches for personal health management: MyPHI for health indexing and SHG-Health for graph-based risk prediction. Both methods demonstrate significant improvements over traditional approaches in handling medical data challenges such as label uncertainty, class imbalance, and heterogeneous health parameters.

The proposed methods address fundamental challenges in health data mining. MyPHI's soft-label optimization effectively handles uncertainty and imbalance in medical datasets, achieving 89.95% AUC under severely imbalanced conditions. SHG-Health's heterogeneous graph structure captures complex relationships between health parameters, reaching over 96% precision in high-risk identification. These approaches contribute to AI-empowered IoT solutions for healthcare by providing core analytical components for health monitoring infrastructures. The methods can integrate with ambient sensing, wearable devices, and remote monitoring systems to support comprehensive health management ecosystems. As aging populations continue to grow globally, such technologies will play an increasingly important role in supporting proactive health monitoring, early risk detection, and personalized health insights for elderly individuals.

Several promising directions emerge from this work, which represent opportunities to enhance AI-empowered health management systems for more effective and personalized healthcare delivery:

- *Multimodal Integration*: Incorporating diverse data sources including wearable sensors, environmental data, and clinical notes for more comprehensive health assessments.
- *Real-time Analytics*: Developing streaming versions for real-time health monitoring and immediate risk assessment.
- *Privacy-Preserving Methods*: Implementing federated learning to enable collaborative model training while protecting sensitive health data.
- *Personalized Modeling*: Advancing toward individualized health trajectory models that account for unique patient characteristics and histories.

References

1. Bright, T.J., Wong, A., Dhurjati, R., Bristow, E., Bastian, L., Coeytaux, R.R., Samsa, G., Hasselblad, V., Williams, J.W., Musty, M.D., Wing, L., Kendrick, A.S., Sanders, G.D., Lobach, D.: Effect of clinical decision-support systems: a systematic review. Ann. Intern. Med. **157**(1), 29–43 (2012)
2. Chen, L., Li, X., Sheng, Q.Z., Peng, W.C., Bennett, J., Hu, H.Y., Huang, N.: Mining health examination records–a graph-based approach. IEEE Trans. Knowl. Data Eng. **28**(9), 2423–2437 (2016)
3. Chen, L., Li, X., Wang, S., Hu, H.Y., Huang, N., Sheng, Q.Z., Sharaf, M.A.: Mining personal health index from annual geriatric medical examinations. In: Proceedings of the IEEE 14th International Conference on Data Mining (ICDM), pp. 761–766. IEEE (2014)
4. Chen, L., Li, X., Yang, Y., Kurniawati, H., Sheng, Q.Z., Hu, H.Y., Huang, N.: Personal health indexing based on medical examinations: a data mining approach. Decis. Supp. Syst. **81**, 30–42 (2016)
5. Prevention, C.: Cdc's vision for public health surveillance in the 21st century, for Disease Control. Technical report, U.S. Department of Health and Human Services (2012)
6. Eichelberg, M., Aden, T., Riesmeier, J., Dogac, A., Laleci, G.B.: A survey and analysis of electronic healthcare record standards. ACM Comput. Surv. **37**(4), 277–315 (2005)
7. Esfandiari, N., Babavalian, M.R., Moghadam, A.M.E., Tabar, V.K.: Knowledge discovery in medicine: current issue and future trend. Expert Syst. Appl. **41**(9), 4434–4463 (2014)
8. Fisher, A., Burke, D.: Critical care scoring systems. In: Contemporary Coloproctology, pp. 513–528. Springer (2012)
9. Ghalwash, M.F., Radosavljevic, V., Obradovic, Z.: Extraction of interpretable multivariate patterns for early diagnostics. In: Proceedings of the 2013 IEEE 13th International Conference on Data Mining, pp. 201–210. IEEE (2013)
10. Glare, P.A., Sinclair, C.T.: Palliative medicine review: prognostication. J. Palliat. Med. **11**(1), 84–103 (2008)
11. Jen, C.H., Wang, C.C., Jiang, B.C., Chu, Y.H., Chen, M.S.: Application of classification techniques on development an early-warning system for chronic illnesses. Expert Syst. Appl. **39**(10), 8852–8858 (2012)
12. Ji, M., Sun, Y., Danilevsky, M., Han, J., Gao, J.: Graph regularized transductive classification on heterogeneous information networks. In: Proceedings of the European Conference on Machine Learning and Knowledge Discovery in Databases (ECML PKDD), pp. 570–586. Springer (2010)
13. Kaplan, R.M., Bush, J.W., Berry, C.C.: Health status: types of validity and the index of well-being. Health Serv. Res. **11**(4), 478–507 (1976)
14. Kontio, E., Airola, A., Pahikkala, T., Lundgrén-Laine, H., Junttila, K., Korvenranta, H., Salakoski, T., Salanterä, S.: Predicting patient acuity from electronic patient records. J. Biomed. Inform. **51**, 8–13 (2014)
15. Mohktar, M.S., Redmond, S.J., Antoniades, N.C., Rochford, P.D., Pretto, J.J., Basilakis, J., Lovell, N.H., McDonald, C.F.: Predicting the risk of exacerbation in patients with chronic obstructive pulmonary disease using home telehealth measurement data. Artif. Intell. Med. **63**(1), 51–59 (2015)
16. Nguyen, Q., Valizadegan, H., Hauskrecht, M.: Learning classification models with soft-label information. J. Am. Med. Inform. Assoc. **21**(3), 501–508 (2014)
17. Nie, F., Xiang, S., Liu, Y., Zhang, C.: A general graph-based semi-supervised learning with novel class discovery. Neural Comput. Appl. **19**, 549–555 (2010)
18. Pan, S., Wu, J., Zhu, X.: Cogboost: boosting for fast cost-sensitive graph classification. IEEE Trans. Knowl. Data Eng. **27**(11), 2933–2946 (2015)
19. Pantelopoulos, A., Bourbakis, N.G.: A survey on wearable sensor-based systems for health monitoring and prognosis. IEEE Trans. Syst. Man Cybern. Part C (Applications and Reviews) **40**(1), 1–12 (2010)

20. Pechenizkiy, M., Tsymbal, A., Puuronen, S., Pechenizkiy, O.: Data mining techniques for disease risk assessment and prediction. In: 19th IEEE Symposium on Computer-Based Medical Systems (CBMS'06), pp. 708–713. IEEE (2006)
21. Sun, Y., Yu, Y., Han, J.: Ranking-based clustering of heterogeneous information networks with star network schema. In: Proceedings of the 15th ACM SIGKDD International Conference on Knowledge Discovery and Data Mining (KDD), pp. 797–806. ACM (2009)
22. Tran, T., Phung, D., Luo, W., Venkatesh, S.: Stabilized sparse ordinal regression for medical risk stratification. Knowl. Inf. Syst. **43**(3), 555–582 (2015)
23. Wang, F., Zhang, P., Qian, B., Wang, X., Davidson, I.: Clinical risk prediction with multilinear sparse logistic regression. In: Proceedings of the 20th ACM SIGKDD International Conference on Knowledge Discovery and Data Mining, pp. 145–154. ACM (2014)
24. Wang, X., Wang, F., Sun, J., Qian, B., Hu, J.: Exploring patient risk groups with incomplete knowledge. In: Proceedings of the 2013 IEEE International Conference on Data Mining, pp. 1223–1228. IEEE (2013)
25. Woodward, M.: Epidemiology: Study Design and Data Analysis, 3rd edn. CRC Press (2013)
26. Yang, Y., Ma, Z., Xu, Z., Yan, S., Hauptmann, A.G.: how related exemplars help complex event detection in web videos? In: Proceedings of the IEEE International Conference on Computer Vision (ICCV), pp. 2104–2111. IEEE (2013)
27. Yi, S.I., So, B.R., Lee, C.S., Lee, S.J., Park, S.K., Park, B.K., Chung, I.W.: Classification of health grade using bio-check unit and health index. J. Biomed. Sci. Eng. **6**(3), 148–155 (2011)
28. Zhao, M., Chan, R.H.M., Chow, T.W.S., Tang, P.: Compact graph based semi-supervised learning for medical diagnosis in alzheimer's disease. IEEE Signal Process. Lett. **21**(10), 1192–1196 (2014)
29. Zhao, Y., Wang, G., Zhang, X., Yu, J.X., Wang, Z.: Learning phenotype structure using sequence model. IEEE Trans. Knowl. Data Eng. **26**(3), 667–681 (2014)

Chapter 12
Identity Management

12.1 Introduction

Identity management plays a critical role in smart aging environments, where secure and reliable authentication is essential for ensuring both safety and personalized care. As aging populations globally continue to increase, there is growing need for robust authentication systems that can protect sensitive information, secure physical spaces, and enable personalized services specifically designed for older adults [7, 41].

Biometric authentication technologies have gained significant popularity due to their reliability and adaptability. These systems generally fall into two categories: physiological and behavioral. Physiological biometrics utilize an individual's unique intrinsic features such as face [13], iris [24], retina [31], voice [14], and fingerprint [35]. Behavioral biometrics, in contrast, analyze an individual's behavior patterns, with gait analysis [4] being among the most prominent examples.

However, traditional biometric authentication systems face growing security challenges. With rapid advancements in manufacturing and technology, conventional biometrics like fingerprints and face recognition have become increasingly vulnerable to spoofing attacks. For instance, fingerprint-based systems can be deceived using fake fingerprint films, while even sophisticated face recognition systems can be fooled by specialized anti-surveillance masks. These vulnerabilities highlight the need for biometric authentication systems with enhanced fake-resistance characteristics, particularly for high-security applications in smart aging contexts.

12.1.1 Challenges and Opportunities

Identity management systems in smart aging environments face significant challenges in balancing security with usability, particularly considering the physical and cognitive limitations of older adults. Traditional unimodal biometric systems

Q. Z. Sheng et al., *Harnessing Artificial Intelligence and Pervasive Internet of Things for an Empowered Aging*, https://doi.org/10.1007/978-3-032-16502-2_12

suffer from limitations including noise susceptibility, low universality, and intra-class variation that restrict their accuracy across diverse applications [20, 21, 33].

Emerging technologies such as Electroencephalography (EEG)-based cognitive biometrics and gait-based authentication systems have attracted increasing attention. EEG signals, which measure the brain's electromagnetic neural oscillations, are unique to each individual and extremely difficult to replicate, offering significant potential for highly secure authentication [7]. Similarly, gait-based authentication leverages an individual's walking patterns determined by intrinsic, temporal, and kinematic factors [5].

Despite their individual promise, both approaches face limitations. EEG-based systems, while offering high fake-resistance, are susceptible to environmental and subjective factors. Gait-based authentication, although more stable across scenarios, typically achieves lower performance levels. Single-modality systems generally obtain insufficient security levels for high-security applications [17].

These challenges create opportunities for multimodal biometric systems that combine complementary traits to achieve higher accuracy, reliability, and security while accommodating the specific needs of older adults in smart aging contexts.

12.1.2 Contributions

This chapter makes several significant contributions to the field of identity management for smart aging. We present a comprehensive overview of biometric authentication technologies with particular focus on smart aging applications, and introduce DeepKey, a novel dual-authentication system that uniquely combines EEG and gait biometrics to achieve enhanced fake-resistance and reliability. The system demonstrates a robust deep learning framework featuring an attention-based RNN that effectively decodes distinctive patterns in brain activities and gait behaviors, achieving superior performance with zero false acceptance rate and minimal false rejection rate.

Our research provides empirical evidence showing that Delta band EEG signals contain the most discriminative information for person identification, offering new insights for developing more effective biometric systems for older adults. Additionally, we explore the practical implications of advanced authentication technologies in smart aging environments, addressing how such systems can balance high security requirements with the specific needs and limitations of older adults, including considerations for usability, privacy, and adaptive authentication approaches.

12.1.3 Chapter Organization

The remainder of this chapter is organized as follows. Section 12.2 introduces the background and related work on biometric authentication technologies, EEG-based and gait-based authentication systems, multimodal biometric approaches, and research gaps in smart aging contexts. Section 12.3 introduces the DeepKey multimodal biometric authentication system and presents our experimental evaluation, including system design, performance analysis, and comparison with state-of-the-art alternatives. Section 12.4 discusses the implications for smart aging applications, current limitations, and directions for future research.

12.2 Background and Related Work

12.2.1 Biometric Authentication Technologies

Biometric authentication has become increasingly prevalent due to the inherent security advantages of using physical or behavioral characteristics that cannot be easily stolen or duplicated. Among the most mature biometric authentication technologies is fingerprint-based authentication, which has demonstrated high matching accuracy and has been utilized for decades [26]. The unique ridge patterns in fingerprints provide a reliable basis for identity verification in various applications.

Iris recognition represents another widely adopted approach for biometric authentication, valued for its unique and stable pattern characteristics [30]. The pioneering work by Daugman [9], which utilizes Gabor phase information and Hamming distance for iris code matching, remains the foundation for most modern iris recognition systems. Building upon this seminal work, researchers have developed numerous enhancements to address various challenges in iris authentication. For instance, Pillai et al. [30] introduced kernel functions to represent transformations of iris biometrics, effectively constraining both intra-class and inter-class variability to address sensor mismatch problems.

Face recognition technologies [12, 16, 42] have gained widespread public acceptance due to their non-invasive nature and the distinctive features they leverage. However, face recognition systems must contend with various challenges including variations in expression, image quality, illumination, and potential disguises. To overcome these limitations, advanced approaches incorporating Infrared Radiation (IR) [16] and 3D scanning technologies [12] have attracted significant research interest. According to Zhang et al. [42], multimodal recognition systems that combine traditional visual textual features with IR or 3D data can achieve substantially higher accuracy than single-modal approaches.

In the context of smart aging, these biometric technologies offer potential advantages for secure authentication without requiring password memorization, which may be particularly beneficial for older adults with cognitive impairments. However, they also present challenges related to age-related physiological changes that may affect biometric features over time.

12.2.2 EEG-Based and Gait-Based Authentication

Electroencephalography (EEG)-based authentication has emerged as a promising approach due to its ability to capture brain signals in a safe and non-invasive manner. Despite the complexity of analyzing these signals, their confidential and fake-resistant nature makes them valuable for high-security applications. Marcel and Millán [29] pioneered this field by employing Gaussian Mixture Models and training client models with Maximum A Posteriori (MAP) adaptation. Building on this foundation, Ashby et al. [3] demonstrated the feasibility of EEG authentication with less expensive devices by extracting five sets of features from EEG electrodes and inter-hemispheric data, combining them, and processing the final features using Support Vector Machines (SVM).

The selection of appropriate features for EEG-based authentication has been a subject of extensive research. Altahat et al. [2] achieved higher accuracy by utilizing Power Spectral Density (PSD) features instead of widely used AutoRegressive (AR) models, and conducted channel selection to identify the most contributive channels among all available EEG channels. Similarly, Thomas and Vinod [34] exploited individual alpha frequency (IAF) and delta band signals to compose specific feature vectors, focusing PSD feature extraction specifically on the gamma band.

Gait-based authentication approaches have also been actively explored, leveraging the most basic human activity of walking. Research in this area has followed two primary paths: model-based approaches [38], which represent gait information using mathematical structures, and appearance-based approaches, which extract features directly without relying on mathematical modeling. Among appearance-based methods, Gait Energy Image (GEI) [27] has gained popularity due to its high efficiency and remarkable performance. Subsequent research has built upon GEIs to investigate external factors and distinguish different body parts in gait analysis.

Cross-view variance remains a significant challenge in gait identification [22, 23]. To address this issue, Wu et al. [37] combined deep Convolutional Neural Networks (CNNs) with techniques for handling cross-view variations to achieve robust gait identification across different viewing angles.

For smart aging applications, EEG-based and gait-based authentication offer potential advantages due to their non-invasive nature and the difficulty of spoofing these biometric traits. However, the practical implementation of these technologies must consider the specific needs and potential physical limitations of older adults.

12.2.3 Multimodal Biometric Systems and AI Integration

As unimodal authentication systems struggle with challenges including environmental noise, limited universality, and intra-class variations, multimodal biometric approaches that combine different biometric traits have gained increasing attention. Most existing multimodal systems combine two biometrics from commonly used modalities such as face, iris, and fingerprints [20, 21, 33]. However, innovative combinations like gait and electrocardiogram (ECG) have also demonstrated effectiveness [10], while Manjunathswamy et al. [28] successfully integrated ECG and fingerprint data at the score level.

Artificial Intelligence (AI) technologies, particularly deep learning approaches, have significantly enhanced the capabilities of biometric authentication systems. Deep neural networks have demonstrated superior performance in extracting discriminative features from complex biometric data, leading to higher accuracy and robustness. For instance, Convolutional Neural Networks (CNNs) have revolutionized face recognition systems by learning hierarchical representations directly from facial images, while Recurrent Neural Networks (RNNs) have shown promising results in analyzing sequential biometric data such as EEG signals and gait patterns.

Recent advances in attention mechanisms [11, 36] have further improved the performance of deep learning models for biometric authentication by allowing the models to focus on the most informative parts of the input data. This capability is particularly valuable for multimodal systems that must integrate information from different biometric sources with varying levels of reliability and discriminative power.

The integration of AI in biometric systems has also enabled adaptive authentication approaches that can account for temporal changes in biometric traits, which is particularly relevant for older adults whose physiological and behavioral characteristics may change more rapidly due to aging or health conditions.

12.2.4 Research Gaps and Opportunities in Smart Aging

In the context of smart aging, several research gaps and opportunities exist in the field of identity management and biometric authentication:

- *Age-Appropriate Authentication System Design*: Most existing authentication systems have not been specifically designed or evaluated with older adults as the target user group, leading to potential usability issues and reduced performance for this demographic. Age-related physiological changes can affect the quality and consistency of biometric traits, potentially compromising the reliability of authentication systems designed primarily for younger populations.
- *Multimodal Biometric Integration*: While multimodal biometric systems offer improved performance compared to unimodal approaches, the specific combination of EEG and gait signals remains largely unexplored, despite the complementary nature of these biometrics. EEG signals provide high fake-resistance but are susceptible to environmental and subjective factors, while gait patterns offer greater stability across different scenarios but typically achieve lower authentication performance when used alone.
- *Usability and Acceptance Challenges*: The practical deployment of biometric authentication systems in smart aging environments faces challenges related to user acceptance, privacy concerns, and the need for non-intrusive, convenient authen-

tication experiences. These challenges are particularly significant for older adults who may have limited technology familiarity or physical/cognitive impairments that affect their interaction with authentication systems.

- *Adaptive Authentication for Changing Biometrics*: Aging brings progressive changes to physiological and behavioral biometric traits, requiring authentication systems that can adapt over time. Traditional static biometric systems may fail to account for these changes, necessitating the development of dynamic models that can evolve alongside the user's aging process while maintaining security and reliability.

These gaps highlight the importance of developing more flexible, secure, and user-friendly authentication systems like DeepKey, which can potentially address many of these challenges through its multimodal approach while specifically addressing the unique needs of elderly users in smart aging environments.

12.3 DeepKey: A Multimodal Biometric Authentication System

12.3.1 Motivation and Overview of DeepKey System

Building upon the research gaps and opportunities identified in the previous section, this section presents DeepKey [40], an innovative multimodal biometric authentication system specifically designed to address the limitations of traditional authentication approaches in smart aging contexts. By combining EEG-based cognitive biometrics with gait-based behavioral biometrics, DeepKey offers enhanced security, reliability, and usability compared to unimodal systems. The following subsections detail the motivation behind DeepKey's development, provide an overview of its architecture and components, and explain how the integration of these complementary biometric modalities creates a robust authentication system particularly well-suited for high-security applications in smart aging environments.

Traditional biometric authentication systems face increasing security challenges as technology advances make spoofing attacks more sophisticated. Fingerprint and face recognition systems, for instance, can be fooled using fake fingerprint films or specialized anti-surveillance masks. These vulnerabilities highlight the need for biometric systems with enhanced fake-resistance properties, particularly for high-security applications in smart aging environments where the protection of vulnerable older adults is paramount.

While EEG and gait-based authentication systems have individually shown promise in addressing these challenges, their true potential emerges when combined in a complementary multimodal system. EEG signals, with their high fake-resistance and unique personal signatures, offer strong security but can be affected by environmental and subjective factors. Gait patterns, while more stable across different scenarios, typically achieve lower performance levels when used alone. The DeepKey system leverages the strengths of both modalities while minimizing their individual limitations.

The DeepKey system addresses these limitations by combining EEG and gait biometrics in a dual-authentication framework. This combination offers superior fake-resistance compared to traditional biometric approaches, making it particularly well-suited for high-security applications in smart aging contexts. DeepKey consists of three main components: (1) an Invalid ID Filter Model to eliminate unauthorized subjects, (2) an EEG Identification Model to identify individuals based on their brain signals, and (3) a Gait Identification Model to identify individuals based on their walking patterns. Access is granted only when a subject passes all authentication components, ensuring a high level of security.

The integration of EEG and gait biometrics in DeepKey represents a significant advance in multimodal biometric authentication, offering enhanced security, reliability, and performance compared to existing approaches.

12.3.2 *DeepKey Authentication System*

This section presents the DeepKey authentication workflow and its core technical components.

System Overview

The DeepKey system is designed for deployment in high-security environments such as confidential facilities. As shown in Fig. 12.1, the authentication workflow consists of four sequential steps: EEG data collection through a headset during relaxation, gait data collection using IMUs during walking, authentication processing where both

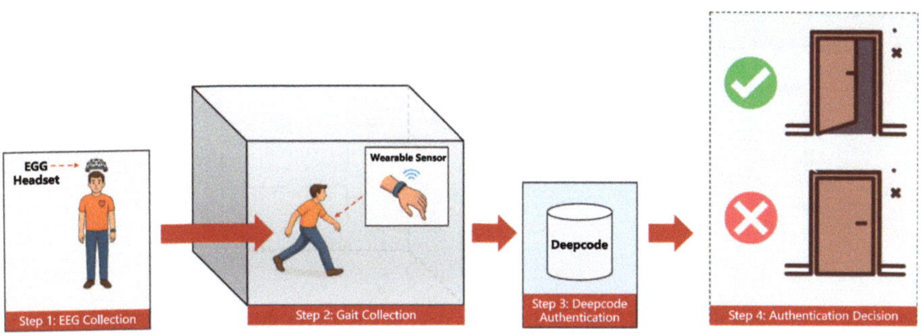

Fig. 12.1 Workflow of DeepKey authentication system. The data collection of EEG and gait are cascade

datasets are fed into the DeepKey algorithm, and final decision making for access approval or denial.

The core authentication process accomplishes two primary goals: authentication and identification. For authentication, we employ EEG signals due to their high fake-resistance and unique characteristics. For identification, we utilize deep learning models to extract distinctive features processed through neighbor-based classifiers. The system implements a three-stage process Fig. 12.2: an Invalid ID Filter based on EEG data determines whether the subject is genuine, followed by parallel EEG

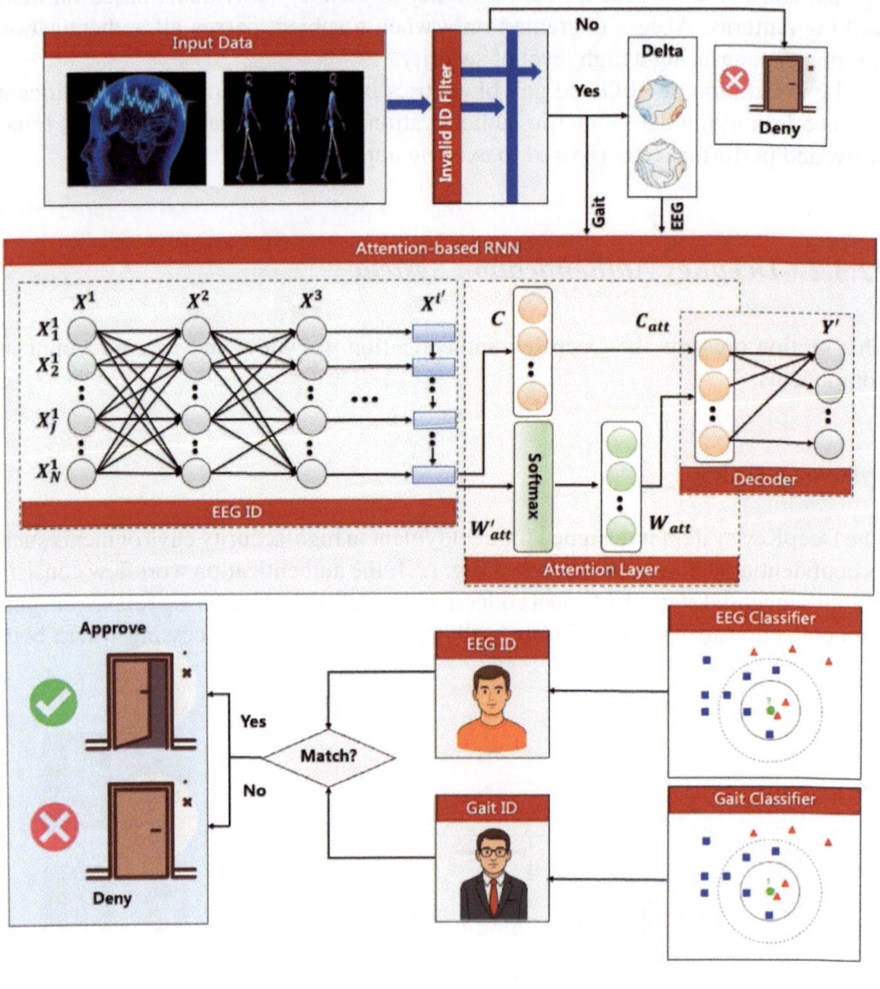

Fig. 12.2 Authentication workflow. If the input data cannot pass the invalid ID filter, it would directly be regarded as an impostor and deny access. If pass, the Delta pattern and gait signals are parallelly fed into an attention-based RNN structure to study the distinctive features C_{att}. The learned features are classified by the EEG and Gait classifier in order to identify the subject's EEG and Gait ID. The subject is approved only if the EEG ID is a match with Gait ID

and Gait Identification Models that generate respective IDs, and finally a consistency check that grants approval only when both IDs match.

Invalid ID Filter Model

Through our preliminary experiments, it has been found that raw EEG signals, compared to raw Gait data, have better characteristics to prevent invalid ID due to the high fake-resistance of EEG data and the richness of distinguishable features in EEG signals. Thus, in this section, we only use EEG for invalid ID filtering.

The subjects in an authentication system are categorized into two classes: *authorized* and *unauthorized*. Since the unauthorized data are not available in the training stage, an unsupervised learning algorithm is required to identify the invalid ID. In this work, we apply a one-class SVM to sort out the unauthorized subjects. Given a set of authorized subjects, $S = \{S_i, i = 1, 2, \ldots, L^o\}$, $S_i \in R^{n_s}$, where L^o denotes the number of authorized subjects and n_s denotes the number of dimensions of the input data. The input data consist of EEG data $E = \{E_i, i = 1, 2, \ldots, L^o\}$, $E_i \in R^{n_e}$ and gait data $\mathcal{G} = \{G_i, i = 1, 2, \ldots, L^o\}$, $G_i \in R^{n_g}$. n_g and n_e denote the number of dimensions of the gait data and EEG data, respectively, and $n_s = n_g + n_e$. The notations can be found in Table 12.1.

For each authentication, the collected EEG data E_i includes a number of samples. Each sample is a vector with shape [1, 14] where 14 denotes the number of

Table 12.1 Notations

Parameters	Explanation
L°	The number of authorized subjects (genuine)
E	The set of EEG signals
G	The set of gait signals
n_s	The number of features in input data sample
G_i	The i-th gait data
n_g	The number of features in per gait sample
E_i	The i-th EEG data
n_e	The number of features in EEG data sample
X^i	The data in the i-th layer of attention RNN
N^i	The number of dimensions in X^i
K	The number of participants (genuine and impostor)
c'_j	The hidden state in the j-th LSTM cell
$T(\cdot)$	The linear calculation of dense neural layers
$\mathcal{L}(\cdot)$	The LSTM calculation process
$\odot$	The elementwise multiplication
C_{att}	Attention-based code

electric-nodes in the Emotiv headset. To trade off the authentication efficiency (less collecting and waiting time) and computational performance, based on the experimental experience, we fed 200 samples ([200, 14]) into the Invalid ID Filter. 200 EEG samples are collected in 1.56 s, which is acceptable. The final filter result is the mean of the results on all the samples.

EEG Identification Model

Compared to gait data, EEG data contain more noise, which is more challenging to handle. Given the complexity of EEG signals, the data pre-processing is necessary. In practical EEG data analysis, the assembled EEG signals can be divided into several different frequency patterns (delta, theta, alpha, beta, and gamma) based on the strong intra-band correlation with a distinct behavioral state. Figure 12.3 reports the topography of EEG signals of different subjects under different frequency bands and demonstrates that the Delta wave, compared to other bands, enriches distinctive features. In detail, we calculate the inter-subject EEG signal cosine-similarity which measures the average similarity among different subjects under all the EEG bands.

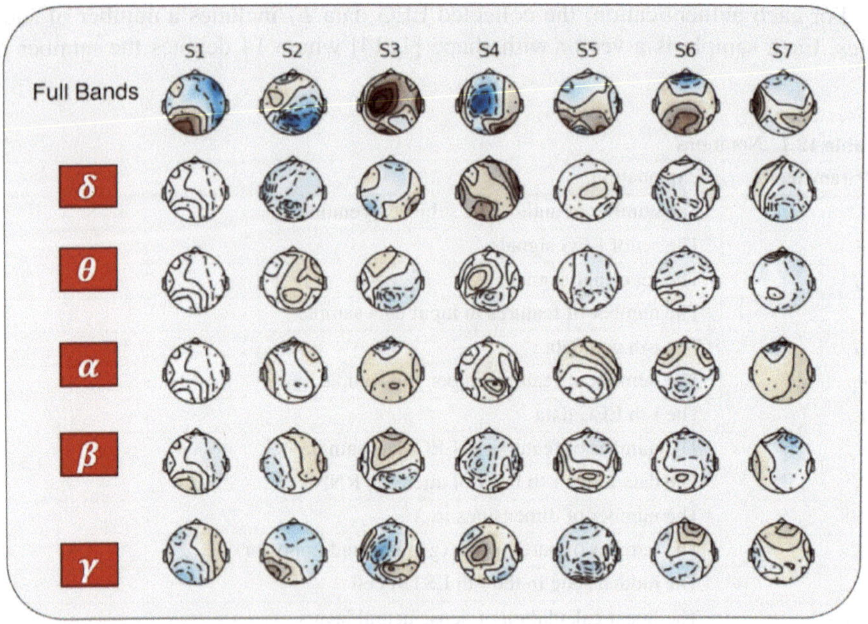

Fig. 12.3 EEG topography of different subjects under different frequency bands. The inter-subject EEG signal cosine-similarity is calculated under each band and the results are reported as 0.1313 (full bands), 0.0722 (Delta band), 0.1672 (Theta band), 0.2819 (Alpha band), 0.0888 (Beta band), and 0.082 (Gamma band). This illustrates that the delta band with the lowest similarity contains the most distinguishable features for person identification

The results are reported as 0.1313 (full bands), 0.0722 (Delta band), 0.1672 (Theta band), 0.2819 (Alpha band), 0.0888 (Beta band), and 0.082 (Gamma band). This illustrates that the delta band with the lowest similarity contains the most distinguishable features for person identification. Our previous work [41] has demonstrated that Delta pattern, compared to other EEG patterns, contains the most distinctive information and is the most stable pattern in different environments by qualitative analysis and empirical experimental results. Thus, in this article, we adopt a bandpass (0.5 Hz–3.5 Hz) Butterworth filter to extract Delta wave signal for further authentication. For simplicity, we denote the filtered EEG data as $\mathcal{E}$.

Since different EEG channels record different aspects of the brain signals, some of which are more representative of the individual, an approach that assumes all dimensions to be equal may not be suitable. Thus, we attempt to develop a novel model which can pay more attention to the most informative signals. In particular, the proposed approach is supposed to automatically learn the importance of the different parts of the EEG signal and focus on the valuable part. The effectiveness of attention-based RNN has been demonstrated in various domains including natural language processing [36] and speech recognition [6]. Inspired by the wide success of an attention mechanism [11], we introduce it to the Encoder-Decoder RNN model to assign varying weights to different dimensions of the EEG data. After EEG filtering, the composed Delta pattern $\mathcal{E}$ is fed into an attention-based Encoder-Decoder RNN structure [36] aiming to learn more representative features for user identification. The general Encoder-Decoder RNN framework regards all the feature dimensions of input sequence as having the same weights, no matter how important the dimension is for the output sequence.

In our approach, the different feature dimensions of the EEG data correspond to the different nodes of the EEG equipment. For example, the first dimension (first channel) collects the EEG data from the $AF3$ node located at the frontal lobe of the scalp while the seventh dimension is gathered from the $O1$ node at the occipital lobe (Both $AF3$ and $O1$ are EEG measurement positions in the International 10–20 Systems). To assign various weights to different dimensions of $\mathcal{E}$, we introduce the attention mechanism to the Encoder-Decoder RNN model. The proposed attention-based Encoder-Decoder RNN consists of three components (Fig. 12.2): the encoder, the attention module, and the decoder. The encoder is designed to compress the input Delta δ wave into a single intermediate code C; the attention module helps the encoder calculate a better intermediate code C_{att} by generating a sequence of the weights W_{att} of different dimensions; the decoder accepts the attention-based code C_{att} and decodes it to the output layer Y'.

The attention-based Encoder-Decoder RNN consists of three main components: the encoder, the attention module, and the decoder. The encoder compresses the input Delta wave patterns into an intermediate representation; the attention module generates weights to focus on the most informative EEG channels; and the decoder produces the final identification output.

Our approach leverages deep learning techniques to automatically learn the importance of different EEG channels, focusing computational attention on the most discriminative brain signals. The attention mechanism helps the model assign varying weights to different EEG measurement locations, such as the frontal lobe ($AF3$ node) versus the occipital lobe ($O1$ node), based on their relevance for individual identification.

The model utilizes standard deep learning components including fully connected layers, LSTM units for sequential processing, attention mechanisms for channel weighting, and softmax normalization for probability calculations. The training process employs cross-entropy loss with L2 regularization to prevent overfitting, optimized using the Adam algorithm.

The Gait Identification Model works similarly to the EEG Identification Model except for the frequency band filtering. The iterations threshold of attention-based RNN is set as n_{iter}^{G}. The Gait Identification Model receives a subject's gait data $\mathcal{G}$ from the input data I and maps to the user's Gait ID G_{ID}. All the model structures, hyper-parameters, optimization, and other settings in the EEG and Gait Identification Models remain the same to keep the lower model complexity of the DeepKey system.

12.3.3 Experiments and Results

In this section, we present a concise overview of our experimental evaluation of the DeepKey system. We focus on three key aspects: (1) comparison with state-of-the-art authentication systems; (2) analysis of critical parameters including single versus multiple sessions; and (3) assessment of authentication latency for practical deployment.

Experimental Settings. Our initial experiments utilized data from seven healthy younger participants (aged 26 ± 2, four males and three females) to establish baseline performance metrics under controlled conditions. While our ultimate target population is older adults, this approach allowed us to first validate the core technical components before addressing the additional complexities associated with age-related variables. EEG data were collected through an EPOC+ Emotiv headset with 14 channels at 128 Hz, while gait data were captured via three IMUs attached to participants' left wrist, back, and left ankle.

To evaluate session impact, which is particularly important for older users who may experience day-to-day variability in physical and cognitive states, we collected both single-session and multi-session datasets across three different days. Table 12.2 presents the detailed characteristics of these datasets. Each EEG or gait sample contains 10 continuous instances without overlapping. The single session datasets (EID-S and GID-S) were collected in a single experiment session, while the multi-session datasets (EID-M and GID-M) were gathered across three sessions conducted in the same place but on three different days. The robust performance across multiple sessions with varying conditions suggests promising adaptability to the variability that would be encountered in older adult populations, though future evaluations will directly involve older adults to validate these initial findings.

Table 12.2 Datasets description

Dataset	Biometric	#-D	Session	Frequency	Samples
EID-S	EEG	14	Single	128 Hz	49,000
EID-M	EEG	14	Multiple	128 Hz	147,000
GID-S	Gait	27	Single	80 Hz	140,000
GID-M	Gait	27	Multiple	80 Hz	420,000

#-D denotes the number of dimensions

For the Invalid ID Filter, we employed a one-class SVM with RBF kernel ($\nu = 0.15$). In our EEG processing pipeline, we focused on the Delta band (0.5-3.5 Hz) based on our preliminary analysis showing its superior discriminative properties for identification. The attention-based RNN model contains two fully connected hidden layers (each with 64 nodes) and one LSTM layer with 64 cells. The learning rate and regularization parameter λ were both set to 0.001, with the weighted code produced after 1,000 iterations. Our evaluation metrics included accuracy, ROC, AUC, false acceptance rate (FAR), and false rejection rate (FRR), with particular emphasis on minimizing FAR for high-security applications.

Overall System Performance. At the system level, DeepKey demonstrated exceptional performance, achieving a FAR of 0 and a FRR of 1%, significantly outperforming existing authentication systems. Table 12.3 presents a comprehensive comparison between DeepKey and other state-of-the-art biometric authentication systems. Our approach achieved 99.96% identification accuracy for EEG and 99.61% for gait over multi-session datasets, substantially outperforming both uni-modal and multi-modal alternatives.

In the Invalid ID Filter component, our approach achieved impressive results with an FAR of 0 and a FRR of 0.006 using one-class SVM on EEG data. For the identification models, detailed performance metrics are presented in Table 12.4, which shows precision, recall, and F1-scores across all seven subjects for both single-session and multi-session datasets. The proposed approach achieves consistently high performance (higher than 99%) on all metrics, with average accuracies of 100% for EID-S, 99.96% for EID-M, 99.83% for GID-S, and 99.61% for GID-M.

Figure 12.4 presents the confusion matrices and ROC curves for all four datasets, demonstrating near-perfect classification performance with AUC scores exceeding 0.99 across all cases. The confusion matrices show minimal misclassification, with the vast majority of predictions falling on the diagonal, while the ROC curves approaching the top-left corner confirm the excellent discriminative capability of our approach.

Table 12.5 provides a comprehensive component-level comparison between our approach and various baseline methods on multi-session datasets. Our method consistently outperforms traditional machine learning approaches (SVM, RF, KNN, AdaB, LDA), deep learning baselines (LSTM, GRU, CNN), and state-of-the-art methods. On the EID-M dataset, our approach achieves 99.96% accuracy compared to 93.24% for Attention-based RNN and 80.29% for the AR+SVM method [19]. On the GID-M

Table 12.3 System-Level comparison between deepkey and other biometric authentication systems

References	Biometric	Method	#-Subj.	Accuracy	FAR	FRR
Uni-modal systems						
[8]	Gait	Semi-supervised + NN	15	97.4	–	–
[1]	Gait	MLP	60	99.01	–	–
[7]	EEG	Customized Threshold	15	–	0	2.2
[15]	EEG	Low-pass filter+wavelets+ANN	32	90.03	–	–
[18]	EEG	CSP+LDA	12	96.97	–	–
[41]	EEG	Attention-based RNN+XGB	8	98.82	–	–
[19]	EEG	AR+SVM	104	97.43	–	–
Multi-modal systems						
[25]	Fingerprint+Face	ZM+RBF Neural Network	40	92.89	4.95	1.12
[39]	Iris+Pupil	Gabor wavelets+Hamming	59	–	2.44	2.44
[28]	ECG+Fingerprint	Score Fusion	50	–	2.5	0
[10]	ECG+Gait	Score Fusion	30	–	1.26	1.26
Ours	**EEG+Gait**	**Attention-based RNN+KNN**	**7**	**99.57**	**0**	**1.0**

The performance of our method is evaluated on multi-session datasets (EID-M, GID-M)

dataset, we achieve 99.61% accuracy, surpassing the MLP method's 99.01% [1] and the semi-supervised approach's 96.53% [8].

In DeepKey, subjects passing the Invalid ID Filter are granted access only if their recognized IDs are consistent, i.e., $E_{ID} = G_{ID}$. The overall FAR remains at 0, while the overall FRR is calculated as approximately $0.006 + 0.994 \times (1 - 0.9961 \times 0.9996) \approx 1\%$. This exceptional performance demonstrates DeepKey's effectiveness in combining EEG and gait biometrics for highly secure authentication.

Key Findings from Parameter Analysis. Our analysis of key parameters revealed several important findings. First, multi-session testing showed slightly lower but still highly competitive performance compared to single-session testing. This demonstrates that our system maintains robust performance despite variations in equipment positioning across different sessions.

Second, our frequency band analysis confirmed that the Delta band (0.5–3.5 Hz) consistently provided higher identification accuracy than other EEG frequency bands. Table 12.6 presents a comprehensive comparison of identification accuracy across different EEG frequency bands (Delta, Theta, Alpha, Beta, Gamma, and Full band) for both single-session and multi-session datasets. The results demonstrate that Delta

Table 12.4 Classification report of the datasets including precision, recall, and F1-Score

Subject	EID-S			EID-M			GID-S			GID-M		
	Prec.	Rec.	F1	Prec.	Rec.	F1	Prec.	Rec.	F1	Prec.	Rec.	F1
0	1.0	1.0	1.0	0.998	1.0	0.999	1.0	1.0	1.0	1.0	1.0	1.0
1	1.0	1.0	1.0	1.0	0.9996	0.9998	0.996	0.996	0.996	0.9915	0.9904	0.9909
2	1.0	1.0	1.0	1.0	1.0	1.0	1.0	1.0	1.0	0.9999	1.0	0.9999
3	1.0	1.0	1.0	1.0	0.9992	0.9996	0.9992	0.9988	0.999	0.9937	0.9948	0.9942
4	1.0	1.0	1.0	1.0	1.0	1.0	0.9976	0.998	0.9978	0.9949	0.996	0.9955
5	1.0	1.0	1.0	0.9996	0.9992	0.9994	0.9969	0.9984	0.9977	0.9963	0.996	0.9961
6	1.0	1.0	1.0	0.9996	0.9993	0.9994	0.9988	0.9972	0.998	0.9962	0.9953	0.9958
Average	**1.0**	**1.0**	**1.0**	**0.9996**	**0.9996**	**0.9996**	**0.9983**	**0.9983**	**0.9983**	**0.9961**	**0.9961**	**0.9961**

The proposed approach gains impressive results (higher than 99%) on all the metrics over all seven subjects

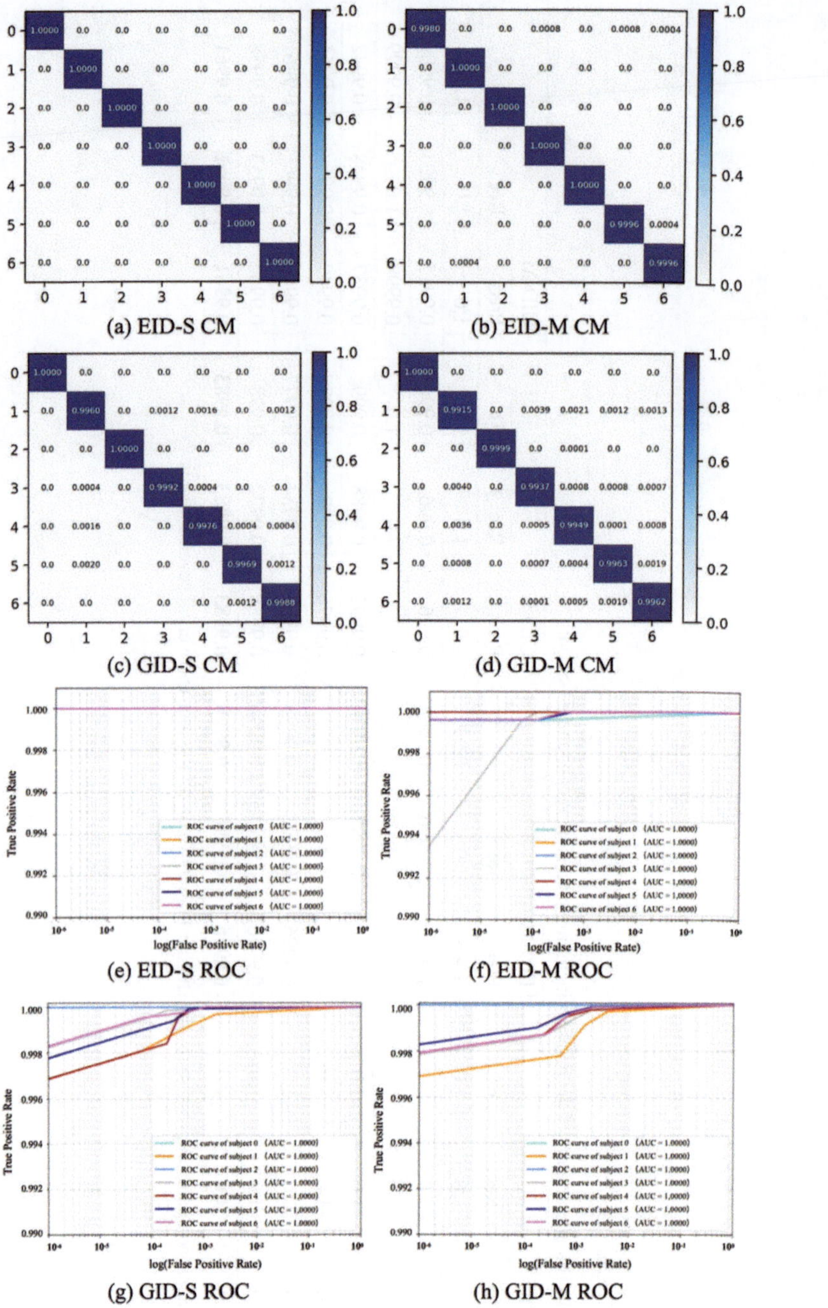

Fig. 12.4 Confusion matrix and ROC curves of the datasets. CM denotes confusion matrix. The AUC scores are provided on the figures, all exceeding 0.99

Table 12.5 Component-Level comparison on multi-session datasets

Baseline	Methods	EID-M				GID-M			
		Acc.	Prec.	Rec.	F1	Acc.	Prec.	Rec.	F1
Non-DL	SVM	0.7796	0.7815	0.7796	0.7796	0.993	0.993	0.993	0.993
	RF	0.8124	0.8139	0.8124	0.8124	0.9954	0.9954	0.9954	0.9954
	KNN	0.8211	0.8232	0.8211	0.8197	0.9953	0.9953	0.9953	0.9953
DL	LSTM	0.8482	0.8509	0.8483	0.8489	0.9935	0.9936	0.9936	0.9936
	GRU	0.862	0.8638	0.8626	0.8629	0.9938	0.9938	0.9938	0.9938
	CNN	0.7647	0.7731	0.7854	0.7625	0.9845	0.9845	0.9845	0.9845
State-of-the-art	[18]	0.5735	0.5721	0.5443	0.5579	–	–	–	–
	[19]	0.8029	0.7986	0.8125	0.8055	–	–	–	–
	[15]	0.8567	0.8533	0.8651	0.8592	–	–	–	–
	[8]	–	–	–	–	0.9653	0.9627	0.9669	0.9648
	[1]	–	–	–	–	0.9901	0.9931	0.9942	0.9936
	[32]	–	–	–	–	0.9875	0.9826	0.9844	0.9835
	Att-RNN	0.9324	0.9343	0.9322	0.9326	0.9894	0.9895	0.9895	0.9895
	Ours	**0.9996**	**0.9996**	**0.9996**	**0.9996**	**0.9961**	**0.9961**	**0.9961**	**0.9961**

DL denotes Deep Learning. Att-RNN denotes attention-based RNN without external classifier

Table 12.6 EEG bands comparison on single and multi-session Datasets

Dataset	Baseline	Methods	Delta	Theta	Alpha	Beta	Gamma	Full
EID-S	Non-DL	SVM	0.4588	0.4682	0.7484	0.5955	0.5239	0.8788
		KNN	0.9897	0.8084	0.7465	0.5553	0.4606	0.8792
	DL	LSTM	0.9596	0.8126	0.8277	0.6906	0.6027	0.9273
		GRU	0.9633	0.7996	0.8082	0.6902	0.6985	0.9251
	State-of-art	[19]	0.8254	0.7935	0.7019	0.6368	0.6621	0.8018
		Att-RNN	0.9384	0.7928	0.8318	0.6854	0.6046	0.9238
		Ours	**1.0**	**0.9285**	**0.8366**	**0.5529**	**0.4558**	**0.9417**
EID-M	Non-DL	SVM	0.7796	0.5424	0.5664	0.6522	0.4915	0.7477
		KNN	0.8211	0.7501	0.7649	0.6611	0.3821	0.8162
	DL	LSTM	0.8482	0.6926	0.7438	0.5726	0.5008	0.8185
		GRU	0.862	0.6935	0.7531	0.5672	0.5072	0.8221
	State-of-art	[19]	0.9931	0.6891	0.6988	0.5124	0.3397	0.7963
		Att-RNN	0.9324	0.6847	0.6846	0.5732	0.4941	0.7976
		Ours	**0.9996**	**0.9013**	**0.8989**	**0.4428**	**0.3661**	**0.8858**

The full band denotes the raw EEG data with full frequency bands. Delta band consistently provides the highest accuracy.

band consistently achieves the highest accuracy across all baseline methods and both datasets, with our approach reaching 100% on EID-S and 99.96% on EID-M using Delta band features.

The superior performance of Delta band can be attributed to its correspondence to fundamental life-support functions and stable brain activity patterns. Delta waves primarily appear during deep relaxation states when higher-level cognitive functions are less active, leaving only the most stable and individual-specific neural patterns related to essential physiological processes. This makes Delta band features highly discriminative for person identification while being relatively stable across different mental states and environmental conditions.

Latency Analysis and Practical Deployment. For practical deployment in smart aging environments, authentication speed is crucial. Figure 12.5 presents the detailed latency breakdown of the DeepKey system. Our system achieved a competitive testing latency of 0.39 s, with the Invalid ID Filter taking 0.06 s and ID Identification requiring 0.33 s. The overall system latency, including data collection, was approximately 10 s, with EEG collection requiring about 4 s and gait collection taking over 6 s.

While our current implementation requires users to wear two different devices sequentially, this trade-off between convenience and security is acceptable for high-security applications in smart aging contexts where precision and fake-resistance are paramount. The total authentication time of approximately 10 s, though longer than traditional methods like fingerprint scanning, is reasonable for high-security access control scenarios. Future improvements could integrate EEG and gait sensors into a single device or leverage environmental sensors to enhance usability without sacrificing security.

In conclusion, our experimental results demonstrate DeepKey's exceptional performance in biometric authentication, achieving near-perfect accuracy with unpar-

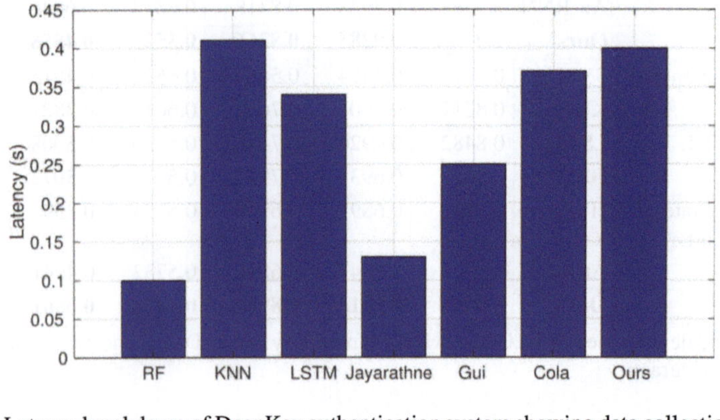

Fig. 12.5 Latency breakdown of DeepKey authentication system showing data collection time and processing time for each component

alleled fake-resistance, making it particularly suitable for high-security applications in smart aging environments.

12.3.4 *Summary of the DeepKey System*

In this section, we presented DeepKey, an innovative multimodal biometric authentication system that combines EEG and gait biometrics. Our system integrates three key components: an Invalid ID Filter using EEG data, an EEG Identification Model focused on Delta band patterns, and a Gait Identification Model—all working together to achieve exceptional security with a 0% False Acceptance Rate and just 1% False Rejection Rate.

The robust performance across multiple sessions suggests promising adaptability for real-world deployment scenarios. Our next steps will include evaluation with diverse user populations and further refinements to enhance both security and usability across different application contexts.

12.4 Discussion and Future Directions

This chapter has presented DeepKey, a novel multimodal biometric authentication system that combines EEG and gait biometrics to achieve enhanced security and reliability. The system demonstrates exceptional performance with 0% False Acceptance Rate and 1% False Rejection Rate, validating the effectiveness of combining complementary biometric modalities in a unified framework.

12.4.1 *Technical Achievements and Deployment Considerations*

Our research reveals several important technical insights. The finding that Delta band (0.5-3.5 Hz) EEG signals provide the most discriminative information for person identification offers valuable guidance for future biometric system design. The attention-based deep learning architecture successfully addresses the challenge of automatically weighting different biometric signal components, enabling the system to focus on the most informative features while maintaining robust performance across multiple sessions.

However, several practical challenges must be addressed for broader adoption. The current implementation requires sequential use of multiple devices and a 10-second total authentication time, which may limit usability in certain deployment contexts. Future research should focus on developing more integrated data collection approaches, such as embedding sensors into wearable devices or leveraging environmental sensing technologies. Additionally, investigating adaptive models that can accommodate gradual changes in biometric signatures over time would enhance long-term system reliability.

Privacy and security considerations are paramount when using EEG data for authentication, as brain signals may contain sensitive information beyond what is necessary for identification. Future implementations should incorporate privacy-by-design principles, extracting only essential features while protecting potentially sensitive neurological information. Security protocols must ensure proper data handling, including secure transmission, storage, and processing of biometric data, with clear policies regarding data ownership, usage limitations, and user consent.

12.4.2 Applications and Future Research Directions

While our initial evaluation focused on younger participants under controlled conditions, the system's characteristics suggest potential applicability to various high-security scenarios, including smart aging environments. The high fake-resistance of the multimodal approach could enhance security for vulnerable populations, while the system's robustness across multiple sessions may accommodate day-to-day variability common in real-world applications. Several important future research directions include:

- Developing less intrusive data collection methods through advanced sensor integration,
- Investigating context-aware authentication that balances security with usability,
- Exploring adaptive algorithms that evolve with changing user characteristics,
- Establishing comprehensive evaluation frameworks for diverse deployment scenarios,
- Addressing ethical and privacy challenges in biometric authentication systems, and
- Evaluating system performance with diverse demographic groups to ensure equitable performance across different user populations.

These advancements will contribute to the development of more practical, secure, and user-friendly identity management solutions suitable for various applications where enhanced security and usability are both critical requirements.

References

1. Al-Naffakh, N., Clarke, N.L., Li, F., Haskell-Dowland, P.S.: Unobtrusive gait recognition using smartwatches. In: A. Brömme, C. Busch, A. Dantcheva, C. Rathgeb, A. Uhl (eds.) International Conference of the Biometrics Special Interest Group (BIOSIG 2017), Darmstadt, Germany, September 20–22 2017, LNI, vol. P-270, pp. 211–218. GI / IEEE (2017)
2. Altahat, S., Chetty, G., Tran, D., Ma, W.: Analysing the robust EEG channel set for person authentication. In: S. Arik, T. Huang, W.K. Lai, Q. Liu (eds.) Neural Information Processing – 22nd International Conference (ICONIP 2015), Istanbul, Turkey, November 9–12 2015, Part IV, Lecture Notes in Computer Science, vol. 9492, pp. 162–173. Springer (2015)
3. Ashby, C., Bhatia, A., Tenore, F., Vogelstein, J.: Low-cost electroencephalogram (EEG) based authentication. In: Proceedings of the 5th International IEEE/EMBS Conference on Neural Engineering (NER'11), pp. 442–445. IEEE (2011)
4. Boulgouris, N.V., Huang, X.: Gait recognition using HMMs and dual discriminative observations for sub-dynamics analysis. IEEE Trans. Image Process. **22**(9), 3636–3647 (2013)
5. Callisaya, M.L., Blizzard, L., Schmidt, M.D., McGinley, J.L., Lord, S.R., Srikanth, V.K.: A population-based study of sensorimotor factors affecting gait in older people. Age Ageing **38**(3), 290–295 (2009)
6. Chan, W., Jaitly, N., Le, Q.V., Vinyals, O., Shazeer, N.M.: Speech recognition with attention-based recurrent neural networks. US Patent 9,799,327 (2017)
7. Chuang, J., Nguyen, H., Wang, C., Johnson, B.: I think, therefore i am: Usability and security of authentication using brainwaves. In: Financial Cryptography and Data Security – FC Workshops 2013, pp. 1–16. Springer (2013)
8. Cola, G., Avvenuti, M., Musso, F., Vecchio, A.: Gait-based authentication using a wrist-worn device. In: Proc. 13th Int. Conf. on Mobile and Ubiquitous Systems (Mobiquitous), pp. 208–217. ACM (2016)
9. Daugman, J.G.: High confidence visual recognition of persons by a test of statistical independence. IEEE Trans. Pattern Anal. Mach. Intell. **15**(11), 1148–1161 (1993)
10. Derawi, M., Voitenko, I.: Fusion of gait and ECG for biometric user authentication. In: International Conference of the Biometrics Special Interest Group (BIOSIG'14), pp. 1–4. IEEE (2014)
11. Dong, M., Yao, L., Wang, X., Benatallah, B., Zhang, X., Sheng, Q.Z.: Dual-stream self-attentive random forest for false information detection. In: 2019 International Joint Conference on Neural Networks (IJCNN'19), pp. 1–8. IEEE (2019)
12. Drira, H., Amor, B.B., Srivastava, A., Daoudi, M., Slama, R.: 3d face recognition under expressions, occlusions, and pose variations. IEEE Trans. Pattern Anal. Mach. Intell. **35**(9), 2270–2283 (2013)
13. Givens, G.H., Beveridge, J.R., Lui, Y.M., Bolme, D.S., Draper, B.A., Phillips, P.J.: Biometric face recognition: From classical statistics to future challenges. Wiley Interdisciplinary Reviews: Computational Statistics **5**(4), 288–308 (2013)
14. Goldstein, S.: Methods and systems for voice authentication service leveraging networking. US Patent 9,282,096 (2016)
15. Gui, Q., Jin, Z., Xu, W.: Exploring EEG-based biometrics for user identification and authentication. In: 2014 IEEE Signal Processing in Medicine and Biology Symposium (SPMB'14), pp. 1–6. IEEE (2014)
16. Guzman, A.M., Goryawala, M., Wang, J., Barreto, A., Andrian, J., Rishe, N., Adjouadi, M.: Thermal imaging as a biometrics approach to facial signature authentication. IEEE J. Biomed. Health Inform. **17**(1), 214–222 (2013)
17. Hoang, T., Choi, D.: Secure and privacy enhanced gait authentication on smart phone. Sci. World J. **2014**, 438254 (2014)
18. Jayarathne, I., Cohen, M., Amarakeerthi, S.: Brainid: Development of an EEG-based biometric authentication system. In: 2016 IEEE 7th Annual Information Technology, Electronics and Mobile Communication Conference (IEMCON'16), pp. 1–6. IEEE (2016)

19. Keshishzadeh, S., Fallah, A., Rashidi, S.: Improved EEG-based human authentication system on large dataset. In: 24th Iranian Conference on Electrical Engineering (ICEE'16), pp. 1165–1169. IEEE (2016)
20. Khiari-Hili, N., Montagne, C., Lelandais, S., Hamrouni, K.: Quality dependent multimodal fusion of face and iris biometrics. In: 6th International Conference on Image Processing Theory Tools and Applications (IPTA'16), pp. 1–6. IEEE (2016)
21. Kumar, P.K., Prasad, P.K., Ramakrishna, M.V., Prasad, B.D.C.N.: Feature extraction using sparse SVD for biometric fusion in multimodal authentication. International Journal of Network Security & Its Applications **5**(4), 83–92 (2013)
22. Kusakunniran, W., Wu, Q., Zhang, J., Li, H., Wang, L.: Recognizing gaits across views through correlated motion co-clustering. IEEE Trans. Image Process. **23**(2), 696–709 (2014)
23. Kusakunniran, W., Wu, Q., Zhang, J., Ma, Y., Li, H.: A new view-invariant feature for cross-view gait recognition. IEEE Trans. Inf. Forensics Secur. **8**(10), 1642–1653 (2013)
24. Latman, N.S., Herb, E.: A field study of the accuracy and reliability of a biometric iris recognition system. Science & Justice **53**(2), 98–102 (2013)
25. Long, T., Thai, L., Hanh, T.: Multimodal biometric person authentication using fingerprint, face features. In: PRICAI 2012: Trends in Artificial Intelligence, pp. 613–624. Springer (2012)
26. Maio, D., Maltoni, D., Cappelli, R., Wayman, J.L., Jain, A.K.: FVC2002: Second fingerprint verification competition. In: 16th International Conference on Pattern Recognition, 2002, Vol. 3, pp. 811–814. IEEE (2002)
27. Man, J., Bhanu, B.: Individual recognition using gait energy image. IEEE Trans. Pattern Anal. Mach. Intell. **28**(2), 316–322 (2006)
28. Manjunathswamy, B.E., Abhishek, A.M., Thriveni, J., Venugopal, K.R., Patnaik, L.M.: Multimodal biometric authentication using ECG and fingerprint. International Journal of Computer Applications **111**(13), 1–6 (2015)
29. Marcel, S., del R. Millán, J.: Person authentication using brainwaves (EEG) and maximum a posteriori model adaptation. IEEE Transactions on Pattern Analysis and Machine Intelligence 29(4), 743–752 (2007)
30. Pillai, J.K., Puertas, M., Chellappa, R.: Cross-sensor iris recognition through kernel learning. IEEE Trans. Pattern Anal. Mach. Intell. **36**(1), 73–85 (2014)
31. Sadikoglu, F., Uzelaltinbulat, S.: Biometric retina identification based on neural network. Procedia Computer Science **102**, 26–33 (2016)
32. Sun, B., Wang, Y., Banda, J.: Gait characteristic analysis and identification based on the iphone's accelerometer and gyrometer. Sensors **14**(9), 17037–17054 (2014)
33. Telgad, R.L., Deshmukh, P.D., Siddiqui, A.M.N.: Combination approach to score level fusion for multimodal biometric system by using face and fingerprint. In: Recent Advances and Innovations in Engineering (ICRAIE 2014), pp. 1–8. IEEE (2014)
34. Thomas, K.P., Vinod, A.P.: Utilizing individual alpha frequency and delta band power in EEG based biometric recognition. In: IEEE International Conference on Systems, Man, and Cybernetics (SMC'16), pp. 4787–4791. IEEE (2016)
35. Unar, J.A., Seng, W.C., Abbasi, A.: A review of biometric technology along with trends and prospects. Pattern Recogn. **47**(8), 2673–2683 (2014)
36. Wang, Y., Huang, M., Zhao, L., et al.: Attention-based LSTM for aspect-level sentiment classification. In: Proc. Conf. Empirical Methods in Natural Language Processing (EMNLP 2016), pp. 606–615. ACL (2016)
37. Wu, Z., Huang, Y., Wang, L., Wang, X., Tan, T.: A comprehensive study on cross-view gait based human identification with deep CNNs. IEEE Trans. Pattern Anal. Mach. Intell. **39**(2), 209–226 (2017)
38. Yam, C.Y., Nixon, M.: Model-based gait recognition. In: Encyclopedia of Biometrics, pp. 633–639. Springer (2009)
39. Yano, V., Zimmer, A., Ling, L.L.: Multimodal biometric authentication based on iris pattern and pupil light reflex. In: 21st International Conference on Pattern Recognition (ICPR'12), pp. 2857–2860. IEEE (2012)

40. Zhang, X., Yao, L., Huang, C., Gu, T., Yang, Z., Liu, Y.: Deepkey: A multimodal biometric authentication system via deep decoding gaits and brainwaves. ACM Trans. Intell. Syst. Technol. 11(4), 49:1–49:24 (2020)
41. Zhang, X., Yao, L., Kanhere, S.S., Liu, Y., Gu, T., Chen, K.: MindID: Person identification from brain waves through attention-based recurrent neural network. Proceedings of the ACM on Interactive, Mobile, Wearable and Ubiquitous Technologies 2(3), 149:1–149:23 (2018)
42. Zhou, H., Mian, A., Wei, L., Creighton, D., Hossny, M., Nahavandi, S.: Recent advances on single-modal and multimodal face recognition: A survey. IEEE Transactions on Human-Machine Systems **44**(6), 701–716 (2014)

Chapter 13
Large Language Models for Medical Report Generation

13.1 Introduction

13.1.1 Overview of Medical Report Generation

Medical report generation (MRG) [21] stands as a core research topic within the medical multi-modal field, aiming to empower models to automatically generate reports that articulate findings from medical examinations. This endeavor seeks to lessen the heavy workload shouldered by radiologists. With the increasing prevalence of complex medical conditions and the growing demand for diagnostic services, accurate and efficient medical reporting becomes increasingly crucial for diverse patient populations.

Deep learning-based MRG models predominantly adopt an encoder-decoder architecture, where the capacity of the decoder to process lengthy sequences is paramount due to the typically extensive nature of medical reports. Initial efforts saw the deployment of LSTM networks, including two-level LSTM configurations, as decoders for generating reports. However, the advent of the Transformer [25] marked a pivotal shift in decoder technology preference, leading to the development of variants like memory-driven Transformers [2, 3], knowledge-enhanced Transformers [8, 16], and those pre-trained on contrastive learning paradigms [15, 18].

More recently, with large language models (LLMs) demonstrating remarkable linguistic processing capabilities, an increasing number of studies have begun utilizing these large models as decoders. By ingeniously crafting prompts infused with prior knowledge [11] and applying fine-tuning techniques, researchers have achieved significant improvements in medical report quality. However, collecting large amounts of paired medical image-report data to support fine-tuning of these models remains expensive and challenging. For example, resource-constrained medical facilities may not be able to gather sufficient paired samples. Additionally, for rare diseases or novel

Q. Z. Sheng et al., *Harnessing Artificial Intelligence and Pervasive Internet of Things for an Empowered Aging*, https://doi.org/10.1007/978-3-032-16502-2_13

conditions, the number of available clinical samples is inherently limited. Therefore, developing MRG models with zero-shot learning capabilities holds greater potential for clinical applications.

13.1.2 Challenges and Opportunities

The field of medical report generation faces several fundamental challenges that limit the widespread adoption of AI-assisted reporting systems in clinical practice. The most critical challenge is the heavy reliance on large amounts of paired image-report data for training effective models. Collecting such paired data is expensive, time-consuming, and often limited by privacy regulations and institutional policies. This limitation becomes particularly pronounced in specialized domains such as aging-related healthcare, where diverse comorbidities and rare geriatric conditions may lack sufficient training samples due to their low prevalence or recent emergence.

Traditional fine-tuning approaches require substantial computational resources and extensive datasets, making them impractical for resource-constrained medical facilities or when dealing with rare diseases where sample sizes are inherently limited. Furthermore, medical centers often have different reporting styles, terminology preferences, and diagnostic protocols, necessitating domain adaptation capabilities that conventional approaches struggle to provide efficiently.

In-context learning [5] emerges as a promising solution by leveraging the zero-shot capabilities of large language models (LLMs), enabling models to generate reports for new scenarios with minimal examples. However, current ICL approaches face significant computational inefficiency when applied to lengthy medical reports, as they require processing all demonstration examples simultaneously. This leads to increased memory consumption, longer inference times, and potential instability in performance, particularly when dealing with the extensive nature of medical reports that often span hundreds of tokens.

The opportunity lies in developing more efficient methods that can harness the power of LLMs for medical report generation while addressing these computational and data scarcity challenges. Such approaches could democratize access to AI-assisted medical reporting, enabling deployment in diverse healthcare settings regardless of their computational resources or available training data.

13.1.3 Contributions

In this chapter, we introduce MCVGen, a novel approach leveraging large language models through Multi-modal Contextual Vectors (MCV) to generate medical reports with zero-shot capabilities. Our methodology captures contextual information from demonstrations and uses it to guide new report generation, particularly valuable in scenarios where specialized medical data may be limited yet accurate reporting is crucial.

Our primary contribution is the development of a zero-shot medical report generation model that fundamentally departs from traditional in-context learning approaches. Instead of directly processing lengthy demonstration sequences, our method compresses contextual information into efficient multi-modal vectors that preserve essential knowledge while reducing computational overhead. Additionally, we develop and validate a pre-trained medical multi-modal model (Med-LMM) that leverages the auto-regressive nature of large language models to extract critical contextual information from the last hidden states of demonstration examples.

Through comprehensive experiments on cross-center and cross-disease evaluation scenarios, we demonstrate exceptional zero-shot capabilities that show significant potential for practical clinical applications. Our approach achieves state-of-the-art zero-shot performance while maintaining computational efficiency, making it particularly suitable for resource-constrained healthcare environments where extensive training data may not be available.

MCVGen offers three key advantages: (1) it maintains computational efficiency without additional processing costs; (2) it enhances report generation control by embedding MCV information within each hidden layer, improving accuracy for complex medical conditions; and (3) it ensures consistent output quality regardless of input template variations. Figure 13.1 depicts the multi-modal in-context learning and our proposed MCVGen.

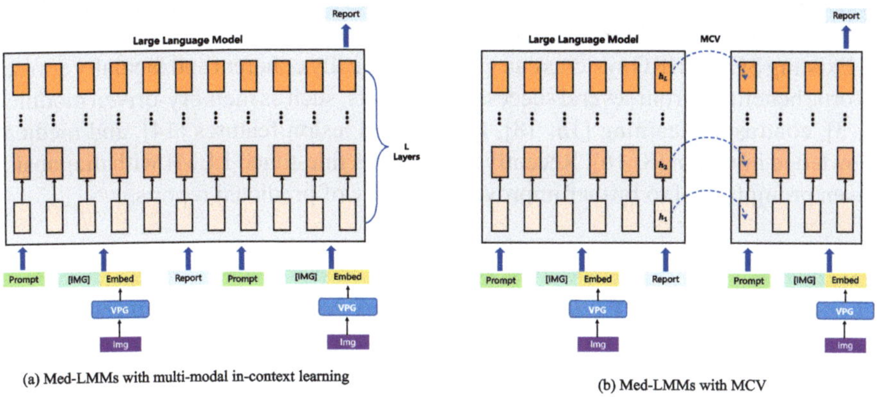

Fig. 13.1 Comparison of multi-modal in-context learning and our proposed MCV. **a** The architecture of adopting multi-modal in-context learning for MRG. **b** The paradigm for our proposed MCV is to alter multi-modal in-context learning. We attain the MCV from the last hidden states of a forward pass on the multi-modal demonstrations. One demonstration consists of a prompt, an example image, and the corresponding report. Img refers to the image features encoded by vision encoders, [IMG] is a specific image proxy for LLMs to differentiate between visual and text embeddings

13.1.4 Chapter Organization

The remainder of this chapter is organized as follows. Section 13.2 presents the background and related work in medical report generation, covering the evolution of deep learning approaches from LSTM-based to Transformer-based architectures, alternative learning paradigms that reduce dependency on large paired datasets, and the fundamentals of in-context learning for large language models. Section 13.3 details our proposed MCVGen approach for zero-shot medical report generation, including the architecture of our medical large multi-modal model (Med-LMM), the construction and application of multi-modal contextual vectors, comprehensive experimental validation on cross-center and cross-disease scenarios, and performance analysis demonstrating state-of-the-art zero-shot capabilities. Section 13.4 discusses the broader implications of our work, including implications for AI-empowered healthcare systems, integration with IoT and smart aging technologies, and future research directions for technological evolution in healthcare reporting.

13.2 Background and Related Work

13.2.1 Medical Report Generation

Medical report generation has emerged as a pivotal research topic in the medical multi-modal field, given its potential to alleviate the heavy workloads of radiologists. Recently, advancements have been made with MRG systems that leverage large multimodal models (LMMs) to generate high-quality reports.

Existing SOTA MRG systems can generate logically coherent and factually correct reports, benefiting from several successful concepts, such as memory-driven modules [2, 3], contrastive learning [15, 18], fine-grained lesion features [14], and medical knowledge injection [8, 16]. Recently, researchers fine-tuned LLMs with diagnosis-driven prompts [11] to further improve the quality of predicted reports.

13.2.2 Alternative Learning Paradigms for Medical Report Generation

To conserve the extensive medical paired data required for training MRG models, another line of research investigating alternative learning paradigms for MRG has attracted increasing attention, due to its potential in clinical practice. These methods can be divided into two categories:

- Knowledge Graph Approaches: Researchers explore extra knowledge graph sharing latent space to bridge the visual and textual domains. For example, Liu et al.

[19] pre-constructed a knowledge graph and integrated it with visual features or linguistic information to predict reports. Similarly, Jia et al. [10] extracted visual features and projected them into node features. Then, a Graph Convolutional Network (GCN) was adopted to model and strengthen the intrinsic correlations among diseases, allowing knowledge transfer from regular diseases to those rare diseases.
- Alternative Supervision Signals: Cheaper and more easily accessible additional annotations are utilized to train the models. Han et al. [6] proposed lesion-guided weakly supervised report generation methods to describe novel chest and retinal diseases. The pre-trained lesion detectors can extract lesion-centric features by detecting abnormal regions to learn correlations between based and novel classes. Adopting lesion detectors also improves the explainability of MRG systems.

13.2.3 In-Context Learning

In-context learning (ICL) has revolutionized the approach to leveraging pre-trained LLMs for a wide array of tasks without the need for explicit retraining or fine-tuning. This paradigm shift is predicated on the model's ability to infer task-specific instructions from very few demonstrations within the same context as the query. This method exploits the inherent capability of LLMs to generate predictions based on the contextual clues provided, making it an efficient strategy for extending the utility of these models to new tasks [5].

However, the performance of ICL highly relies on the selections of templates and demonstrates, especially in the multi-modal domain. Recent works explore the underlying mechanism behind ICL and propose several kinds of vectors [7, 23] to alter the ICL. Due to the auto-regressive mechanism, the last hidden state can contain essential contextual information. For instance, Hendel et al. [7] compresses a training set into a single task vector, which then modulates the LLM to generate outputs. Furthermore, Todd et al. [23] reveals that LLMs possess a neural mechanism for encapsulating input-output functions as compact and distinct from task vectors, being robust across contexts and capable of semantic vector composition, thus enabling the execution of complex new tasks.

13.2.4 Research Gaps and Opportunities in Smart Aging

The intersection of large language models and medical reporting presents unique opportunities for advancing smart aging technologies and elderly healthcare services. Traditional medical report generation systems face particular challenges when applied to aging populations, where complex comorbidities, medication interactions, and age-related physiological changes require nuanced interpretation and reporting.

Current medical AI systems often lack the contextual understanding necessary to address the specific needs of elderly patients, who may present with atypical symptoms or require specialized attention to quality of life factors. The development of zero-shot learning capabilities in medical reporting becomes especially relevant for aging-related conditions, where training data may be scarce for rare geriatric syndromes or emerging age-related disorders.

The integration of medical report generation with Internet of Things (IoT) devices commonly used in smart aging applications—such as continuous monitoring systems, fall detection sensors, and medication adherence trackers—requires adaptive AI systems that can synthesize information from multiple sources without extensive retraining. Large language models with zero-shot capabilities offer particular promise for elderly care applications, where the ability to generate contextually appropriate medical interpretations from diverse data streams could significantly enhance healthcare delivery in resource-constrained settings where specialized geriatric expertise may be limited.

Furthermore, the computational efficiency requirements for edge computing in smart aging applications align well with the objectives of developing more efficient medical report generation systems. As aging populations increasingly rely on home-based monitoring and remote healthcare services, the need for AI systems that can provide accurate medical insights without requiring extensive computational infrastructure becomes critical for ensuring equitable access to healthcare technologies.

13.3 MCVGen: A Zero-Shot Medical Report Generation System

13.3.1 Motivation and Overview of MCVGen System

To address the challenge of collecting large amounts of paired medical image-report data for training, we propose MCVGen [20], a zero-shot report generation model based on in-context learning. Rather than directly feeding all demonstrations to a pre-trained large model, our approach innovates by employing a multi-modal contextual vector (MCV) to represent the contextual information of demonstrations.

Initially, we pre-train a medical large multi-modal model (Med-LMM) and extract the last hidden state of each demonstration through a forward pass in Med-LMM. Benefiting from the auto-regressive mechanism, the last hidden state captures critical information for the targeted scenarios. Subsequently, we average the multiple MCVs and integrate them with the first hidden state on the new query, thereby shifting the latent states and guiding the model toward acquiring previously unlearned multi-modal contextual information. This approach has the advantage of regulating the number of prompts, thus reducing computational costs.

We conducted experiments on the publicly available IU-Xray [4] and MIMIC [12] benchmarks and propose two zero-shot settings, namely cross-center and cross-disease, to validate the model's zero-shot capabilities. For the cross-center experiments, we first trained a Med-LMM model capable of report generation using data from one center and then tested it on data from another center. For the cross-disease tests, we utilized CheXpert [9] to label diseases and employed a leave-one-out approach, selecting 13 disease types for training and the remaining disease type for testing in each iteration. The experimental results demonstrate that our MCVGen exhibits exceptional zero-shot MRG capabilities. It can generate reports with different writing styles or describe novel diseases based on a few demonstrations, achieving state-of-the-art (SOTA) zero-shot MRG performances and comparable performance compared to existing fully supervised MRG systems.

13.3.2 MCVGen: A Zero-Shot Approach

The detailed pipeline of our MCVGen is presented in Fig. 13.2, it has three critical steps to harness the zero-shot capabilities of LLMs to generate new writing-style reports or describe novel diseases. First, we pre-train a Medical Large Multi-modal Model (Med-LMM) that can achieve comparable report generation performances with existing SOTA methods. Second, we use a forward pass on each multi-modal demonstration to attain MCV from the last hidden state of the Med-LMM. Last, MCV is employed to shift the latent space of the Med-LMM on a new query.

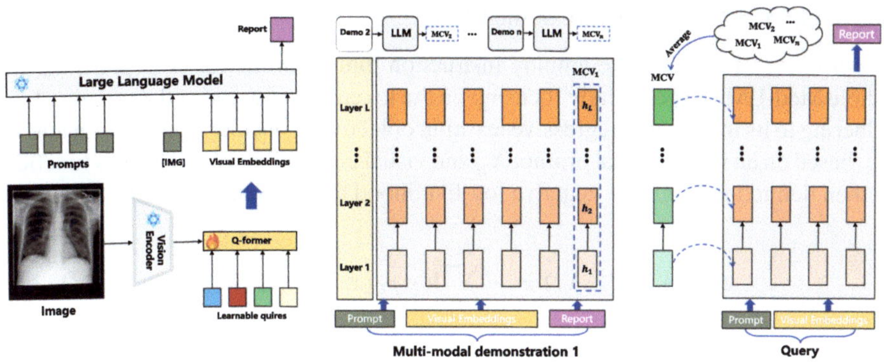

(a) Med-LMM (b) Generate MCV (c) Apply MCV

Fig. 13.2 Overview of our proposed MCVGen, which contains three key steps. **a** The architecture of our proposed Med-LMM. It utilizes the MedCLIP-ViT to encode image representations and adopts the LLaMa-2 to generate medical reports. **b** The illustration for generating MCV on a forward pass on multi-modal demonstrations. h_i refers to outputs of the i-th transformer hidden layer at the last token position. **c** Applying MCV for new queries to generate new writing-style reports or describe novel diseases

Medical Large Multi-modal Model

Unlike the natural domain, which boasts numerous open-source Visual Language Models (VLMs) with exemplary multi-modal reasoning and generation capabilities, existing open-source Medical VLMs (Med-VLMs) tend to focus primarily on Medical Visual Question Answering (Med-VQA) capabilities. In response, we first pre-train a Medical Large Multi-modal Model (Med-LMM) with report generation capabilities and then validate the zero-shot capability of our proposed MCV.

Med-LMMs typically feature a straightforward and cohesive design, incorporating a vision encoder, a Visual-Prompt Generator (VPG), and a pre-trained Large Language Model (LLM) to furnish LLMs with the capability to generate multimodal content. The role of the VPG involves translating the image features processed by the vision encoder into visual embeddings. These embeddings are then utilized to bridge the understanding between LLMs and the visual context presented. Our Med-LMM architecture, detailed in Fig. 13.2a, utilizes the MedCLIP-ViT [27] model for vision encoding to convert images into representations, labeled *Img*. Subsequently, these representations are processed by the Q-former [13] to transform image data into a format that LLMs can interpret, optimizing the number of visual tokens to enhance computational efficiency and aligning the dimension of visual embeddings with that of the text embedding of the LLM. In this study, we integrate the LLaMa-2 [24] model as our LLM choice. A special token $[IMG]$ is introduced to the middle of prompts and visual embeddings, aiding the LLM in differentiating between visual and textual inputs. In this manner, image and text embeddings can be directly fed into the LLM and treated equally, without employing extra gated cross-attention layers and modifying the architecture of the LLM.

Pre-training Paradigm. We employ instruction tuning on the LLM to pre-train the whole Med-LMM, specifically focusing on the tokens that comprise the report, while adhering to its initial auto-regressive learning objective. Consider a report with length L_r, based on an instructional prompt X_p and visual embeddings X_v. The loss function is then defined through the negative log-likelihood as follows:

$$\mathcal{L}(\theta; X_p, X_v, X_r) = -\sum_{i=1}^{L_r} \log p_\theta(x_i | X_p, X_v, X_{r,<i}), \tag{13.1}$$

where θ represents the parameters subject to training, and $X_{r,<i}$ denotes the sequence of report tokens preceding the current token x_i to be predicted. During training, we use the instructional prompt "Generate a comprehensive and precise report for this Chest X-ray image." We froze both MedCLIP-ViT and LLaMa-2 during pre-training, and all trainable parameters only come from the Q-former.

Multi-modal Contextual Vector

After preparing a Med-LMM that harnesses the power of the LLM to generate reports, the next step is to construct MCV from given demonstrations. The auto-regressive nature of LLMs ensures that the hidden states at any given token position encapsulate the contextual relationships among all preceding tokens. This principle forms the foundation of ICL, enabling the effective generation of MCV that are rich in contextual information derived from multimodal data inputs.

The pre-trained Med-LMM can be represented as $f(\cdot)$. Given a multimodal demonstration X, which includes prompts X_p, images X_v, and the corresponding report X_r, the Multimodal Contextual Vector is generated as: $h_{MCV} = f([X_p, X_v, X_r])$. More precisely, an MCV encapsulates the outputs from each hidden layer of the large language model at the position of the last token. Thus, the MCV can be expressed as $h_{MCV} = \{h_1, h_2, \ldots, h_L\}$, where L denotes the number of hidden layers in the LLM, $h_i \in \mathbb{R}^d$. For this study, we employ LLaMa-7B, which comprises a total of $L = 32$ hidden layers, and $d = 4096$ is the dimension of text embeddings.

Medical reports are typically more extensive than captions for natural images, resulting in multi-modal demonstrations that can span 450–700 tokens, encompassing prompts, visual, and textual elements. Generating a single MCV for multiple demonstrations is inefficient and necessitates the use of larger backbone networks. Therefore, we generate one MCV for each demonstration and compute the average output of each layer to obtain the final task-specific MCV. This MCV offers three primary advantages. Firstly, it is more efficient and conserves computational resources, enabling the use of a greater number of demonstrations. Secondly, it prevents the model from overly relying on the contextual information from the most recent demonstrations when generating new reports, ensuring a more balanced and comprehensive understanding of the task at hand. Finally, we employ the outputs from each hidden layer, opting to bypass the selection of activations within the multi-head self-attention modules. This approach is straightforward and readily adaptable to a variety of tasks.

MCV Guides New Query

As discussed in previous work, the rationale for utilizing vector representations to alter in-context learning can be formulated as:

$$Att(x_{query}W_q, XW_k, XW_0) =: \alpha h(X_{query}) + (1-\alpha)h(X_{demo}), \tag{13.2}$$

where $Att(\cdot)$ refers to the multi-head self-attention module in each layer, $X = [X_{demo}; X_{query}]$ denotes the inputs and x_{query} is the token in X_{query}. Then, $h(X_{demo})$ can be replaced by the proposed MCV. Therefore, the overview process of employing MCV to control the new query generation can be written as follows:

$$Att(x_{query}W_q, XW_k, XW_0) =: \alpha h(X_{query}) + (1-\alpha)h_{MCV}, \tag{13.3}$$

More specifically, after securing the MCV, we execute a forward pass on the query example and add the MCV to the hidden states at the first query token position at all layers $l = 1, 2, \ldots, L$ as:

$$\tilde{h}_I = h_I + h^l_{MCV}. \tag{13.4}$$

To retain the model's inherent capabilities to the fullest extent, we normalize the adjusted hidden states to align with the ℓ_2 norm of the hidden states prior to modification:

$$\tilde{h}_I = \tilde{h}_I \cdot \frac{\|h_I\|_2}{\|\tilde{h}_I\|_2}. \tag{13.5}$$

This normalization ensures that the adjusted latent state vectors maintain a magnitude compatible with the expectations of the model's subsequent processing stages.

13.3.3 Experimental Validation and Performance Analysis

Implementation Details and Zero-Shot Settings

Datasets and Metrics. Our experimental evaluation employs two public MRG datasets: the *IU-Xray* dataset [4] (3,955 reports with 7,470 chest X-rays, split into 2069/296/590 train/validation/test) and the *MIMIC-CXR* database [12] (222,758 reports with 368,960 images, split into 270790/2130/3858 train/validation/test).

For evaluation, we utilize two categories of metrics: *Natural Language Generation Metrics* (NLG) including BLEU-4 [22], CIDEr [26], ROUGE-L [17], and METEOR [1]; and *Clinical Efficacy Metrics* (CE) that assess clinical correctness through F1-score, Precision, and Recall using the CheXPert [9] labeling tool. BLEU calculates similarity between generated text and reference reports based on word n-gram overlap, while CIDEr emphasizes topic-specific terminology critical in MRG tasks while downplaying common phrases.

Model Architecture and Training. We implement Med-LMM by combining MedCLIP-ViT for image encoding, Q-former with 32 learnable queries for visual embedding extraction, and LLaMa-2 for report generation. During pre-training, we freeze MedCLIP-ViT and LLaMa-2, with only the Q-former and projection layer (192M parameters) being trainable. We used mixed-precision training with Adam optimizer (learning rate 1e-4, weight decay 0.02) for 5 and 15 epochs on IU-Xray and MIMIC respectively, using 4 NVIDIA RTX A5000 GPUs. Training requires 0.18 s per batch with batch size 8, implemented in Python 3.11.

Zero-shot Evaluation Settings. To evaluate MCVGen's zero-shot capabilities, we designed two clinically relevant scenarios that simulate real-world challenges in medical practice. For cross-center evaluation, we addressed the practical challenge of medical centers having insufficient paired data and variations in report writing styles across institutions. This evaluation stems from the realistic consideration that smaller medical centers often lack resources to gather sufficient paired data for fine-tuning, and significant disparities exist in report writing styles and terminology across different centers. We tested how our Med-LMM, pre-trained on one dataset (IU-Xray), could describe images from another dataset (MIMIC) guided by MCV, and vice versa.

Our cross-disease evaluation simulated scenarios where healthcare facilities encounter novel diseases with insufficient samples for model training. Using the MIMIC dataset, we implemented a leave-one-out approach where one disease was withheld from training and used exclusively for testing, challenging the model to generalize to previously unseen conditions without disease-specific data.

Supervised Performance Evaluation

We evaluated Med-LMM's fully supervised performance to establish a ceiling for our zero-shot learning approach, comparing it with state-of-the-art MRG systems including R2Gen [3], R2GenCMN [2], and PromptMRG [11]. Notably, the primary goal of introducing Med-LMM is not to claim state-of-the-art results in MRG but to present a medical vision large model with the potential for zero-shot learning. Hence, existing works have not been strictly replicated; instead, a general comparison with the results presented in their original publications is provided, showcasing the capabilities of the Med-LMM.

Table 13.1 presents a general comparison of fully supervised MRG performance across NLG metrics on the IU-Xray and MIMIC datasets. The proposed Med-LMM exhibits competitive performance, almost matching the best-reported BLEU-4 score of 0.128 versus 0.134 on the MIMIC dataset, a notable achievement. While Med-LMM's performance on the IU-Xray dataset does not reach the peak in any single metric, it shows a robust balance across all considered NLG metrics, with scores closely trailing the best in METEOR (0.209 vs. 0.211) and nearly matching the top performance in ROUGE (0.381 vs. 0.383). On the MIMIC dataset, Med-LMM ties for the highest METEOR score and demonstrates commendable performance in ROUGE (0.289) and BLEU-4 (0.128), underscoring its effectiveness in generating descriptively correct reports.

In addition, Table 13.2 presents a comparison of fully supervised MRG performance across CE metrics within the context of the MIMIC dataset. Notably, the PromptMRG outperforms other approaches, securing the highest metrics across the board. The proposed Med-LMM exhibits a balanced performance with a Precision of 0.412, Recall of 0.373, and a macro F1-score of 0.395. Such results reflect its capability to accurately generate clinically relevant content.

When compared to the R2GenGPT variants, the observation across these tables underscores an intriguing point about the performance of the Med-LMM model. It holds its ground against the R2GenGPT-D (Deep) and significantly surpasses the R2GenGPT-S (Shallow). The R2GenGPT framework integrates the Swin Transformer as its vision encoder, a simple linear layer as the mapper, and LLaMa-2 for decoding. In its shallow configuration, both the Swin Transformer and LLaMa-2 are

Table 13.1 Comparison of fully supervised MRG performance across NLG metrics on IU-Xray and MIMIC datasets. The results are quoted from their original papers. The highest performances for each metric are highlighted in bold

Method	IU-Xray				Method	MIMIC-CXR			
	BLEU-4	ROUGE	METEOR	CIDEr		BLEU-4	ROUGE	METEOR	CIDEr
R2Gen	0.165	0.371	0.187	–	R2Gen	0.103	0.277	0.142	–
PPKED	0.168	0.376	0.190	0.351	PPKED	0.106	0.284	0.149	0.237
DCL	0.163	**0.383**	0.193	**0.586**	DCL	0.109	0.284	0.150	**0.281**
MET	0.172	0.380	0.192	0.435	PromptMRG	0.112	0.268	0.157	–
R2GenGPT-S	0.156	0.370	0.202	0.405	R2GenGPT-S	0.117	0.277	0.136	0.145
R2GenGPT-D	**0.173**	0.377	**0.211**	0.438	R2GenGPT-D	**0.134**	**0.297**	0.160	0.269
Med-LMM (ours)	0.168	0.381	0.209	0.427	Med-LMM (ours)	0.128	0.289	**0.161**	0.265

Table 13.2 Comparison of fully supervised MRG performance across CE metrics on MIMIC dataset. The highest performances for each metric are highlighted in bold

Method	Precision	Recall	F1-score
R2Gen	0.333	0.273	0.276
DCL	0.471	0.352	0.373
PromptMRG	**0.501**	**0.509**	**0.476**
R2GenGPT-S	0.341	0.312	0.325
R2GenGPT-D	0.392	0.387	0.389
Med-LMM	0.412	0.373	0.395

frozen, with only the mapper's 4.2 million parameters being trainable. Conversely, the deep model allows full training of both the Swin Transformer and the mapper, engaging a total of 90.9 million parameters. This difference in approach between the shallow and deep models of R2GenGPT highlights the significance of training depth in achieving higher performance metrics. The Med-LMM model, leveraging the MedCLIP-ViT as its foundation with a trainable Q-former, demonstrates that it doesn't require additional training on the data of downstream tasks to achieve competitive results.

Zero-Shot Learning Results

Cross-center Performance. Tables 13.3 and 13.4 showcase a detailed comparison of cross-center zero-shot learning performance across NLG and CE metrics, respectively. Notably, the incorporation of the proposed MCV, denoted as "+ MCV" in the table, significantly enhances the performance across all metrics for baseline models engaged in this study. For instance, in the IU-Xray to MIMIC-CXR adaptation, the R2GenGPT-D model improved from a BLEU-4 score of 0.071 to 0.101, ROUGE from 0.218 to 0.251, METEOR from 0.113 to 0.122, and CIDEr from 0.072 to 0.134 after incorporating MCV. This indicates a substantial enhancement, particularly in the CIDEr metric, which nearly doubled. Similarly, for the MIMIC-CXR to IU-Xray direction, the same model with MCV added saw improvements in BLEU-4 from 0.083 to 0.112, ROUGE from 0.275 to 0.308, METEOR from 0.163 to 0.177, and CIDEr from 0.231 to 0.236.

The most striking advancement is observed with the model, MCVGen (Med-LMM + MCV), which achieves the highest performance improvements in both directions. Specifically, for IU-Xray to MIMIC-CXR, MCVGen boosts the BLEU-4 score from 0.068 to 0.106, ROUGE from 0.215 to 0.256, METEOR from 0.115 to 0.128, and CIDEr from 0.069 to 0.142. For the reverse direction, the enhancements are even more pronounced, with BLEU-4 jumping from 0.087 to 0.125. The enhancements across NLG metrics illustrate that incorporating the MCV can foster the generation of reports with a new writing style, due to greater word overlap that stems from

Table 13.3 Comparison of cross-center zero-shot learning performance across NLG metrics on the IU-Xray and MIMIC dataset. The datasets on the left and right of → indicate the pre-training and testing sets, respectively

Method	IU-Xray→MIMIC-CXR				Method	MIMIC-CXR→IU-Xray			
	BLEU-4	ROUGE	METEOR	CIDEr		BLEU-4	ROUGE	METEOR	CIDEr
R2Gen	0.067	0.201	0.108	0.072	R2Gen[a]	0.059	0.253	0.131	–
R2GenCMN	0.061	0.213	0.105	0.069	DCL[a]	0.074	0.267	0.152	–
DCL	0.064	0.208	0.105	0.063	PromptMRG[a]	0.098	0.281	0.160	–
R2GenGPT-S	0.064	0.211	0.108	0.066	R2GenGPT-S	0.051	0.229	0.114	0.196
+ MCV	0.088	0.247	0.118	0.083	+ MCV	0.083	0.291	0.149	0.207
R2GenGPT-D	0.071	0.218	0.113	0.072	R2GenGPT-D	0.083	0.275	0.163	0.231
+ MCV	0.101	0.251	0.122	0.134	+ MCV	0.112	0.308	0.177	0.236
Med-LMM	0.068	0.215	0.115	0.069	Med-LMM	0.087	0.279	0.137	0.252
+ MCV (MCVGen)	**0.106**	**0.256**	**0.128**	**0.142**	+ MCV (MCVGen)	**0.125**	**0.313**	**0.185**	**0.280**

[a] Indicates the results are quoted from their original papers

Table 13.4 Comparison of cross-center zero-shot learning performance across CE metrics in the IU-Xray to MIMIC-CXR adaptation

Method	Precision	Recall	F1-score
R2Gen	0.139	0.134	0.135
R2GenCMN	0.145	0.132	0.134
DCL	0.156	0.143	0.146
R2GenGPT-S	0.128	0.116	0.119
+ MCV	0.181	0.169	0.173
R2GenGPT-D	0.208	0.193	0.197
+ MCV	0.242	0.226	0.234
Med-LMM	0.211	0.206	0.208
+ MCV (MCVGen)	**0.249**	**0.235**	**0.237**

similar writing styles. Comparable improvements are observed across CE metrics in the IU-Xray to MIMIC-CXR adaptation. By integrating MCV with R2GenGPT-S, R2GenGPT-D, and Med-LMM, the precision is increased by 5.3%, 3.4%, and 3.8%, respectively. These enhancements highlight that the generated reports can capture accurate medical terminologies, thereby enhancing clinical factual correctness.

Overall, these results demonstrate that the MCVGen achieves SOTA zero-shot MRG performances on both datasets and even surpasses some fully supervised MRG systems. The impact of incorporating MCV underscores its ability to leverage the unique strengths of LLMs. When comparing MCVGen and R2GenGPT-D+MCV, the advantages of utilizing Q-former, which provides stronger visual embedding capabilities, become evident.

Cross-disease Performance. The cross-disease evaluation results are presented across both NLG and CE metrics on the MIMIC in Table 13.5. It is observed that incorporating MCV can enhance the baseline models on both NLG and CE metrics. In terms of NLG metrics, integrating MCV with R2GenGPT-S improved BLEU-4 scores from 0.098 to 0.105. For R2GenGPT-D, the introduction of MCV resulted in an increase in

Table 13.5 Comparison of cross-disease zero-shot learning performance across NLG and CE metrics on MIMIC dataset

Method	NLG metric				CE metric		
	BLEU-4	METEOR	ROUGE	CIDEr	Precision	Recall	F1-score
R2GenGPT-S	0.098	0.253	0.122	0.093	0.173	0.161	0.163
+ MCV	0.105	0.267	0.132	0.121	0.192	0.179	0.180
R2GenGPT-D	0.117	0.277	0.136	0.144	0.253	0.238	0.244
+ MCV	0.124	0.285	0.145	0.187	0.289	0.267	0.275
Med-LMM	0.113	0.269	0.141	0.140	0.261	0.232	0.246
+ MCV (MCVGen)	**0.129**	**0.291**	**0.148**	**0.203**	**0.294**	**0.277**	**0.281**

BLEU-4 scores from 0.117 to 0.124 and CIDEr from 0.144 to 0.187. The MCVGen demonstrated the most pronounced gains, with BLEU-4 scores rising from 0.113 to 0.129 and CIDEr from 0.140 to 0.203. On the CE front, the incorporation of MCV into R2GenGPT-S and R2GenGPT-D boosted the precision from 0.173 to 0.192 and 0.253 to 0.289, respectively. MCVGen also achieved significant improvements in precision from 0.261 to 0.294, recall from 0.232 to 0.277, and F1-score from 0.246 to 0.281. These results clearly illustrate the significant impact that MCV has on enhancing the performance of MRG systems in cross-disease zero-shot learning contexts. The enhancements in CE metrics that are more important in the cross-disease evaluation highlight MCV's role in increasing the clinical factual correctness of the reports, crucial for practical medical applications. It shows the potential of deploying MCVGen in clinical practice to describe novel diseases with a few demonstrations.

13.3.4 Summary of MCVGen

In this chapter, we introduced MCVGen, a novel approach for zero-shot medical report generation that harnesses large language models' capabilities through multi-modal contextual vectors (MCV). Our method adapts traditional in-context learning by averaging hidden states from demonstrations to guide the generation process. Through experiments on the IU-Xray and MIMIC datasets, we demonstrated that MCVGen effectively produces high-quality medical reports in new writing styles and for novel diseases without specific training, achieving state-of-the-art zero-shot performance across both linguistic and clinical efficacy metrics.

MCVGen addresses several critical challenges in medical reporting, including the need for accurate reporting of complex conditions, adaptation to rare diseases, and efficient deployment in resource-constrained healthcare settings. The ability to generate clinically accurate reports with minimal training examples is particularly valuable for improving diagnostic efficiency and clinical decision-making across diverse patient populations.

While promising, our approach currently relies on LLaMa-2 7B due to computational constraints. We are investigating methods to leverage more powerful LLMs efficiently. Additionally, our current evaluation is limited to chest radiology; future work will explore cross-modality zero-shot capabilities across different medical imaging types.

13.4 Discussion and Future Directions

13.4.1 Implications for AI-Empowered Healthcare Systems

The MCVGen approach presents significant opportunities for advancing AI-empowered healthcare delivery, particularly in contexts where computational efficiency and data scarcity present challenges. The zero-shot capabilities demonstrated in this work address fundamental barriers to implementing AI-assisted medical reporting across diverse healthcare environments, from resource-rich academic medical centers to community hospitals and specialized care facilities.

The computational efficiency of our MCV approach enables deployment on modest hardware configurations, making AI-assisted reporting accessible to smaller healthcare facilities that may lack extensive computational infrastructure. This democratization of AI capabilities is particularly relevant for aging populations, who often receive care across diverse settings including home-based care, assisted living facilities, and specialized geriatric clinics where computational resources may be limited.

Our cross-disease evaluation methodology demonstrates the potential for handling novel medical conditions with minimal training data—a capability that becomes increasingly important as healthcare systems encounter emerging health challenges and rare conditions. For aging populations, this flexibility is especially valuable given the heterogeneity of age-related conditions and the frequent co-occurrence of multiple chronic diseases that may require specialized reporting approaches.

13.4.2 Integration with IoT and Smart Aging Technologies

The intersection of large language models with Internet of Things (IoT) technologies opens new possibilities for comprehensive health monitoring and reporting systems. MCVGen's demonstrated ability to adapt across different clinical contexts suggests natural extensions to IoT-enabled healthcare applications, where diverse data streams from connected devices require intelligent interpretation and synthesis.

In smart aging scenarios, the integration of MCVGen with IoT sensor networks could enable automated generation of comprehensive health reports that combine traditional medical imaging with continuous monitoring data from wearable devices, environmental sensors, and smart home technologies. The zero-shot learning capabilities would allow the system to adapt to new sensor types or monitoring protocols without requiring extensive retraining, supporting the evolving landscape of IoT healthcare technologies.

The computational efficiency of the MCV approach aligns well with edge computing requirements in IoT networks, where local processing capabilities may be limited. This enables real-time health assessment and reporting generation directly at the point of care, reducing dependence on cloud-based processing and supporting privacy-preserving healthcare applications—considerations that are particularly important for aging populations who may have concerns about data privacy and security.

13.4.3 Future Research Directions and Technological Evolution

The foundation established by MCVGen opens several promising avenues for future research that could significantly advance the application of large language models in healthcare reporting and smart aging technologies:

- *Multi-modal Healthcare Integration*: Future developments should explore the integration of MCVGen with diverse data sources beyond medical imaging, including laboratory results, vital signs from IoT devices, and structured clinical data. This would create a more comprehensive zero-shot reporting capability that could synthesize information from multiple healthcare data streams, particularly valuable for aging populations where comprehensive geriatric assessments require integration of functional, cognitive, and medical indicators.
- *Temporal and Longitudinal Analysis*: Extending MCVGen to incorporate temporal information from sequential healthcare encounters could significantly enhance its utility for monitoring chronic disease progression and treatment response—critical capabilities for managing the complex health trajectories common in aging populations. This could include integration with IoT-based continuous monitoring systems to provide longitudinal health insights.
- *Personalized and Context-Aware Reporting*: Adapting the MCV approach to incorporate patient-specific historical data and contextual factors could enable more personalized report generation. This is particularly relevant for aging care, where individual health trajectories, functional status, and quality of life considerations require personalized attention in medical reporting and care planning.
- *Explainable AI and Clinical Trust*: Combining MCVGen with explainable AI techniques would enhance transparency and trust in generated reports—a critical consideration for clinical adoption, especially in aging care where clinical decisions often have significant implications for quality of life and functional independence.

These research directions collectively represent opportunities to enhance the application of large language models in healthcare reporting while supporting the broader goals of AI-empowered IoT solutions for smart aging and improved healthcare delivery across diverse patient populations.

References

1. Banerjee, S., Lavie, A.: METEOR: an automatic metric for MT evaluation with improved correlation with human judgments. In: Proceedings of the ACL Workshop on Intrinsic and Extrinsic Evaluation Measures for Machine Translation and/or Summarization, pp. 65–72. Association for Computational Linguistics (2005)
2. Chen, Z., Shen, Y., Song, Y., Wan, X.: Cross-modal memory networks for radiology report generation. In: Proceedings of the 59th Annual Meeting of the Association for Computational Linguistics, pp. 5904–5914. Association for Computational Linguistics (2021)
3. Chen, Z., Song, Y., Chang, T., Wan, X.: Generating radiology reports via memory-driven transformer. In: Proceedings of the 2020 Conference on Empirical Methods in Natural Language Processing, pp. 1439–1449. Association for Computational Linguistics (2020)
4. Demner-Fushman, D., Kohli, M.D., Rosenman, M.B., Shooshan, S.E., Rodriguez, L., Antani, S., Thoma, G.R., McDonald, C.J.: Preparing a collection of radiology examinations for distribution and retrieval. J. Am. Med. Inform. Assoc. **23**(2), 304–310 (2016)
5. Dong, Q., Li, L., Dai, D., Zheng, C., Wu, Z., Chang, B., Sun, X., Xu, J., Sui, Z.: A survey on in-context learning. arXiv:2301.00234 (2022)
6. Han, Z., Wei, B., Leung, S., Chung, J., Li, S.: Towards automatic report generation in spine radiology using weakly supervised framework. In: Medical Image Computing and Computer Assisted Intervention—MICCAI 2018, LNCS 11073, pp. 185–193. Springer (2018)
7. Hendel, R., Geva, M., Globerson, A.: In-context learning creates task vectors. In: Proceedings of the 2023 Conference on Empirical Methods in Natural Language Processing, pp. 9318–9333. Association for Computational Linguistics (2023)
8. Huang, Z., Zhang, X., Zhang, S.: KIUT: knowledge-injected U-transformer for radiology report generation. In: Proceedings of the IEEE/CVF Conference on Computer Vision and Pattern Recognition, pp. 19809–19818 (2023)
9. Irvin, J., Rajpurkar, P., Ko, M., Yu, Y., Ciurea-Ilcus, S., Chute, C., Marklund, H., Haghgoo, B., Ball, R., Shpanskaya, K., et al.: Chexpert: a large chest radiograph dataset with uncertainty labels and expert comparison. In: Proceedings of the AAAI Conference on Artificial Intelligence, vol. 33, pp. 590–597 (2019)
10. Jia, X., Xiong, Y., Zhang, J., Zhang, Y., Zhu, Y.: Few-shot radiology report generation for rare diseases. In: Proceedings of the 2020 IEEE International Conference on Bioinformatics and Biomedicine, pp. 601–608. IEEE (2020)
11. Jin, H., Che, H., Lin, Y., Chen, H.: Promptmrg: Diagnosis-driven prompts for medical report generation. In: Proceedings of the AAAI Conference on Artificial Intelligence, vol. 38, pp. 2607–2615 (2024)
12. Johnson, A.E.W., Pollard, T.J., Berkowitz, S.J., Greenbaum, N.R., Lungren, M.P., Deng, C.Y., Mark, R.G., Horng, S.: MIMIC-CXR: a large publicly available database of labeled chest radiographs. arXiv:1901.07042 (2019)
13. Li, J., Li, D., Savarese, S., Hoi, S.C.H.: Blip-2: Bootstrapping language-image pre-training with frozen image encoders and large language models. In: Proceedings of the 40th International Conference on Machine Learning, pp. 19730–19742 (2023)
14. Li, M., Cai, W., Liu, R., Weng, Y., Zhao, X., Wang, C., Chen, X., Liu, Z., Pan, C., Li, M., et al.: FFA-IR: towards an explainable and reliable medical report generation benchmark. In: NeurIPS Datasets and Benchmarks Track (2021)
15. Li, M., Lin, B., Chen, Z., Lin, H., Liang, X., Chang, X.: Dynamic graph enhanced contrastive learning for chest x-ray report generation. In: Proceedings of the IEEE/CVF Conference on Computer Vision and Pattern Recognition, pp. 3334–3343 (2023)
16. Li, M., Liu, R., Wang, F., Chang, X., Liang, X.: Auxiliary signal-guided knowledge encoder–decoder for medical report generation. World Wide Web **26**(1), 253–270 (2023)
17. Lin, C.: ROUGE: A package for automatic evaluation of summaries. In: Text Summarization Branches Out (2004)

18. Lin, Z., Zhang, D., Shi, D., Xu, R., Tao, Q., Wu, L., He, M., Ge, Z.: Contrastive pre-training and linear interaction attention-based transformer for universal medical reports generation. J. Biomed. Inform. **138**, 104281 (2023)
19. Liu, F., You, C., Wu, X., Ge, S., Sun, X.: Auto-encoding knowledge graph for unsupervised medical report generation. In: Advances in Neural Information Processing Systems, vol. 34, pp. 16266–16279 (2021)
20. Liu, R., Li, M., Zhao, S., Chen, L., Chang, X., Yao, L.: In-context learning for zero-shot medical report generation. In: Proceedings of the 32nd ACM International Conference on Multimedia, MM 2024, Melbourne, VIC, Australia, 28 October 2024–1 November 2024, pp. 8721–8730. ACM (2024)
21. Messina, P., Pino, P., Parra, D., Soto, A., Besa, C., Uribe, S., Andía, M., Tejos, C., Prieto, C., Capurro, D.: A survey on deep learning and explainability for automatic report generation from medical images. ACM Comput. Surv. **54**(10s), 1–40 (2022)
22. Papineni, K., Roukos, S., Ward, T., Zhu, W.: Bleu: a method for automatic evaluation of machine translation. In: Proceedings of the 40th Annual Meeting of the Association for Computational Linguistics, pp. 311–318 (2002)
23. Todd, E., Li, M.L., Sharma, A.S., Mueller, A., Wallace, B.C., Bau, D.: Function vectors in large language models. arXiv:2310.15213 (2023)
24. Touvron, H., Martin, L., Stone, K., Albert, P., Almahairi, A., Babaei, Y., Bashlykov, N., Batra, S., Bhargava, P., Bhosale, S., et al.: LLaMA 2: open foundation and fine-tuned chat models. arXiv:2307.09288 (2023)
25. Vaswani, A., Shazeer, N., Parmar, N., Uszkoreit, J., Jones, L., Gomez, A.N., Kaiser, Ł., Polosukhin, I.: Attention is all you need. In: Advances in Neural Information Processing Systems, vol. 30, pp. 5998–6008 (2017)
26. Vedantam, R., Zitnick, C.L., Parikh, D.: CIDEr: Consensus-based image description evaluation. In: Proceedings of the IEEE Conference on Computer Vision and Pattern Recognition, pp. 4566–4575 (2015)
27. Wang, Z., Wu, Z., Agarwal, D., Sun, J.: Medclip: contrastive learning from unpaired medical images and text. In: Proceedings of the 2022 Conference on Empirical Methods in Natural Language Processing (2022)

Chapter 14
Emergent Capabilities of Large Foundation Models for Intelligent Navigation

14.1 Introduction

14.1.1 Overview of Emergent Capabilities in Large Foundation Models

The emergence of large foundation models, particularly Large Language Models (LLMs) and Vision-Language Models (VLMs), has marked a transformative era in artificial intelligence, characterized by the manifestation of emergent capabilities that are not explicitly programmed during training. These emergent properties represent qualitatively new abilities that arise from the complex interactions within large-scale neural architectures, enabling models to perform tasks and exhibit behaviors beyond their initial training objectives [6, 29, 47].

One of the most remarkable emergent capabilities is zero-shot learning, where models demonstrate competency in novel tasks without explicit task-specific training. This phenomenon has been particularly evident in language models that can adapt to new domains and modalities through carefully designed prompts and context. In the realm of embodied AI and intelligent navigation, these capabilities have opened unprecedented opportunities for developing agents that can understand and execute complex navigation instructions based on natural language commands.

Visual Language Navigation (VLN) exemplifies a domain where emergent capabilities of large foundation models can be effectively leveraged. VLN represents a fundamental task within Embodied AI, focusing on agents' ability to navigate complex environments based on natural language instructions [15]. The integration of pre-trained LLMs and VLMs into VLN systems has demonstrated that effective navigation agents can be produced with minimal training by harnessing the rich multimodal knowledge embedded within these foundation models.

In the context of smart aging environments, such emergent capabilities hold particular promise for developing intuitive and adaptive assistance systems that can help elderly individuals navigate both physical and digital spaces through natural lan-

Q. Z. Sheng et al., *Harnessing Artificial Intelligence and Pervasive Internet of Things for an Empowered Aging*, https://doi.org/10.1007/978-3-032-16502-2_14

guage interactions, potentially revolutionizing how aging populations interact with their living environments.

14.1.2 Challenges and Opportunities

Despite the remarkable progress enabled by large foundation models, several fundamental challenges persist when attempting to harness their emergent capabilities for specific applications such as intelligent navigation. The primary challenges lie in the gaps between the general knowledge encoded in these models and the specialized requirements of domain-specific tasks.

First, while pre-trained foundation models exhibit impressive zero-shot capabilities, their performance often falls short of task-specific trained methods due to the absence of domain-specific knowledge [6, 29, 47]. In navigation scenarios, this manifests as difficulties in understanding spatial relationships, environmental dynamics, and the nuanced requirements of following navigation instructions in real-world settings. Second, the computational requirements for fine-tuning large foundation models on specific tasks are often prohibitive, requiring substantial computational resources and extensive datasets [25, 32, 45]. This limitation is particularly pronounced in resource-constrained environments or when dealing with specialized domains where training data are scarce. Third, existing approaches often rely on pre-trained visual perception backbones that struggle with dynamic scenarios inherent in navigation tasks, such as constantly changing viewpoints and environmental contexts [13]. This limitation highlights the need for novel approaches that can effectively bridge the gap between general-purpose foundation models and task-specific requirements.

These challenges also present significant opportunities. The emergent capabilities of foundation models, particularly their ability to perform cross-modal reasoning and adapt to new contexts, provide a foundation for developing more efficient and effective approaches to intelligent navigation. For smart aging applications, these capabilities can enable the development of personalized assistance systems that adapt to individual needs and preferences without requiring extensive retraining.

14.1.3 Contributions

This chapter makes several key contributions to understanding and leveraging the emergent capabilities of large foundation models for intelligent navigation, with particular relevance to smart aging environments. Our primary contributions are threefold:

- We introduce a novel causal perspective for understanding navigation tasks that reveals how emergent capabilities of foundation models can be effectively harnessed. We analyze the association structure within observation histories and design a partial contrastive learning framework that leverages the zero-shot object recognition capabilities of VLMs while mitigating their limitations in domain-specific scenarios.

- We present a weakly-supervised learning paradigm that integrates knowledge from pre-trained large foundation models into navigation systems without requiring computationally expensive fine-tuning. This approach demonstrates how emergent capabilities can be channeled through carefully designed supervisory signals, effectively bridging the gap between general-purpose foundation models and specialized navigation requirements.
- We provide comprehensive empirical evidence demonstrating the effectiveness and robustness of our approach across multiple benchmarks, showcasing how emergent capabilities of different VLMs can be consistently leveraged for navigation tasks. Our analysis reveals insights into the transferability and generalizability of emergent capabilities across different foundation models.

Through the lens of a specific case study involving Weakly-supervised VLM-guided Partial Contrastive Learning (WPCL) for Visual Language Navigation, we illustrate how emergent capabilities can be systematically identified, understood, and leveraged to create more effective and efficient intelligent systems suitable for diverse applications, including smart aging environments.

14.1.4 Chapter Organization

The remainder of this chapter is organized as follows. Section 14.2 provides comprehensive background on large foundation models and their emergent capabilities, with particular focus on vision-language models and their applications in navigation tasks, as well as research gaps and opportunities in smart aging contexts. Section 14.3 presents our case study on Weakly-supervised VLM-guided Partial Contrastive Learning for Visual Language Navigation, demonstrating how emergent capabilities can be effectively leveraged through detailed methodology and comprehensive experimental validation. Section 14.4 discusses the broader implications of our findings for intelligent navigation and outlines future research directions, particularly focusing on applications in smart aging environments and the continued evolution of emergent capabilities in foundation models.

14.2 Background and Related Work

14.2.1 Large Foundation Models and Emergent Capabilities

Large foundation models have revolutionized the landscape of artificial intelligence by demonstrating emergent capabilities that arise from scale and architectural sophistication. These models, trained on vast datasets with billions or trillions of parameters, exhibit behaviors and competencies that are not explicitly programmed during their training phase. The emergence of such capabilities represents a fundamental shift in how we understand and develop AI systems.

Emergent capabilities in foundation models manifest in various forms, most notably through zero-shot and few-shot learning abilities. When pre-trained Large Language Models (LLMs) and Vision-Language Models (VLMs) are presented with novel tasks, they can often perform competently without additional training, drawing upon the rich representations learned during their pre-training phase. This phenomenon has been particularly evident in models such as GPT-4 [1], where the model demonstrates competency across diverse domains ranging from natural language understanding to complex reasoning tasks.

The integration of vision and language modalities in VLMs has further expanded the scope of emergent capabilities. Models such as CLIP [34], LLaVA [27], BLIP-2 [23], and OpenFlamingo [5] have demonstrated remarkable ability to understand and reason about visual content in conjunction with textual instructions. These capabilities emerge from the models' ability to learn rich cross-modal representations that capture complex relationships between visual and linguistic information.

The utilization of these emergent capabilities presents both opportunities and challenges. While zero-shot performance can be impressive, it often falls short of task-specific training methods, particularly in specialized domains. This gap highlights the need for approaches that can effectively leverage emergent capabilities, while addressing domain-specific requirements.

14.2.2 Vision-Language Models in Navigation Tasks

The application of foundation models to navigation tasks represents a natural convergence of emergent capabilities with practical embodied AI challenges. Vision-and-Language Navigation (VLN) tasks [4, 33] require agents to follow human instructions to reach specific destinations, making them ideal testbeds for evaluating how well foundation models can transfer their general knowledge to specialized spatial reasoning tasks. Early approaches to VLN focused on end-to-end training methods [4, 14, 36] or incorporated VLN-specific pre-training and fine-tuning steps [17, 19]. These methods, while effective, require substantial computational resources and task-specific data collection efforts. The emergence of large foundation models has provided alternative pathways that can potentially reduce these requirements while maintaining or improving performance.

Recent studies have explored various strategies for integrating foundation models into VLN systems. Some approaches leverage the zero-shot capabilities of pre-trained models directly [6, 29, 47], demonstrating that effective navigation agents can be developed with minimal training by carefully designing prompts and input representations. These methods showcase the potential of emergent capabilities but often exhibit performance gaps compared to specialized approaches.

Other approaches focus on fine-tuning foundation models for VLN-specific tasks [25, 32, 45], typically adapting medium-sized models such as LLaMA-7B [37] or similar architectures. While these methods can achieve strong performance, they require substantial computational resources for fine-tuning, making them less accessible for many research groups and practical applications.

To enhance action planning in navigation tasks, existing methods often incorporate additional techniques such as historical action tracking [20, 43], self-correction mechanisms [21, 31], navigation map generation [8, 28, 42], and external knowledge integration [24, 30, 44]. The challenge lies in effectively combining these techniques with the emergent capabilities of foundation models to create systems that are both effective and computationally efficient.

14.2.3 Research Gaps and Opportunities in Smart Aging

The intersection of emergent capabilities in foundation models and smart aging applications presents a largely unexplored but highly promising research area. Smart aging environments require sophisticated yet intuitive interfaces that can adapt to the changing needs and capabilities of aging individuals. The emergent capabilities of foundation models, particularly their ability to understand natural language instructions and perform cross-modal reasoning, align well with the requirements of such environments.

Current smart aging research has focused primarily on sensor-based monitoring, health management systems, and basic assistive technologies. However, the potential for leveraging emergent capabilities of foundation models to create more intelligent and adaptive assistance systems remains largely untapped. For instance, navigation assistance systems that can understand complex spatial instructions, adapt to individual mobility constraints, and provide personalized guidance represent a significant opportunity for improving the quality of life for aging populations.

The challenges in this domain are multifaceted. Aging individuals may have varying levels of technological literacy, diverse physical and cognitive capabilities, and different environmental constraints. Foundation models' emergent capabilities, such as their ability to adapt communication styles and reasoning approaches based on context, could be particularly valuable in addressing these diverse needs.

Furthermore, the considerations on computational efficiency that we explore in this chapter are particularly relevant for smart aging applications, where deployment may occur in resource-constrained environments or require real-time responsiveness. Approaches that can leverage emergent capabilities without requiring extensive fine-tuning or computational resources are therefore especially valuable in these contexts. The research presented in this chapter, while focused on general navigation tasks, provides insights and methodologies that can be readily adapted to smart aging scenarios. The principles of leveraging emergent capabilities through weakly-supervised approaches, minimizing computational requirements, and maintaining robustness across different foundation models are all directly applicable to developing next-generation smart aging assistance systems.

14.3 Emergent Capability Utilization Through Weakly-Supervised Learning

14.3.1 Motivation and Overview of the WPCL Method

The development of the Weakly-supervised VLM-guided Partial Contrastive Learning (WPCL) method [39] emerges from the recognition that emergent capabilities of large foundation models can be systematically leveraged to address fundamental challenges in Visual Language Navigation, while simultaneously demonstrating broader principles applicable to intelligent systems in smart aging contexts.

Visual Language Navigation represents a fundamental task within the field of Embodied AI, focusing on the ability of agents to navigate complex environments based on natural language instructions. Despite the progress made by the existing methods, these approaches often encounter common limitations that highlight the need for more effective utilization of foundation models' emergent capabilities. First, they rely on pre-trained backbone models for visual perception, which struggle with the dynamic viewpoint changes inherent in VLN scenarios. Second, their performance is constrained when using pre-trained LLMs or VLMs without fine-tuning, due to the absence of VLN domain knowledge. Third, while fine-tuning LLMs and VLMs can improve results, their computational costs are significantly higher than approaches that leverage zero-shot capabilities.

The WPCL method addresses these limitations by demonstrating how emergent capabilities of foundation models can be effectively channeled through carefully designed weakly-supervised mechanisms. Our approach enhances an agent's ability to identify objects from dynamic viewpoints in VLN scenarios by integrating pre-trained VLM knowledge into the perception process without requiring computationally expensive VLM fine-tuning. This represents a concrete example of how emergent zero-shot object recognition capabilities can be leveraged to solve domain-specific challenges while maintaining computational efficiency.

The key insight underlying our approach is that the emergent capabilities of VLMs for object recognition and cross-modal understanding can be harnessed through weak supervision signals, effectively bridging the gap between general-purpose foundation models and specialized navigation requirements. By leveraging the zero-shot capability of pre-trained Vision-Language Models to guide positive sample selection in a contrastive learning framework, we demonstrate how emergent capabilities can be systematically integrated into task-specific learning paradigms.

Over the years, various methods have been developed to advance VLN, ranging from end-to-end training approaches [4, 14, 36] to methods incorporating VLN-specific pre-training and fine-tuning steps [17, 19]. The rise of pre-trained Large Language Models and Vision-Language Models has fueled interest in leveraging these models for VLN, with studies showing that effective agents can be produced with minimal training [6, 29, 47] by integrating pre-trained knowledge into VLN systems.

However, these methods often present common challenges that our WPCL approach specifically addresses. Traditional approaches using pre-trained backbone models such as ResNet [18] or CLIP [34] for visual perception are not ideally suited for VLN scenarios due to constant viewpoint changes [13]. When incorporating pre-trained LLMs or VLMs without fine-tuning, performance often falls short of traditional methods due to the lack of VLN-specific information [6, 29, 47]. Conversely, while fine-tuning LLMs or VLMs can enhance performance, it is computationally expensive [25, 32, 45] and not always feasible.

To overcome these limitations, our WPCL method demonstrates how emergent capabilities can be leveraged through three key innovations: 1) enhancing environmental understanding by identifying objects from dynamic viewpoints, addressing shortcomings of pre-trained visual perception backbones, 2) introducing a weakly-supervised mechanism to reduce reliance on potentially biased LLM/VLM outputs while leveraging their zero-shot capabilities; and 3) integrating pre-trained large VLMs into VLN without fine-tuning, avoiding associated computational costs while maintaining effectiveness.

The broader implications of this approach extend beyond navigation tasks to intelligent assistance systems for smart aging environments, where similar principles of leveraging emergent capabilities through efficient, weakly-supervised mechanisms could enable the development of adaptive and personalized assistance systems that understand natural language instructions and adapt to individual needs without requiring extensive computational resources or task-specific training data.

14.3.2 WPCL: A Weakly-Supervised Framework

Causal Framework and Theoretical Foundation

Our approach is grounded in a novel causal understanding of the navigation process that reveals how emergent capabilities of foundation models can be systematically leveraged to address fundamental challenges in visual perception under dynamic viewpoint conditions.

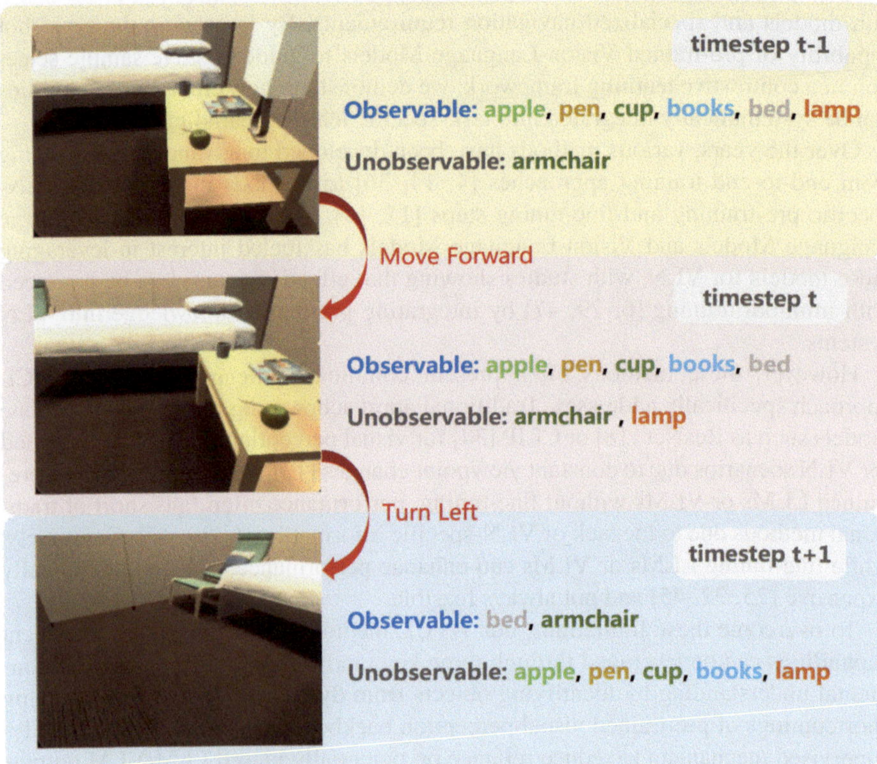

Fig. 14.1 Illustrative example of our motivation. The agent's actions do not alter the environment but only change its viewpoint, resulting in different observations. The agent should recognize the same object from different angles by identifying common elements across observations

Understanding Viewpoint Dynamics Through Causal Analysis. In navigation scenarios, an agent's actions do not alter the environment but only shift its viewpoint, changing the perspective from which objects are observed. As illustrated in Fig. 14.1, when an agent moves from timestep $t-1$ to t via "Move Forward", most objects remain visible from a different angle, except for certain objects like the lamp, which may disappear due to the viewpoint change. After performing "Turn Left" at $t+1$, new objects such as an armchair may enter the field of view while previously visible objects like books become unobservable. Although all objects persist in the environment, the agent's viewpoint dictates their observability.

This observation leads to a fundamental insight: an ideal agent with comprehensive environmental understanding should recognize the same objects from different angles, leveraging the emergent cross-modal understanding capabilities of foundation models. However, many VLN methods rely on pre-trained vision models like ResNet [18] or CLIP [34], which have been shown to be highly sensitive to viewpoint changes, making it difficult to consistently recognize the same object from different perspectives [13].

To address this challenge, we introduce a generalizable causal framework, where Obs represents the agent's observations, Obj denotes the objects in the environment, and vw stands for the viewpoint. The Obj layer remains static over time, while the Obs and vw layers are fully connected, indicating that all objects can potentially appear in an observation, depending on the viewpoint. At each timestep, the agent's action induces an intervention on the viewpoint vw, which does not causally affect the environment but influences how the agent perceives it, thus determining how objects are represented in that observation.

Within this causal framework, objects act as confounders between observations, especially when two observations share the same object. To enable the agent to consistently identify the same object from various viewpoints, we employ a contrastive learning framework that leverages the emergent object recognition capabilities of VLMs to extract mutual information between observations.

Leveraging Contrastive Learning for Emergent Capability Integration. The causal framework reveals the data generation process of an agent's observations, and contrastive learning can be leveraged to encourage better environmental understanding by extracting mutual information between positive samples [50]. Traditional contrastive learning frameworks generate positive samples through random augmentations [9, 10] and train encoders to bring them closer in the latent space through specialized loss functions that encourage similar representations for related inputs while pushing apart dissimilar ones.

To adapt this framework to our navigation scenario, we select pairs of images from the observation history that contain common objects as positive samples. This approach allows the framework to extract mutual information representing the shared objects between samples, effectively inverting the data generation process and enhancing the agent's understanding of the environment. The key insight is that by identifying and leveraging these common visual elements across different viewpoints, the agent develops more robust object recognition capabilities that are crucial for consistent navigation performance.

VLM-Guided Weak Supervision for Emergent Capability Utilization. We choose a VLM-guided weakly-supervised mechanism to harness emergent capabilities for two key reasons. First, the standard contrastive learning framework assumes that positive samples share mutual information, which is typically valid when positive samples are generated through image augmentation [9]. However, in our case, randomly selecting two observations from the observation history does not guarantee mutual information sharing. Therefore, we leverage the emergent zero-shot object recognition capability of VLMs to guide the selection of positive samples. Second, as established in our analysis of foundation model applications in navigation, methods relying heavily on pre-trained LLMs or VLMs often underperform VLN-tailored training due to lacking task-specific information. Therefore, we minimize reliance on pre-trained models by using a weakly-supervised approach instead of a fully-supervised one, potentially enhancing performance while circumventing the computational costs of

VLM fine-tuning and demonstrating how emergent capabilities can be efficiently leveraged without extensive model adaptation.

Weakly-Supervised VLM Integration

As elaborated in our theoretical foundation, we leverage the emergent zero-shot capability of pre-trained Vision-Language Models to assist in positive sample selection, demonstrating how emergent capabilities can be systematically harnessed for domain-specific applications. Specifically, given an observation history $O = \{o_i\}_{i=1}^N$ where N is the number of historical observations, we independently input each o_i into the pre-trained LLaVA v1.5 [27], asking it to identify objects in the image using the following prompt to extract a list of objects contained in each image:

> Give me a list of objects that appear in the given image. Ignore the general environmental objects such as walls, floors or rooftops. Please only answer with a list of objects, and separate each object by a comma.

We specify the expected output format in the prompt to ensure consistency across all images in the observation history. The same prompt and output templates are applied uniformly. Below is a sample output:

> desk, chair, television, sofa, coffee table, fruits

We process this output sentence by splitting it at commas to obtain a set of objects for each observation. We then construct a sample selection matrix, which serves as a symmetric binary matrix that indicates when two observations share sufficient common objects based on a tunable threshold parameter. This matrix formation process creates the foundation for our weakly-supervised learning approach by systematically identifying which observation pairs contain meaningful shared visual content.

This sample selection matrix is subsequently incorporated as the weak supervisory signal into the agent's training process, providing guidance for the contrastive learning framework without requiring extensive manual annotation or expensive fine-tuning of the foundation models.

Partial Contrastive Learning

We employ a Partial Contrastive Learning framework to encourage the agent to recognize objects from different angles as it navigates the environment. The core principle is to identify positive sample pairs from the observation history based on shared object content, while designating observations with insufficient common objects as negative samples.

Unlike traditional contrastive learning frameworks that assume entire representations between positive samples should be fully invariant, our approach relaxes this assumption to better accommodate the emergent capabilities of foundation models. We recognize that only a portion of the visual representation should remain consistent across positive sample pairs, specifically the part encoding common objects, while other aspects of the representation may legitimately differ due to viewpoint changes, environmental variations, or the presence of unique objects in each observation.

Our framework introduces a learnable mechanism that divides visual features into two complementary segments: one dedicated to encoding shared object information that should remain consistent across different viewpoints, and the other a flexible component that captures viewpoint-specific and unique visual elements. This architectural design enables the model to maintain object recognition consistency while preserving the ability to encode important environmental details that vary across observations.

The training process applies contrastive objectives specifically to the object-focused feature segment, encouraging the model to develop robust representations for identifying the same objects from different perspectives. This targeted approach enables more effective utilization of the emergent capabilities in foundation models while avoiding the computational overhead associated with full model fine-tuning.

Overall Workflow

The overall workflow of our proposed method is depicted in Fig. 14.2, which consists of three key modules: (1) Visual Perception, (2) Instruction Understanding, and (3) Action Prediction. Our primary contribution lies in the Visual Perception module.

The observation history is first processed through a pre-trained CLIP model to generate initial image features. We select CLIP for image processing due to its proven effectiveness in navigation tasks [22] and its computational efficiency. These features are then refined through our trainable Partial Contrast Module, which produces enhanced visual representations segmented into object-focused and flexible

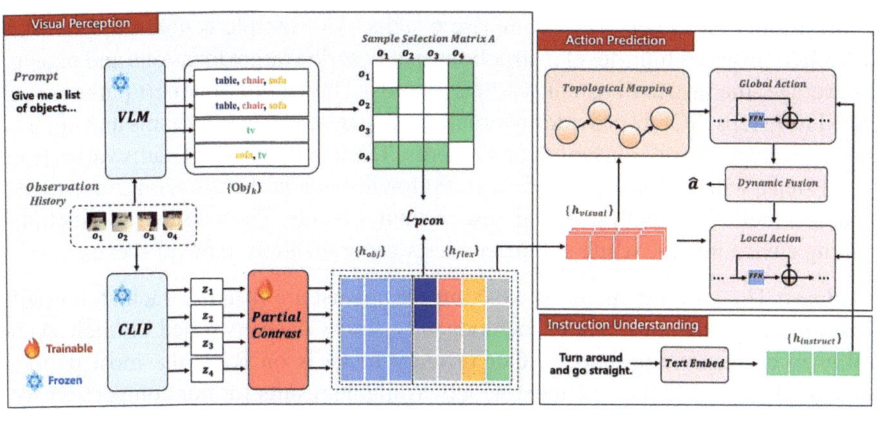

Fig. 14.2 The overall workflow of our method. The observation histories are first processed by the pre-trained CLIP model. And a VLM is used to generate the Sample Selection Matrix A. The final visual features are subsequently integrated into the DUET framework for VLN

components as described in our partial contrastive learning framework. Simultaneously, the observation history is processed by the pre-trained VLM to generate object lists for each observation, which are used to construct the sample selection matrix that provides supervisory signals for guiding the agent's ability to identify objects from changing viewpoints.

In the Instruction Understanding Module, we employ text embedding layers to convert input instructions into feature representations. The enhanced visual features and instruction features are then integrated in the Action Prediction Module, which adapts the Dual-Scale Graph Transformer (DUET) architecture [8]. This module incorporates both Global Action prediction with topological mapping and Local Action prediction based on immediate visual and instruction inputs. A Dynamic Fusion component consolidates these predictions to generate the final action decision.

During training, the system employs a multi-objective approach that combines traditional VLN training objectives with our partial contrastive learning objective. The training process includes single-step action prediction using expert demonstrations, object grounding when annotations are available, and supervision from pseudo interactive demonstrators. The overall training objective balances these components through carefully tuned weighting parameters to ensure effective learning while maintaining computational efficiency.

14.3.3 Experimental Validation and Performance Analysis

Experimental Settings

Datasets: We evaluate our method on three widely used VLN benchmarks: R2R [4], REVERIE [33] and SOON [48]. R2R provides step-by-step instructions that guide the agent to navigate to a specified location. On average, the instructions consist of 32 words, and the expert paths comprise 6 steps. An example is given in Fig. 14.3. REVERIE provides high-level instructions that describe target locations and objects. On average, the instructions consist of 21 words. The length of expert paths ranges from 4 to 7 steps. SOON provides instructions that describe target rooms and objects, with an average instruction length of 49 words. The length of expert paths varies from 2 to 21 steps, with an average of 9.5 steps. Following standard evaluation conventions, we assess methods in both seen and unseen environments. The val seen split includes training environments, while val unseen tests generalization to novel scenes.

Baselines: The baseline methods we compare against are listed in each result table across the three datasets. These methods vary across datasets based on their availability in corresponding papers. Our primary focus is on R2R, the most popular benchmark, as it provides the most widely available results for our comparison. We broadly categorize existing methods into three groups: those without pre-trained large models, those using pre-trained large models with fine-tuning, and those using pre-trained large models without fine-tuning. Our method leverages the knowledge

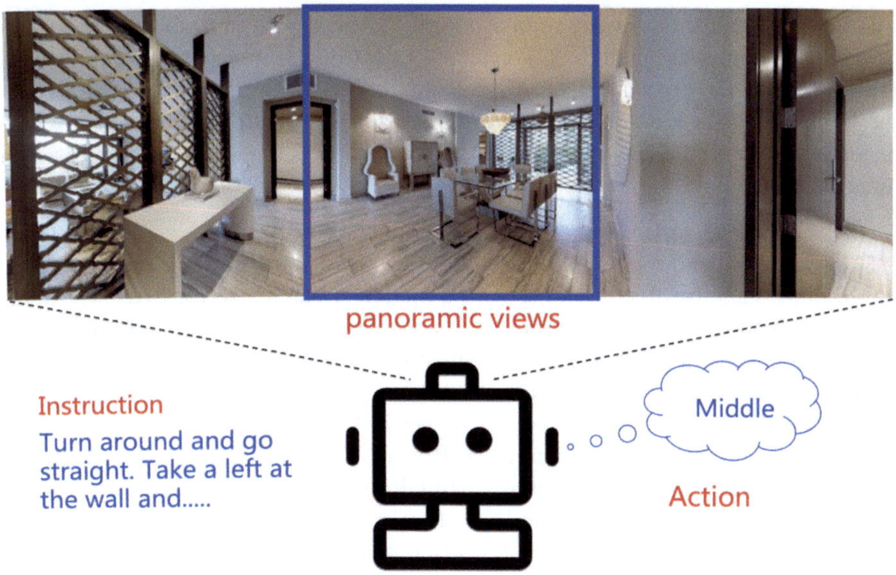

Fig. 14.3 An example of the Visual Language Navigation task. The agent follows a natural language instruction and navigates from an initial viewpoint within the given environment. At each time step, the agent chooses one view from its surrounding panoramic options to move towards

from the pre-trained VLM without fine-tuning it, thus lies in the third category and directly comparable to the methods in that category.

- Methods without LLMs/VLMs: This type of method does not leverage any pre-trained knowledge from foundation models. Some can be trained in an end-to-end manner such as Seq2Seq [4], RCM [40], Speaker-Follower [14], and EnvDrop [36], while others involve VLN-specific pre-training and fine-tuning steps, such as PREVALENT [17], VLNBERT [19], HAMT [7], BEVBERT [2], GridMM [42], DUET [8], and GOAT [38]. While ScaleVLN [41] and MiniVLN [49] demonstrated strong performance through dataset scaling, we focus on comparing methods that use the same amount of data and do not directly compare with them.
- Methods with LLMs/VLMs fine-tuning: These methods leverage pre-trained large foundation models by fine-tuning them on VLN-specific datasets, including NavCoT [25], LangNav [32], NaviLLM [45], and NaviCoT [46]. They typically use small or medium-sized LLMs/VLMs such as LLAMA-7B [37], Vicuna-7B, Vicuna-13B [11], and FlanT5 [12]. Fine-tuning these models is computationally intensive, requiring substantial hardware resources.
- Methods with pre-trained LLMs/VLMs: These methods leverage the zero-shot capability of pre-trained LLMs or VLMs such as GPT-4 [1], reducing computational costs. The methods include NavGPT [47], MapGPT [6], and Discuss-Nav [29].

Evaluation Metrics: Following prior work [3, 8, 46], we adopt a comprehensive set of navigation metrics, including Trajectory Length (TL), measuring average path length; Navigation Error (NE), the average distance to the target; Success Rate (SR), the frequency of task completion; Success weighted by Path Length (SPL), which accounts for path efficiency; and Oracle Success Rate (OSR), the success rate under an ideal stop policy.

Implementation Details: For the implementation, we utilize pre-trained LXMERT [35] as the initialization foundation and employ a two-stage training approach. The pre-training stage involved training with a moderate batch size for extensive iterations, followed by policy fine-tuning with a smaller batch size for additional iterations. Model selection was based on achieving optimal performance on validation data using path-length-weighted success metrics.

For feature extraction, we employ CLIP ViT-B/16 [34] due to its balance of effectiveness and computational efficiency. The Partial Contrast Module is implemented as a single-layer feed-forward network to maintain simplicity while providing the necessary feature transformation capabilities. Key hyperparameters are carefully tuned, including the weighting parameters for different loss components, the feature allocation ratio for object-focused representations, and the threshold parameter for constructing the sample selection matrix. These values are selected based on validation performance and maintained consistently across all experiments.

Overall Results

Our experimental evaluation demonstrates the effectiveness and robustness of the WPCL approach across multiple benchmark datasets. The comprehensive evaluation is conducted on three widely-used VLN benchmarks: R2R, REVERIE, and SOON, each presenting unique challenges and evaluation criteria.

Performance on the R2R Dataset: On the R2R benchmark (Table 14.1), our method achieves substantial improvements across most evaluation metrics. When compared with other methods that leverage pre-trained foundation models without fine-tuning, our approach demonstrates significant performance gains. Specifically, on the validation unseen split, WPCL achieves a Success Rate (SR) of 78% and SPL of 70%, substantially outperforming NavGPT (SR: 34%, SPL: 29%), MapGPT (SR: 39%, SPL: 26%), and DiscussNav (SR: 43%, SPL: 40%). This represents improvements of over 35% points in SR and 30% points in SPL compared to these zero-shot methods, demonstrating the effectiveness of our weakly-supervised approach in leveraging emergent capabilities.

Moreover, our method achieves competitive performance compared to approaches involving VLN-specific pre-training or even LLM fine-tuning. On validation unseen, WPCL surpasses several strong baselines including VLN-BERT (SR: 63%), HAMT (SR: 66%), and NaviLLM (SR: 67%). While GOAT achieves slightly higher performance (SR: 77%, SPL: 68%), it requires extensive VLN-specific pre-training. Our approach also demonstrates superior Navigation Error (NE) of 2.69 m on validation

Table 14.1 Results on the R2R benchmark. The top section lists methods that do not utilize any pre-trained large models, the middle section lists methods that involve LLM fine-tuning, and the bottom section lists methods that incorporate pre-trained large models. Our method belongs to the bottom section and outperforms not only other methods in this category but also those in the other sections. A—indicates unavailable performance data for that metric in the corresponding paper

	Val seen					Val unseen				
	TL	NE ↓	OSR ↑	SR ↑	SPL ↑	TL	NE ↓	OSR ↑	SR ↑	SPL ↑
Seq2Seq [4]	11.33	6.01	53	39	–	8.39	7.81	28	21	–
Speaker-Follower [14]	–	3.36	74	66	–	–	6.62	45	36	–
EnvDrop [36]	11.00	3.99	–	62	59	10.70	5.22	–	52	48
PREVALENT [17]	10.32	3.67	–	69	65	10.19	4.71	–	58	53
VLN-BERT [19]	11.13	2.90	–	72	68	12.01	3.93	–	63	57
HAMT [7]	11.15	2.51	–	76	72	11.46	2.29	–	66	61
BEVBert [2]	13.56	2.17	88	81	74	14.55	2.81	84	75	64
DUET [8]	12.32	2.28	86	79	73	13.94	3.31	81	72	60
GOAT [38]	–	1.79	88	83	79	–	2.40	84	77	68
GridMM [42]	–	–	–	–	–	–	2.83	–	75	64
NavCoT [25]	10.08	6.46	48	41	38	9.95	6.26	48	40	37
LangNav [32]	–	–	–	56	–	–	–	–	46	–
NaviLLM [45]	–	–	–	–	–	12.81	3.51	–	67	59
NavGPT-2 [46]	13.08	2.98	79	74	65	13.25	3.18	80	71	60
NavGPT [47]	–	–	–	–	–	11.45	6.46	42	34	29
MapGPT [6]	–	–	–	–	–	–	6.92	58	39	26
DiscussNav [29]	–	–	–	–	–	9.69	5.32	61	43	40
WPCL (Ours)	11.26	1.91	89	82	80	12.83	2.69	86	78	70

unseen, indicating more accurate navigation to target locations. On validation seen, WPCL achieves an impressive SR of 82% and SPL of 80%, demonstrating strong performance in familiar environments while maintaining excellent generalization capabilities.

Performance on the REVERIE and SOON Datasets: On both REVERIE (Table 14.2) and SOON (Table 14.3) datasets, our method outperforms baseline approaches by considerable margins across all evaluation metrics. The consistent improvements across these diverse benchmarks highlight the robustness and generalizability of our approach.

On the REVERIE dataset, which requires agents to follow high-level instructions describing target locations and objects, WPCL achieves an SR of 79.41% and SPL of 71.39% on validation seen, outperforming the strong GOAT baseline (SR: 78.64%, SPL: 71.40%). More importantly, on validation unseen, our method achieves SR of 54.03% and SPL of 37.41%, surpassing GOAT (SR: 53.37%, SPL: 36.70%) and demonstrating superior generalization to novel environments. Compared to DUET,

Table 14.2 Results on REVERIE. Our method demonstrates superior performance compared to existing approaches.

	Val seen			Val unseen		
	OSR ↑	SR ↑	SPL ↑	OSR ↑	SR ↑	SPL ↑
Seq2Seq [4]	35.70	29.59	24.01	8.07	4.20	2.84
RCM [40]	29.44	23.33	21.82	14.23	9.29	6.97
Airbert [16]	48.98	47.01	42.34	34.51	27.89	21.88
HAMT [7]	47.65	43.29	40.19	36.84	32.95	30.20
DUET [8]	73.86	71.75	63.94	51.07	46.98	33.73
GOAT [38]	–	78.64	71.40	–	53.37	36.70
WPCL (Ours)	75.31	79.41	71.39	53.94	54.03	37.41

Table 14.3 Results on SOON. Our method demonstrates superior performance compared to existing approaches.

	Val seen			Val unseen		
	OSR ↑	SR ↑	SPL ↑	OSR ↑	SR ↑	SPL ↑
GBE [48]	28.54	19.52	13.34	21.45	12.90	9.23
DUET [8]	50.91	36.28	22.58	43.00	33.44	21.42
GOAT [38]	54.69	40.35	28.05	50.63	40.50	25.18
WPCL (Ours)	55.13	41.24	28.53	52.21	42.92	26.57

which uses similar architectural components, WPCL shows substantial improvements of over 7% points in SR and nearly 4% points in SPL on validation unseen.

On the SOON dataset, which presents challenges with longer instruction lengths and more complex navigation paths, WPCL continues to demonstrate strong performance. On validation seen, our method achieves SR of 41.24% and SPL of 28.53%, outperforming GOAT (SR: 40.35%, SPL: 28.05%). The performance advantage is even more pronounced on validation unseen, where WPCL achieves SR of 42.92% and SPL of 26.57%, representing improvements of 2.42 and 1.39% points respectively over GOAT. These results are particularly significant given that SOON presents different challenges in terms of instruction complexity and navigation task requirements, with expert paths ranging from 2 to 21 steps.

Comparative Analysis: Our experimental results reveal several important insights. First, when compared with methods that do not utilize pre-trained large models, our approach demonstrates the clear benefits of leveraging emergent capabilities from foundation models. Second, among methods that incorporate pre-trained models, our weakly-supervised approach achieves competitive or superior performance while avoiding the computational overhead associated with fine-tuning. Third, the consistent performance improvements across different datasets and metrics indicate

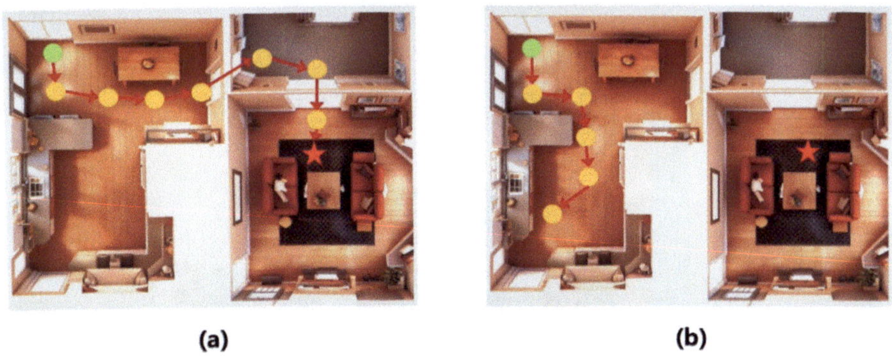

Fig. 14.4 Case study on R2R with the instruction: Walk through the kitchen and into the living area with two red sofas facing each other. Stop just when you reach the black rug. **a** Our method successfully completes the task. **b** DUET deviates in the wrong direction and fails to complete the task

that our approach effectively addresses fundamental challenges in visual language navigation.

The case study analysis further validates our approach's practical effectiveness. As illustrated in Fig. 14.4, in challenging navigation scenarios where agents must follow complex instructions like "Walk through the kitchen and into the living area with two red sofas facing each other. Stop just when you reach the black rug", our method successfully completes the task while traditional approaches failed, demonstrating improved spatial understanding and instruction following capabilities. This success can be attributed to the enhanced object recognition consistency achieved through our partial contrastive learning framework.

Further Analysis

Sensitivity to Prompt Design: Our analysis of different prompt designs reveals crucial factors for effective object information extraction from images. We have found that specifying criteria for desired objects is essential for system performance. Without such specificity, VLMs often identify irrelevant environmental elements that are ubiquitous across observations, which would undermine the effectiveness of our contrastive learning approach. Therefore, our prompt explicitly instructs the model to focus on meaningful objects while ignoring general environmental elements.

Additionally, specifying the expected output format proves critical for consistent processing. Clear formatting instructions ensure that VLM outputs maintain structural consistency, facilitating reliable post-processing and integration into our learning framework. This attention to prompt engineering demonstrates the importance of careful interface design when leveraging emergent capabilities of foundation models.

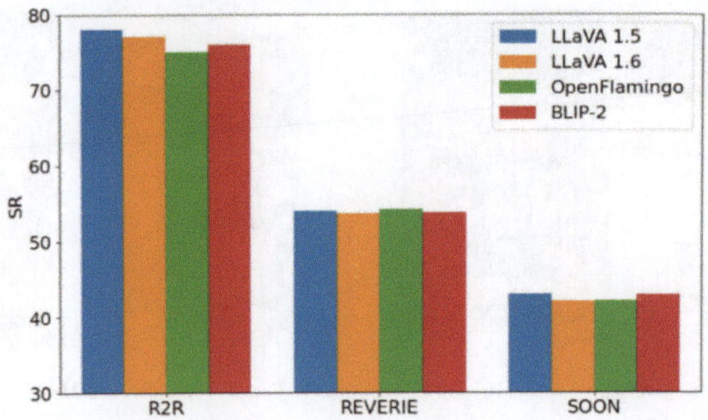

Fig. 14.5 Sensitivity to VLM choice. We report the Success Rate (SR) on the validation unseen set for all tasks, using various Vision-Language Models (VLMs). The results indicate that the choice of VLM has minimal impact on performance, highlighting the robustness of our method

Robustness Across Different VLMs: We conduct comprehensive experiments using various Vision-Language Models, including LLaVA 1.5 [27], LLaVA 1.6 [26], OpenFlamingo [5], and BLIP-2 [23], applying consistent prompting strategies across all models. The outputs from these different models are largely consistent, and performance variations are minimal across different VLM choices.

As visualized in Fig. 14.5, our experimental results demonstrate that the choice of VLM has minimal impact on overall navigation performance across all three benchmark datasets (R2R, REVERIE, and SOON). The Success Rate variations remain within a narrow range regardless of which VLM is used to generate the supervisory signals, highlighting the robustness of our approach. This consistency is observed despite the different architectural designs and training procedures of these VLMs, suggesting that our weakly-supervised framework effectively captures common emergent capabilities shared across well-trained vision-language models.

This finding has significant implications for practical deployment, as it demonstrates that our method minimizes reliance on specific VLM implementations. The consistency across different foundation models suggests that our approach captures fundamental emergent capabilities that are shared across well-trained vision-language models, rather than exploiting model-specific artifacts. This robustness is particularly valuable for real-world applications where VLM availability and computational constraints may dictate the choice of foundation model.

Object Detection Accuracy: Through case study analysis, we observe that VLM-based object detection achieves high accuracy in our navigation contexts. While direct quantitative evaluation of detection accuracy is limited by the absence of object-level annotations in standard VLN datasets, qualitative analysis and the consistency of results across different VLMs provide strong evidence for the reliability of the object recognition capabilities we leverage.

Computational Efficiency: Our method demonstrates significant computational efficiency compared to approaches requiring foundation model fine-tuning. The WPCL framework operates effectively on standard consumer-grade hardware, requiring only a single GPU with moderate memory capacity, while fine-tuning-based methods typically demand substantially more computational resources including high-end GPUs with larger memory capacities or multi-GPU configurations. This efficiency advantage stems from our core design principle of leveraging emergent capabilities through weak supervision rather than expensive model adaptation. By using VLMs only for inference-time object recognition rather than full model fine-tuning, we maintain the benefits of foundation model capabilities while avoiding the associated computational overhead. This approach makes our method more accessible for research groups and practical applications with limited computational resources, which is particularly relevant for smart aging deployments where edge computing constraints may apply.

To summarize, the Weakly-supervised VLM-guided Partial Contrastive Learning (WPCL) framework demonstrates how emergent capabilities of large foundation models can be systematically leveraged for Visual Language Navigation tasks. Our approach effectively integrates pre-trained Vision-Language Models into the perception process of navigation agents without requiring computationally expensive fine-tuning, thereby maintaining computational efficiency while reducing reliance on potentially biased outputs.

Through our novel causal analysis framework and tailored partial contrastive learning approach, we have shown that emergent capabilities such as zero-shot object recognition can be channeled through carefully designed weak supervision signals to address domain-specific challenges. Our method achieves strong performances across multiple benchmarks, highlighting its potential to advance VLN while offering a balanced solution that leverages pre-trained models' strengths without their associated limitations.

The robustness of our approach across different VLMs further demonstrates the generalizability of our framework for harnessing emergent capabilities, providing insights that extend beyond navigation tasks to broader applications in intelligent assistance systems, particularly those relevant to smart aging environments.

14.4 Discussion and Future Directions

14.4.1 Implications for Emergent Capabilities Research

The WPCL framework presented in this chapter provides several important insights into the nature and utilization of emergent capabilities in large foundation models. Our work demonstrates that emergent capabilities are not merely emergent properties to be observed, but can be systematically identified, understood, and leveraged through carefully designed methodological frameworks.

The success of our weakly-supervised approach highlights a critical insight: emergent capabilities can be effectively channeled through weak supervision signals that respect the pre-trained models' existing knowledge structures while guiding them toward domain-specific requirements. This finding has broader implications for how we approach the integration of foundation models into specialized applications, suggesting that the binary choice between zero-shot deployment and expensive fine-tuning may not be necessary.

Our causal framework provides a theoretical foundation for understanding how emergent capabilities can be leveraged in scenarios involving temporal and spatial dependencies. The insight that objects act as confounders between observations in navigation scenarios, and that this can be leveraged through contrastive learning, suggests that similar approaches might be applicable to other domains where emergent capabilities need to be harnessed for structured prediction tasks.

14.4.2 Relevance to Smart Aging Applications

The principles demonstrated through our WPCL framework have direct relevance to the development of intelligent assistance systems for smart aging environments. The ability to leverage emergent capabilities efficiently, without requiring extensive computational resources or specialized training data, aligns well with the practical constraints often encountered in smart aging deployments. Smart aging environments would benefit significantly from navigation assistance systems that can understand natural language instructions, adapt to individual mobility patterns, and operate efficiently on resource-constrained devices. Our demonstration that emergent object recognition capabilities can be leveraged through weak supervision suggests that similar approaches could be developed for understanding and responding to the specific needs of aging individuals.

The robustness of our approach across different VLMs is particularly relevant for smart aging applications, where system reliability and consistency are paramount. The ability to achieve stable performance across different foundation models suggests that such systems could be deployed with confidence, even as the underlying foundation models continue to evolve. Furthermore, the computational efficiency of our approach makes it practical for deployment in smart home environments, where real-time responsiveness is crucial but computational resources may be limited. The fact that our method runs on a single consumer-grade GPU while maintaining competitive performance suggests that similar approaches could be integrated into edge computing devices commonly used in smart aging systems.

14.4.3 Future Research Directions

Several promising research directions have emerged from our work on leveraging emergent capabilities for intelligent navigation and their broader applications:

- *Expanding the Framework to Multimodal Interactions*: While our current work focuses on vision-language navigation, the principles could be extended to incorporate additional modalities relevant to smart aging, such as audio input for voice commands, tactile feedback for mobility assistance, or biometric monitoring for adaptive behavior.
- *Personalization and Adaptation*: Future research could explore how emergent capabilities can be leveraged to create personalized assistance systems that adapt to the needs, preferences, and capabilities of individual users over time. This is particularly relevant for smart aging applications where individuals may have varying and changing requirements.
- *Causal Reasoning in Complex Environments*: Our causal framework provides a foundation for more sophisticated reasoning about environmental dynamics. Future work could expand this to handle more complex scenarios involving multiple agents, dynamic environments, or long-term planning tasks.
- *Efficient Foundation Model Integration*: The success of our weakly-supervised approach suggests that more research is needed into efficient methods for integrating foundation models into specialized applications without expensive fine-tuning. This could include exploring different types of weak supervision signals, alternative architectural approaches, or novel training paradigms.
- *Evaluation Frameworks for Emergent Capabilities*: As the field moves toward more systematic utilization of emergent capabilities, there is a need for better evaluation frameworks that can assess not just task performance but also the efficiency, robustness, and transferability of approaches that leverage these capabilities.
- *Ethical and Safety Considerations*: As intelligent assistance systems become more prevalent in smart aging environments, research into ensuring their safety, reliability, and ethical deployment becomes increasingly important. This includes understanding potential biases in foundation models and developing approaches to mitigate their impact in sensitive applications.

The convergence of emergent capabilities in foundation models with practical applications in smart aging represents a rich area for future research that could significantly impact how we support aging populations through intelligent technology. Our work provides a foundation for this research by demonstrating how emergent capabilities can be systematically leveraged to create more effective and efficient intelligent systems.

References

1. Achiam, J., Adler, S., Agarwal, S., Ahmad, L., Akkaya, I., Aleman, F.L., Almeida, D., Altenschmidt, J., Altman, S., Anadkat, S., et al.: Gpt-4 technical report. arXiv preprint arXiv:2303.08774 (2023)
2. An, D., Qi, Y., Li, Y., Huang, Y., Wang, L., Tan, T., Shao, J.: Bevbert: Topo-metric map pre-training for language-guided navigation. arXiv preprint arXiv:2212.04385 (2022)
3. Anderson, P., Chang, A., Chaplot, D.S., Dosovitskiy, A., Gupta, S., Koltun, V., Kosecka, J., Malik, J., Mottaghi, R., Savva, M., et al.: On evaluation of embodied navigation agents. arXiv preprint arXiv:1807.06757 (2018)
4. Anderson, P., Wu, Q., Teney, D., Bruce, J., Johnson, M., Sünderhauf, N., Reid, I., Gould, S., Hengel, A.V.D.: Vision-and-language navigation: Interpreting visually-grounded navigation instructions in real environments. In: Proceedings of the IEEE/CVF Conference on Computer Vision and Pattern Recognition, CVPR, pp. 3674–3683. IEEE (2018)
5. Awadalla, A., Gao, I., Gardner, J., Hessel, J., Hanafy, Y., Zhu, W., Marathe, K., Bitton, Y., Gadre, S., Sagawa, S., et al.: Openflamingo: An open-source framework for training large autoregressive vision-language models. arXiv preprint arXiv:2308.01390 (2023)
6. Chen, J., Lin, B., Xu, R., Chai, Z., Liang, X., Wong, K.K.: Mapgpt: Map-guided prompting for unified vision-and-language navigation. arXiv preprint arXiv:2401.07314 (2024)
7. Chen, S., Guhur, P.L., Schmid, C., Laptev, I.: History aware multimodal transformer for vision-and-language navigation. In: Advances in Neural Information Processing Systems, NeurIPS, vol. 34, pp. 5834–5847 (2021)
8. Chen, S., Guhur, P.L., Tapaswi, M., Schmid, C., Laptev, I.: Think global, act local: Dual-scale graph transformer for vision-and-language navigation. In: Proceedings of the IEEE/CVF Conference on Computer Vision and Pattern Recognition, CVPR, pp. 16537–16547. IEEE (2022)
9. Chen, T., Kornblith, S., Norouzi, M., Hinton, G.: A simple framework for contrastive learning of visual representations. In: Proceedings of the International Conference on Machine Learning, ICML, pp. 1597–1607. PMLR (2020)
10. Chen, X., Fan, H., Girshick, R., He, K.: Improved baselines with momentum contrastive learning. arXiv preprint arXiv:2003.04297 (2020)
11. Chiang, W.L., Li, Z., Lin, Z., Sheng, Y., Wu, Z., Zhang, H., Zheng, L., Zhuang, S., Zhuang, Y., Gonzalez, J.E., Stoica, I., Xing, E.P.: Vicuna: An open-source chatbot impressing gpt-4 with 90% chatgpt quality. https://lmsys.org/blog/2023-03-30-vicuna/ (2023)
12. Chung, H.W., Hou, L., Longpre, S., Zoph, B., Tay, Y., Fedus, W., Li, Y., Wang, X., Dehghani, M., Narang, S., et al.: Scaling instruction-finetuned language models. J. Mach. Learn. Res. **25**(70), 1–53 (2024)
13. Fan, L., Zhou, J., Xing, X., Wu, Y.: Active open-vocabulary recognition: Let intelligent moving mitigate clip limitations. In: Proceedings of the IEEE/CVF Conference on Computer Vision and Pattern Recognition, CVPR, pp. 16394–16403. IEEE (2024)
14. Fried, D., Hu, R., Cirik, V., Rohrbach, A., Andreas, J., Morency, L.P., Berg-Kirkpatrick, T., Saenko, K., Klein, D., Darrell, T.: Speaker-follower models for vision-and-language navigation. In: Advances in Neural Information Processing Systems, vol. 31 (2018)
15. Gu, J., Stefani, E., Wu, Q., Thomason, J., Wang, X.E.: Vision-and-language navigation: A survey of tasks, methods, and future directions. arXiv preprint arXiv:2203.12667 (2022)
16. Guhur, P.L., Tapaswi, M., Chen, S., Laptev, I., Schmid, C.: Airbert: In-domain pretraining for vision-and-language navigation. In: Proceedings of the IEEE/CVF International Conference on Computer Vision, ICCV, pp. 1634–1643. IEEE (2021)
17. Hao, W., Li, C., Li, X., Carin, L., Gao, J.: Towards learning a generic agent for vision-and-language navigation via pre-training. In: Proceedings of the IEEE/CVF Conference on Computer Vision and Pattern Recognition, CVPR, pp. 13137–13146. IEEE (2020)
18. He, K., Zhang, X., Ren, S., Sun, J.: Deep residual learning for image recognition. In: Proceedings of the IEEE Conference on Computer Vision and Pattern Recognition, CVPR, pp. 770–778. IEEE (2016)

19. Hong, Y., Wu, Q., Qi, Y., Rodriguez-Opazo, C., Gould, S.: A recurrent vision-and-language bert for navigation. arXiv preprint arXiv:2011.13922 (2020)
20. Kareer, S., Yokoyama, N., Batra, D., Ha, S., Truong, J.: Vinl: Visual navigation and locomotion over obstacles. In: 2023 IEEE International Conference on Robotics and Automation, ICRA, pp. 2018–2024. IEEE (2023)
21. Ke, L., Li, X., Bisk, Y., Holtzman, A., Gan, Z., Liu, J., Gao, J., Choi, Y., Srinivasa, S.: Tactical rewind: Self-correction via backtracking in vision-and-language navigation. In: Proceedings of the IEEE/CVF Conference on Computer Vision and Pattern Recognition, CVPR, pp. 6741–6749. IEEE (2019)
22. Khandelwal, A., Weihs, L., Mottaghi, R., Kembhavi, A.: Simple but effective: Clip embeddings for embodied ai. In: Proceedings of the IEEE/CVF Conference on Computer Vision and Pattern Recognition, CVPR, pp. 14829–14838. IEEE (2022)
23. Li, J., Li, D., Savarese, S., Hoi, S.: Blip-2: Bootstrapping language-image pre-training with frozen image encoders and large language models. In: Proceedings of the International Conference on Machine Learning, ICML, pp. 19730–19742. PMLR (2023)
24. Li, X., Wang, Z., Yang, J., Wang, Y., Jiang, S.: Kerm: Knowledge enhanced reasoning for vision-and-language navigation. In: Proceedings of the IEEE/CVF Conference on Computer Vision and Pattern Recognition, CVPR, pp. 2583–2592. IEEE (2023)
25. Lin, B., Nie, Y., Wei, Z., Chen, J., Ma, S., Han, J., Xu, H., Chang, X., Liang, X.: Navcot: Boosting llm-based vision-and-language navigation via learning disentangled reasoning. arXiv preprint arXiv:2403.07376 (2024)
26. Liu, H., Li, C., Li, Y., Li, B., Zhang, Y., Shen, S., Lee, Y.J.: Llava-next: Improved reasoning, ocr, and world knowledge. https://llava-vl.github.io/blog/2024-01-30-llava-next/ (2024)
27. Liu, H., Li, C., Wu, Q., Lee, Y.J.: Visual instruction tuning. arXiv preprint arXiv:2304.08485 (2023)
28. Liu, R., Wang, X., Wang, W., Yang, Y.: Bird's-eye-view scene graph for vision-language navigation. In: Proceedings of the IEEE/CVF International Conference on Computer Vision, ICCV, pp. 10968–10980. IEEE (2023)
29. Long, Y., Li, X., Cai, W., Dong, H.: Discuss before moving: Visual language navigation via multi-expert discussions. In: 2024 IEEE International Conference on Robotics and Automation, ICRA, pp. 17380–17387. IEEE (2024)
30. Lyons, D.M., Rahouti, M.: Wavn: Wide area visual navigation for large-scale, gps-denied environments. In: 2023 IEEE International Conference on Robotics and Automation, ICRA, pp. 2039–2045. IEEE (2023)
31. Ma, C.Y., Wu, Z., AlRegib, G., Xiong, C., Kira, Z.: The regretful agent: Heuristic-aided navigation through progress estimation. In: Proceedings of the IEEE/CVF Conference on Computer Vision and Pattern Recognition, CVPR, pp. 6732–6740. IEEE (2019)
32. Pan, B., Panda, R., Jin, S., Feris, R., Oliva, A., Isola, P., Kim, Y.: Langnav: Language as a perceptual representation for navigation. arXiv preprint arXiv:2310.07889 (2023)
33. Qi, Y., Wu, Q., Anderson, P., Wang, X., Wang, W.Y., Shen, C., van den Hengel, A.: Reverie: Remote embodied visual referring expression in real indoor environments. In: Proceedings of the IEEE/CVF Conference on Computer Vision and Pattern Recognition, CVPR, pp. 9982–9991. IEEE (2020)
34. Radford, A., Kim, J.W., Hallacy, C., Ramesh, A., Goh, G., Agarwal, S., Sastry, G., Askell, A., Mishkin, P., Clark, J., et al.: Learning transferable visual models from natural language supervision. In: Proceedings of the International Conference on Machine Learning, ICML, pp. 8748–8763. PMLR (2021)
35. Tan, H., Bansal, M.: Lxmert: Learning cross-modality encoder representations from transformers. arXiv preprint arXiv:1908.07490 (2019)
36. Tan, H., Yu, L., Bansal, M.: Learning to navigate unseen environments: Back translation with environmental dropout. In: Proceedings of the 2019 Conference of the North American Chapter of the Association for Computational Linguistics (Human Language Technologies), NAACL, pp. 2610–2621. Association for Computational Linguistics (2019)

37. Touvron, H., Lavril, T., Izacard, G., Martinet, X., Lachaux, M.A., Lacroix, T., Rozière, B., Goyal, N., Hambro, E., Azhar, F., et al.: Llama: Open and efficient foundation language models. arXiv preprint arXiv:2302.13971 (2023)
38. Wang, L., He, Z., Dang, R., Shen, M., Liu, C., Chen, Q.: Vision-and-language navigation via causal learning. In: Proceedings of the IEEE/CVF Conference on Computer Vision and Pattern Recognition, CVPR, pp. 13139–13150. IEEE (2024)
39. Wang, R., Yu, T., Wu, J., Liu, Y., McAuley, J., Yao, L.: Weakly-supervised vlm-guided partial contrastive learning for visual language navigation. In: 2025 IEEE/RSJ International Conference on Intelligent Robots and Systems, IROS. IEEE (2025)
40. Wang, X., Huang, Q., Celikyilmaz, A., Gao, J., Shen, D., Wang, Y., Wang, W.Y., Zhang, L.: Reinforced cross-modal matching and self-supervised imitation learning for vision-language navigation. In: Proceedings of the IEEE/CVF Conference on Computer Vision and Pattern Recognition, CVPR, pp. 6629–6638. IEEE (2019)
41. Wang, Z., Li, J., Hong, Y., Wang, Y., Wu, Q., Bansal, M., Gould, S., Tan, H., Yiqiao: Scaling data generation in vision-and-language navigation. In: Proceedings of the IEEE/CVF International Conference on Computer Vision, ICCV, pp. 12009–12020. IEEE (2023)
42. Wang, Z., Li, X., Yang, J., Liu, Y., Jiang, S.: Gridmm: Grid memory map for vision-and-language navigation. In: Proceedings of the IEEE/CVF International Conference on Computer Vision, ICCV, pp. 15625–15636. IEEE (2023)
43. Wasserman, J., Chowdhary, G., Gupta, A., Jain, U.: Exploitation-guided exploration for semantic embodied navigation. In: 2024 IEEE International Conference on Robotics and Automation, ICRA, pp. 2901–2908. IEEE (2024)
44. Zhao, Q., Zhang, L., He, B., Qiao, H., Liu, Z.: Zero-shot object goal visual navigation. In: 2023 IEEE International Conference on Robotics and Automation, ICRA, pp. 2025–2031. IEEE (2023)
45. Zheng, D., Huang, S., Zhao, L., Zhong, Y., Wang, L.: Towards learning a generalist model for embodied navigation. In: Proceedings of the IEEE/CVF Conference on Computer Vision and Pattern Recognition, CVPR, pp. 13624–13634. IEEE (2024)
46. Zhou, G., Hong, Y., Wang, Z., Wang, X.E., Wu, Q.: Navgpt-2: Unleashing navigational reasoning capability for large vision-language models. arXiv preprint arXiv:2407.12366 (2024)
47. Zhou, G., Hong, Y., Wu, Q.: Navgpt: Explicit reasoning in vision-and-language navigation with large language models. In: Proceedings of the AAAI Conference on Artificial Intelligence, pp. 7641–7649. AAAI (2024)
48. Zhu, F., Liang, X., Zhu, Y., Yu, Q., Chang, X., Liang, X.: Soon: Scenario oriented object navigation with graph-based exploration. In: Proceedings of the IEEE/CVF Conference on Computer Vision and Pattern Recognition, CVPR, pp. 12689–12699. IEEE (2021)
49. Zhu, J., Qiao, Y., Zhang, S., He, X., Wu, Q., Liu, J.: Minivln: Efficient vision-and-language navigation by progressive knowledge distillation. arXiv preprint arXiv:2409.18800 (2024)
50. Zimmermann, R.S., Sharma, Y., Schneider, S., Bethge, M., Brendel, W.: Contrastive learning inverts the data generating process. In: Proceedings of the International Conference on Machine Learning, ICML, pp. 12979–12990. PMLR (2021)

Chapter 15
Conclusion and Future Directions

This monograph begins in Chap. 1 with Fiona's father making tea in an apartment where tiny sensors quietly monitored his actions, providing timely prompts when needed and peace of mind to his family through unobtrusive support. From this motivating scenario, we set out to examine how the convergence of artificial intelligence (AI) and the Internet of Things (IoT) can transform aging support from traditional reactive care models to proactive, predictive, and personalized systems. Across Chaps. 2–14, we have developed a coherent framework that integrates device-free environmental intelligence, wearable and physiological sensing, interactive ambient systems, and AI-empowered solutions into a privacy-preserving, adaptive, and human-centered ecosystem. We synthesize the technical and translational contributions, reflect on evidence and limitations, and outline a forward-looking research and deployment agenda that remains faithful to the goals articulated at the outset: dignified, independent, and safe aging supported by trustworthy ambient intelligence.

15.1 Synthesis Across the Four Strands

Device-free Sensing and Environmental Intelligence (Chaps. 4 **and** 5**).** We demonstrate how device-free localization, tracking, and human activity recognition transform the built environment into an unobtrusive sensing platform. By leveraging radio frequency, acoustic, and depth modalities together with contextual Human–Object Interaction cues, the system infers spatial trajectories, daily routines, and safety-critical events (e.g., falls) without placing burden on older adults. This strand emphasizes privacy-preserving sensing, continuous operation, and resilience to the annotation scarcity that is characteristic of aging applications.

Wearable and Physiological/Cognitive Monitoring (Chaps. 6 **and** 7**).** Wearable sensors complement environmental intelligence by adding fine-grained kinematic and physiological signals for physical and cognitive state estimation. These chapters

Q. Z. Sheng et al., *Harnessing Artificial Intelligence and Pervasive Internet of Things for an Empowered Aging*, https://doi.org/10.1007/978-3-032-16502-2_15

address fundamental problems of inter-activity similarity, heterogeneous populations, and distribution shift through semi-supervised learning, transfer learning, and personalized modeling. Cognitive activity recognition and brain–computer interfaces (BCIs) demonstrate how thought-driven interaction can extend accessibility and autonomy in daily living.

Interactive Ambient Intelligence (Chaps. 8–10). We integrate recognition capabilities with Web-based IoT management, intent-aware reasoning, and robotic actuation. The resulting systems coordinate perception, semantics, and action to anticipate needs, reduce cognitive load, and provide physical assistance. Direct brain-to-device communication further broadens interaction modalities, aligning system behavior with user intent while maintaining safety and transparency.

AI-empowered IoT Solutions (Chaps. 11–14). The final strand concretizes application-level capabilities: personal health management through longitudinal data mining; secure identity management via multimodal biometrics; conversational interfaces powered by large language models (LLMs); and the emergent capabilities of vision–language models (VLMs) for instruction following and navigation. Together, these advances move the field from isolated prototypes toward integrated, end-to-end solutions deployable in homes, clinics, and community settings.

15.2 Cross-Cutting Principles

Privacy-Preserving Intelligence. From the outset, we prioritize privacy and autonomy. Device-free sensing reduces the capture of personally identifiable information. Edge computation, federated learning, and differential privacy enable adaptive models with local control of sensitive data. These techniques allow systems to improve collectively while keeping raw signals appropriately contained. This aligns with the core principles of smart aging technologies that must balance comprehensive monitoring with ethical considerations of dignity and privacy rights.

Adaptive and Personalized Systems. Aging trajectories are diverse and dynamic. Models must adapt across individuals and over time. We employ semi- and self-supervised representation learning, transfer and domain adaptation, and lightweight on-device personalization to mitigate annotation scarcity, handle distribution shifts, and sustain performance as users' capabilities evolve. The highly individual nature of aging requires systems that can accommodate not only person-to-person differences, but also temporal changes in capabilities, preferences, and needs over extended periods.

Multimodal Integration and Interpretability. Robust performance arises from principled fusion of environmental, wearable, and contextual signals. Attention mechanisms, graph-based modeling, and uncertainty-aware fusion allocate reliance to the most informative modalities given quality and availability. Interpretability and explanation link sensor evidence to human-understandable rationales—an essential feature for clinicians, caregivers, and users. This approach embraces the Cognitive Internet of Things (CIoT) paradigm introduced in Chap. 2, where systems learn, reason, and adapt to both physical and social contexts rather than simply connecting devices.

Reliability, Safety, and Human Factors. In safety-critical contexts, reliability and clarity of failure modes matter as much as accuracy. We emphasize monitoring for out-of-distribution inputs, fallbacks to conservative behaviors, and human-in-the-loop control consistent with Consumer Directed Care (CDC). Interfaces are designed to be simple, familiar, and inclusive, with options spanning voice, touch, and brain-computer interfaces. This emphasis on dependability acknowledges that aging support technologies must earn and maintain trust through consistent, transparent, and predictable operation, especially when serving vulnerable populations.

Evidence, Validation, and Limitations. This monograph intentionally described empirical findings at a high level. While many components have been validated on public datasets and controlled trials, some experiments necessarily have used non-elderly cohorts due to data scarcity—a common challenge in aging-related research. The methodological choices reflect our commitment to develop techniques that can generalize across varied populations despite these constraints. To address the data gap, we have proposed and implemented evaluation practices that emphasize:

- *Generalization under Distribution Shift*: person-independent splits, cross-site validation, and temporal robustness to bridge the gap between available data sources and target populations.
- *Rare-event Sensitivity*: class-imbalance handling and clinically meaningful error trade-offs, particularly critical for safety events like falls that occur infrequently but require high detection accuracy.
- *Multi-occupant and Multi-activity Settings*: disentangling overlapping behaviors in realistic homes, moving beyond simplified laboratory scenarios to complex domestic environments.
- *Longitudinal Reliability*: stability over weeks to months, with graceful degradation and recovery to accommodate the extended timeframes characteristic of aging support applications.

Our models incorporate domain adaptation techniques specifically designed to transfer knowledge from available datasets to aging-specific contexts, while our evaluation methodologies prioritize robustness across diverse user populations rather than optimization for homogeneous test sets. Nonetheless, limitations remain. Dataset representativeness, consistency of annotation across sites, and standardization of deployment metrics need continued attention. Ethical review, consent management, and data governance must be embedded from design through operation—particularly important when technologies are deployed with vulnerable populations.

15.3 From Architecture to Deployment

Real-world impact requires more than algorithms. We outline an implementation path that couples technical architecture with service design and governance:

- *Architectures*: hybrid edge–cloud processing; on-device inference for latency-critical functions; privacy-preserving federated updates; and secure key management for identity.
- *Interoperability*: semantic device models, open APIs, and standardized ontologies enabling plug-and-play integration across vendors and care providers.
- *Security and Identity*: multimodal authentication calibrated for aging-related changes in physiology and motor control, with robust anti-spoofing.
- *Care Models and Policy*: alignment with Consumer Directed Care, clinical pathways, and reimbursement; auditability for safety and accountability; equity-by-design to ensure access in rural and resource-constrained communities.

Economic analyses suggest that early detection, fall prevention, medication adherence support, and streamlined reporting can reduce avoidable utilization while improving quality of life and caregiver capacity. Procurement and maintenance strategies should favor modular systems, remote updates, and clear total-cost-of-ownership models.

15.4 A Research and Innovation Agenda

To fulfill the promise of AI-empowered IoT for smart aging, we identify the following priorities:

- *Learning with Less*: self-supervised pretraining on unlabeled ambient data; active learning to focus limited annotation; continual and federated learning to personalize safely.
- *Trustworthy Intelligence*: uncertainty estimation, calibration, and causal reasoning to support reliable recommendations and transparent decision-making.
- *Multimodal Sensing at the Edge*: RF and radar sensing, smart textiles, and energy-efficient compute for 24/7 operation.
- *Human–AI Interaction*: intent-aware assistance that reduces cognitive load; adaptive interfaces spanning voice, gesture, and BCI; and rigorous usability evaluation with older adults and caregivers.
- *Foundation Models for Healthcare Contexts*: domain-adapted LLMs/VLMs that respect privacy constraints, operate under resource limits, and provide grounded explanations.
- *Evaluation Science*: longitudinal field studies, fairness and accessibility audits, and standardized benchmarks tailored to aging-in-place scenarios.

15.5 From Aspiration to Achievement: The Future of Smart Aging

We begin this monograph with a simple aspiration encapsulated in Fiona's story: that ambient intelligence could quietly safeguard daily life of an older person, providing timely assistance while preserving privacy, autonomy, and dignity. The journey through Chaps. 2–14 demonstrates that this aspiration is technically achievable and socially meaningful when pursued with rigor and empathy. The most compelling systems amplify human capability—they do not replace it. They learn from the rhythms of everyday living, intervene sparingly yet effectively, and communicate in forms users can understand and control.

Revisiting the scenario that opens Chap. 1, we can now see how each component we have developed contributes to making it a reality: device-free sensing monitors tea-making without requiring wearable devices; activity recognition algorithms detect potential difficulties and incidents; intent-aware systems provide contextual reminders precisely when needed; and secure Web-based interfaces allow family members to maintain awareness while respecting privacy. For Fiona's father, the technology remains largely invisible, supporting his independence rather than highlighting his limitations. For Fiona, it provides reassurance without requiring constant check-ins or intrusive monitoring.

Realizing this vision at scale will require interdisciplinary collaborations among engineers, clinicians, caregivers, designers, and policy makers. It will also require sustained investment in privacy-preserving methods, standards and interoperability, and inclusive evaluation in the populations we aim to serve. If we meet these challenges, AI-empowered IoT will help deliver the future we have envisioned at the outset of this monograph: aging that is independent yet connected, safeguarded yet private, and supported by technology that is as respectful as it is intelligent—technology that serves human needs rather than technological imperatives, embodying the paradigm shift from reactive care to proactive, predictive, and personalized support that maintains dignity throughout the aging journey.

Live longer, aging well. We are looking forward to the day, like how Fiona's father lives, to come!

MIX
Papier aus verantwortungsvollen Quellen
Paper from responsible sources
FSC® C105338

If you have any concerns about our products,
you can contact us on
ProductSafety@springernature.com

In case Publisher is established outside the EU,
the EU authorized representative is:
Springer Nature Customer Service Center GmbH
Europaplatz 3, 69115 Heidelberg, Germany

Printed by Libri Plureos GmbH
in Hamburg, Germany